Nursing Law and Ethics

Nursing Law and Ethics

Third Edition

Edited by John Tingle and Alan Cribb

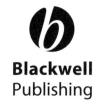

Blackwell
Publishing

Blackwell Publishing editorial offices:
Blackwell Publishing Ltd, 9600 Garsington Road, Oxford OX4 2DQ, UK
Tel: +44 (0)1865 776868
Blackwell Publishing Inc., 350 Main Street, Malden, MA 02148-5020, USA
Tel: +1 781 388 8250
Blackwell Publishing Asia Pty Ltd, 550 Swanston Street, Carlton, Victoria 3053, Australia
Tel: +61 (0)3 8359 1011

First published 1995 by Blackwell Science Ltd
Second edition published 2002 by Blackwell Publishing Ltd
Third edition published 2007

ISBN-13: 978-1-4051-3228-2

Library of Congress Cataloging-in-Publication Data
Nursing law and ethics / edited by John Tingle and Alan Cribb. — 3rd ed.
p. ; cm.
Includes bibliographical references and index.
ISBN–13: 978–1–4051–3228–2 (pbk. : alk. paper)
ISBN–10: 1–4051–3228–0 (pbk. : alk. paper) 1. Nursing—Law and legislation—
Great Britain. 2. Nursing ethics—Great Britain. I. Tingle, John. II. Cribb, Alan.
[DNLM: 1. Ethics, Nursing—Great Britain. 2. Legislation,
Nursing—Great Britain. WY 33 FA1 N974 2007]

KD2968.N8N87 2007
344.4104′14—dc22
2007012913

A catalogue record for this title is available from the British Library

Set in 10/12pt Palatino
by Graphicraft Limited, Hong Kong
Printed in United Kingdom by TJ International Ltd, Padstow, Cornwall

For further information on Blackwell Publishing, visit our website:
www.blackwellnursing.com

Contents

Preface to the Third Edition

We are pleased to have been given the chance to update and revise this book into a third edition. Health care legal and ethical issues continue to dominate social and political agendas and the courts. Since the last edition a myriad of ethical and legal dilemmas have flowed through the media and the courts and we have tried to reflect many of these in this new edition. Such dilemmas arise in the context of an NHS that appears to be in a constant state of reform and subject to a number of increasingly contentious and competing political agendas. This unstable platform brings about its own problems as NHS organisations struggle to implement government health quality, risk and patient safety policies and at the same time manage root and branch change. Nursing law and ethics, as an academic discipline, continues to develop and is now often seen to sit alongside these patient safety, quality and risk topics. The focus now, practically speaking, is the practical and holistic integration of these topics (the government, for example, currently puts all this under the umbrella of 'Integrated Governance'). We suggest that nursing law and ethics, to be understood properly, should been see in this broader context, which includes the wider policy context of the NHS. The nursing law and ethics student cannot ignore the work of NHS organisations such as the NPSA, NHSLA and Healthcare Commission and the related governance agendas. An understanding of these broader institutional and policy frameworks is essential for a fully informed discussion, and we hope this book helps to support such a discussion as well as to properly represent the more focused and disciplinary demands of law and ethics.

The preface to the first edition sets out the rationale for, and the structure of, the book. We hold true to this for the third edition as we did for the second. There have been changes, particularly to the law, and we have tried to capture these up to August 2006. That health care law is in a fairly constant state of flux is a self-evident truth, and it is simply impossible, for practical reasons, to represent all the legal changes that took place before the book went to press. We would note, however, that the NHS Redress Act 2006 was eventually passed into law. Positive changes were made to it as it progressed through Parliament, and it now has the potential to make a real difference to patients who have been harmed through lack of care in the NHS.

We, once again, very much hope that this new edition of the book will prove to be of practical benefit – and theoretical interest – to the nursing community.

Alan Cribb and John Tingle
London and Nottingham

Preface to the Second Edition

We are, of course, pleased that the first edition of this book was so well received; and we are delighted to have had the chance to update and revise it. There is comparatively little to add to the Preface produced for the first edition; this sets out the rationale for, and the structure of, the book, and these remain the same. But there are many changes to the content of the book. The last six years have seen an extraordinary amount of change in many aspects of health care law and ethics, in the regulation and management of health services, and in conceptions of health professional accountability. The contributors to this new edition have sought to reflect and illuminate these changes and also to provide clear overviews of their subject matter.

There is a new chapter in the first part of the book which summarises the changing policy context and legal environment of nursing; and in the second part there is a new 'pair' of chapters on clinical governance. We are grateful to all the authors who have updated their work and/or written material for the first time in this edition. We very much hope that this new edition will prove to be of practical benefit – and theoretical interest – to the nursing community.

Acknowledgements

We would like to thank Professor Jean McHale, Faculty of Law, University of Leicester and Mr Harry Lesser, Centre for Philosophy, University of Manchester, for acting as editorial advisers.

Alan Cribb and John Tingle

Preface to the First Edition

One of the key indicators of the maturation of nursing as a profession and as a discipline is the growing importance of nursing law and ethics. A profession which seeks not only to maintain, and improve on, high standards but also to hold each of its individual members accountable for an increasing range of responsibilities is inevitably concerned with legal and ethical matters. It is not surprising that these matters have come to prominence in nurse education, and to enjoy a central place along with clinical and social sciences in the disciplinary bases of nursing. There is now a substantial body of literature devoted to nursing law and to nursing ethics.

This book is distinctive because it is about both law *and* ethics. We believe it is of practical benefit, and academic value, to consider these two subjects together. Put simply we need to be able to discuss 'what the law requires' and 'what is right', and to decide, amongst other things, whether these two are always the same.

The book is divided into two parts. The first part is designed to be an overview of the whole subject and includes introductions to the legal, ethical and professional dimensions of nursing, as well as a special chapter on patient complaints. The second part looks at a selection of issues in greater depth. These chapters contain two parts or perspectives – one legal and one ethical. The legal perspectives take the lead – the authors were invited to introduce the law relating to the subject at hand. The ethics authors were invited to write a complementary (and typically shorter) piece in which they took up some of the issues but then went on to make any points they wished. Thus the terms of invitation for the ethics authors were different, and more flexible, than those for the lawyers. This difference in treatment of the two perspectives is quite deliberate.

The essential difference is this: it makes good sense to ask lawyers for an authoritative account of the law, but it is not sensible to ask authors for an authoritative account of what is good or right – which is the subject matter of ethics. An account of the law will not simply be factual; it will inevitably include some discussion of the complexity and uncertainties involved in identifying and interpreting the implications of the law. But it is in the nature of the law that lawyers should be able to give expert guidance about legal judgments. There are no equivalent authorities on ethical judgement. Instead some nurses with an interest in ethics and some philosophers with an interest in nursing ethics were invited to discuss some of the issues and/or cases raised in the first part of the chapter. Clearly these responses are of different styles and are written from different standpoints. Each author is responsible for his or her piece and any of the views or opinions expressed within them. This difference between the two sets of perspectives is indicated (indeed rather exaggerated) by giving the former the definite, and the latter an indefinite, article – 'The Legal Perspective' but 'An Ethical Perspective'!

These differences in presentation reflect deeper differences between the two subjects. In short, law and ethics are concerned with two contrasting kinds of 'finality' – in principle ethics is final but in practice law is final. It is important to appreciate the need for both open-ended debate and for practical closure. When it comes to making judgements about what is right and wrong, acceptable or unacceptable, the law is not the end of the matter. Although it is reasonable to expect a considerable convergence of the legal and the ethical, it is perfectly possible to criticise laws or legal judgments as unethical (this is the central impetus behind legal reform). On the other hand society cannot organise itself as if it were a never-ending philosophy seminar. There are many situations in which we need some authoritative system for decision making, and mechanisms for closing debate and implementing decisions – this is the role of the law. Any such system will be less than perfect but a society without such a system will be less perfect still.

Of course there are also areas in which there is little or no role for the law. The way in which nurses routinely talk to their patients raises ethical issues, and may also raise legal issues (e.g. informed consent, negligence) but unless some significant harm is involved these ethical issues can fall outside the scope of the law. For example, it is a reasonable ideal for a nurse to aim to empathise with someone she is advising or counselling; she might even feel guilty for failing to meet this ideal, but she could hardly be held legally guilty. Laws which cannot be enforced, or which are unnecessary, could be harmful in a number of ways. They could detract from respect for the law and its legitimate role, and they could create an oppressive and inflexible climate in which no-one benefited. So even if we are clear that a certain practice is ethically unacceptable it does not follow that it should be made illegal. However, the opposite can also be true. The overall consequences of legalising something which many people regard as ethically acceptable (e.g. voluntary euthanasia) may be judged, *by these same people*, to be unacceptable – as raising too many serious ethical and legal complications. Both lawyers and ethicists have to consider the proper boundaries of the law.

Even these few examples show that the relationship between the law and ethics is complicated. Professional values, such as those represented in the UKCC Code of Conduct, act as a half-way house between the two. They provide a means of enabling public discussion of public standards. They address the individual conscience but, where necessary, they are enforceable by disciplinary measures. We hope that this book will illustrate the importance of considering all of these matters together, and will help to provide nurses with insight into what is expected of them, and the skills to reflect on what they expect of themselves.

Alan Cribb and John Tingle

Notes on Contributors

Richard E. Ashcroft Professor of Biomedical Ethics, Institute of Health Sciences Education, Queen Mary, University of London, 2 Newark Street, London, E1 2AT

Professor Robert Campbell Director of Professional Research Development, University of Bolton, Deane Road, Bolton, BL3 15AB

Alan Cribb Director, Centre for Public Policy Research, King's College London, Cornwall House, London, SE1 8WA

Fiona Culley Independent Consultant, formerly Training and Liaison Manager, NMC, London

Linda Delany Principal Lecturer, School of Law, Manchester Metropolitan University, Sandra Burslem Building, Lower Ormond Street, Manchester, M15 6HB

Bobbie Farsides Professor of Clinical and Biomedical Ethics, Medical Research, Building 2.09, University of Sussex, Falmer, Brighton, BN1 9PH

Charles Foster Barrister, Outer Temple Chambers, London, WC2R 1BA

Marie Fox Professor of Law, School of Law, University of Keele, Staffordshire, ST5 5BG

Lucy Frith Lecturer in Health Care and Ethics, Division of Primary Care, The University of Liverpool, Whelan Building, Liverpool, L69 3BX

Professor Michael Gunn Pro Vice Chancellor (Learning, Teaching and Scholarship), University of Derby, Kedleston Road, Derby, DE22 1GB

John Hodgson Learning and Teaching Co-ordinator, Nottingham Law School, Nottingham Trent University, Burton Street, Nottingham, NG1 1BU

Professor Robert Lee Professor of Law and Co-Director ESRC Research Centre for Business, Responsibility, Accountability, Sustainability and Society (BRASS), Cardiff University, CF10 3AT

Harry Lesser Senior Lecturer in Philosophy, Centre for Philosophy, University of Manchester, M13 9PL

Dr Vanessa L. Mayatt Director Mayatt Risk Consulting Ltd, Rose Tree Cottage, Flaxmere, Norley, Frodsham, Cheshire, WA6 6PF and HPA Board Member, Health Protection Agency, 7th Floor Holborn Gate, 330 High Holborn, London WC1V 7PP

Professor Jean V. McHale Professor of Law, Faculty of Law, University of Leicester, Leicester, LE1 7RH

M.E. Rodgers Senior Lecturer in Law, Nottingham Trent University, Nottingham and Legal Member of the Mental Health Review Tribunal

David Seedhouse Professor of Health and Social Ethics at Auckland University of Technology and Visiting Professor of Values Transparency at Staffordshire University in the UK

Arnold Simanowitz OBE Commissioner, Commission for Patient and Public Safety in Health, Non-Executive Director, National Patient Safety Agency

John Tingle Reader in Health Law, Nottingham Law School, Nottingham Trent University, Burton Street, Nottingham, NG1 4BU

Part One: The Dimensions

1 The Legal Dimension: Legal System and Method

John Hodgson

We live in a society dominated to an increasing – some would say excessive – extent by legal rules and processes. Many of these apply to all of us, for instance the rules relating to use of the road as driver, passenger, cyclist or pedestrian, while others apply only to specific groups. In this chapter we will concentrate on the law as it affects the provision of health care. It is easier to do this than to look at the law relating to nurses or nursing, since for many purposes there is no legal distinction between different health care professionals and their contributions to the overall health care system. Before we do this, however, it is necessary to look briefly at the main features of the legal system in which health care operates. This system is the English and Welsh one; Scotland and Northern Ireland have their own systems and rules, although there are some common areas. It is also possible to draw valuable illustrations and guidance from other countries, although these are influential rather than decisive.

1.1 The law and its interpretation

In this section we will look briefly at the various sources of law operating in England and Wales and at some of the methods used by judges when they have to interpret and apply the law.[1]

1.1.1 Statute law

Most English law is in the form of statutes. These are made by the Crown in Parliament. Since 1688 the Crown in Parliament has been the supreme legislative body in England, and subsequently in the United Kingdom. A statute, or Act of Parliament, results from a bill or proposal for a statute. The bill may be proposed by the government or by any individual MP or member of the House of Lords. It is debated and approved, with or without amendment, in both Houses.[2] Once approved in Parliament, the bill receives formal Royal Assent. Statutes have been passed on almost every topic imaginable. Among those of direct relevance to the health care professions are:

- The series of statutes establishing the NHS and subsequently modifying its structure and organisation. The original Act was the National Health Service Act 1946 which carried through Nye Bevan's project to secure a national, public, health service. Today the principal Act is the National Health Service Act 1977, but this has been amended and supplemented many times, for example by the National Health Service and Community Care Act 1990, which introduced NHS Trusts and the internal market; the Health Act 1999, which introduced Primary Care Trusts and the Commission for Health Improvement; the Health and Social Care Act 2001, which made numerous changes to community health provision; and the Health and Social Care (Community Health and Standards) Act 2003, which among other things created Foundation Trusts.
- The Acts regulating the health care professions, such as the Medical Act 1983 for doctors and the Nurses, Midwives and Health Visitors Act 1997.[3]

Statutes generally provide the broad framework of rules. Thus section 1(1) of the National Health Service Act 1977 provides:

> It is the Secretary of State's duty to continue the promotion in England and Wales of a comprehensive health service designed to secure improvement – (a) in the physical and mental health of the people of those countries, and (b) in the prevention, diagnosis and treatment of illness, and for that purpose to provide or secure the effective provision of services in accordance with this Act.

This is called 'primary legislation' because it sets out basic rules. More detailed regulations are contained in statutory instruments, which are made by ministers (or in practice by their civil servants) under powers conferred by a relevant statute. This is called 'secondary legislation' because it deals with matters of detail dependent on the general powers given by primary legislation. So, for instance, the provision of general medical services is governed by sections 28Q to 28W of the National Health Service Act 1977, and these provide for regulations on a variety of topics, including the manner in which, and standards to which, services are to be provided; the persons who perform services; the persons to whom services are to be provided; and the adjudication of disputes.

The Welsh Assembly has powers to make secondary legislation of this kind for Wales, but no powers to pass primary legislation.[4]

In theory the Crown in Parliament can pass a statute on any subject whatever, and may also repeal any existing legislation. In theory Parliament can accordingly legislate for the execution of people on some arbitrary ground, such as having red hair. This is subject to three very different qualifications:

(1) Parliament can only operate within the scope of what is politically and socially acceptable. This not only means that the Red-haired Persons (Compulsory Slaughter) Act will never see the light of day, but more importantly that

legislation on such contentious issues as abortion or euthanasia is not undertaken lightly.

(2) By virtue of the European Communities Act 1972, Parliament has granted supremacy to the legislation of the European Community and Union in those areas covered by the Treaty of Rome and the Treaty of the European Union. This can mean that existing parliamentary legislation is found to be incompatible with EC law, although the courts will always try to interpret the two pieces of legislation consistently with each other, and it can even mean that new legislation must be disregarded.[5] In practice EC law does not really have much specific bearing on medico-legal and ethical issues, although since it does deal with recognition of qualifications and many equal pay and equal opportunity issues in employment law, it may have an impact on the professional life of many nurses. EC free trade and competition rules apply to drugs and medicines as they do to any other products, and they feature in much of the case law.

(3) The Human Rights Act 1998 came into full effect on 2 October 2000. This Act is designed to give effect in English law to the rights conferred by the European Convention on Human Rights and Fundamental Freedoms ('Convention rights'). This has been in effect since 1954, and was originally binding on the UK internationally, but not as part of our own legal system. So even if rules of English law, whether in statutes or otherwise, were inconsistent with the Convention, the English rule prevailed, although the UK might then be held to be in default by the European Court of Human Rights. This has now changed:

- Each new bill must be certified by the Minister responsible to comply with the Convention rights, or an explanation given as to why it is appropriate to legislate incompatibly.
- English law must be construed so far as possible to be compatible with the Convention rights. The courts have now made it clear that they will exercise this power robustly, as explained later.
- If an Act is found by the courts to be incompatible, the judges will make a declaration to that effect and it will be up to the government to invite Parliament to make the necessary changes.
- The courts will have regard to decisions of the European Court of Human Rights when interpreting English law.
- All public bodies must act in accordance with the Convention. This includes the health service.

Judges must interpret all statutes to conform to Convention rights 'so far as it is possible to do so'. Although the full implications of this are still being worked through, the approach of the judges is to first consider what the social or other policy purpose of the legislation is, then whether there is a breach of Convention rights if it is interpreted naturally. If there is, but this was clearly intended because of the overall structure of the Act, or the issues are complex and far-reaching, the judges will be reluctant to impose an alternative interpretation. Where they can work 'with the grain' of the legislation, especially where the incompatibility appears accidental, and there is no need to review policy issues, the courts will 'read down' the actual words used and substitute a form of words that secures respect for Convention rights.[6] The Convention confers a number of rights on people. Some of them are substantive in nature, such as the right to life and the right to freedom of expression, while others are procedural, such as the guarantee of a fair trial. This applies to disciplinary proceedings and requires that there be an independent and impartial tribunal. This may be problematic for bodies such as the Nursing and Midwifery Council (NMC) which have been responsible for the investigation and adjudication of complaints and do not seem to provide for the necessary degree of independence.

It is too soon to predict exactly how the Act will operate, but some areas of medico-legal significance are likely to be affected. One example is the detention of the mentally impaired. This is permitted in principle under Article 5 where it is necessary for the protection of the patient or others and there is the safeguard of an appeal to an independent judicial body independent of the executive government.[7]

In 1998 in the case of *L* v. *Bournewood NHS Trust* the House of Lords approved under the doctrine of necessity the use of informal measures to keep 'compliant' patients in hospital without using the powers under the Mental Health Act. In *HL* v. *United Kingdom* (2004) the European Court of Human Rights ruled that this did not provide adequate safeguards.[8] The right to life would appear to be of direct concern to the health care community, but in practice it focuses on negative aspects (preventing officially sanctioned killing), rather than positive ones (requiring states to provide resources and facilities to cure the sick).[9] In *D* v. *United Kingdom* (1997) it was held that, while deporting an HIV-positive prisoner to St Kitts, where treatment was not available, amounted to inhuman and degrading treatment, it was not necessary to consider whether the state was failing to ensure the right to life. Indeed recent decisions of the UK courts have held that deportation of HIV-positive patients will not even amount to inhuman or degrading treatment in the absence of extreme circumstances.[10]

It is also, however, clear as a result of one of the first cases under the Act that withdrawal of hydration and nutrition from a patient in PVS (persistent vegetative state) does not entail a breach of the right to life (*NHS Trust A* v. *Mrs M., NHS Trust B* v. *Mrs H.* (2000)).

Both the UK courts and the European Court of Human Rights have held that the refusal of the state to allow assisted suicide is neither an infringement of the right to life (this was a rather convoluted argument that the right to life included a right to terminate one's own life) nor a failure of proper respect for the privacy and autonomy of the patient. In this latter instance it was held that while there was a right to die, safeguards might be necessary against abuse and coercion, and the existing rules were not disproportionate for achieving this.[11]

1.1.2 Common law

The rules of the common law predate statute. However, there are now so many statutes in so many areas of law that the common law rules are normally of secondary importance. These rules are legal principles laid down over the centuries by the judges in deciding the cases that came before them. In theory the judges were simply isolating the relevant principles from a body of law that already existed and which represented the common view of the English people as to what was right and lawful, but in practice the judges were really developing a coherent and technical set of rules based on their own understanding of legal principle. We will look at the techniques the judges currently use later. For the moment it is important to recognise that there are some areas where, despite the rise of statute, the common law remains of considerable importance.

The best example is tort, in particular negligence. This is important to nurses, as this branch of the law deals with whether a patient who has suffered harm while being treated will be able to recover compensation because the treatment he received was inadequate.

The judges also have the task of interpreting statutes and statutory instruments and giving effect to them. They have developed their own techniques and principles for this task, which are themselves part of the common law.

An important function of the judges today is controlling the activity of central and local government and other public bodies by means of judicial review. This is now the responsibility of the Administrative Court, which is part of the High Court. Judicial review is essentially a means of ensuring that decisions and policies are made lawfully and by the correct procedures. The judges themselves have developed the rules on which decisions can be challenged and what grounds of challenge are available.[12] In principle, the judges accept that they have not been given responsibility for making the decisions in question, and so do not consider the merits. In R v. *Central Birmingham Health Authority ex parte Walker* (1987) the court had to consider a failure to provide treatment to a particular patient, as a result of decisions not to allocate funds to this particular aspect of the health authority's operations. It was held that the authority was responsible for planning and delivering health care within a given budget and the resulting decisions on priorities. The court could not substitute its own, inexpert, judgment, particularly as it would only hear detailed arguments about the needs of this one patient and not about the whole range of demands. The issue of health care resources is more fully discussed in Chapter 8.

1.1.3 European Union/Community Law

Throughout the post-World War II period, the states of western Europe have been engaged in a complex and long-term project of economic cooperation and integration. The first major stage in this was the Treaty of Rome, which established the European Economic Community in the 1950s. The United Kingdom joined this Community in 1974. The initial objective was the establishment of a common market, an area within which there was to be free movement of the various factors of production of goods and provision of services, namely goods, labour, management and professional skills and capital. Initially this meant the removal of obvious barriers, such as customs duties, immigration controls, exchange controls on money and other restrictions. Subsequently other objectives, such as environmental protection, have been added, although the main impact of the Community is still on economic affairs.

Free movement of workers, guaranteed by Article 39 of the European Community Treaty, implied many additional social policies, as workers would not, in practice, move around the Community unless their social security entitlements were ensured and they were allowed to bring their families with them. Genuine freedom of movement also required a common approach to qualifications, with no discrimination on grounds of nationality, and also equal opportunity, at least between men and women. This has resulted in much legislation and many decisions of the European Court of Justice. Article 47 of the Treaty specifically gives power to regulate mutual recognition of diplomas and qualifications. Directives 77/452 and 80/154 have made provision for general nurses and midwives respectively, and there are also general frameworks for the recognition of degree-level and other vocational qualifications (covering a number of professions allied to medicine) in Directives 89/48 and 92/51 respectively. The case of *Marshall* v. *Southampton and SW Hants AHA* (1986) established that UK law permitting differential retirement ages as between men and women in the health service was incompatible with EC law requiring equal treatment, and as a result the UK law had to be disregarded.

The member states of the Community have agreed, in effect, to transfer their sovereign rights to make and apply laws to the Community institutions in those areas for which the Community is to be responsible. As a result EC law prevails over national law in these areas where they are in conflict. However, there are a number of different mechanisms for securing this, and it is not simply a question of ignoring national legal provisions. The European Union, introduced in the Maastricht Treaty of 1992, operates somewhat differently. It is an agreement by the member states to cooperate and collaborate in relation to foreign affairs and aspects of criminal justice and home affairs, but action is by the states acting through the European Council and no rights are transferred to the other institutions, although one of the Commissioners has responsibility for the common foreign policies determined by the European Council.

The European Council, which comprises the heads of government of the member states together with the president of the European Commission, is also the principal policy-making and legislative body for the Community. In some cases it can legislate itself, after consultation with the European Parliament. In most cases, however, the legislation is made jointly by the Council and the Parliament. In many cases the Council can act by a majority, and thus legislate against the wishes of one or more member states. The majority is usually a 'qualified' or weighted majority designed to ensure that there is very substantial support for the measure. In practice great efforts are made to ensure a consensus of opinion. The Parliament does not initiate legislation but, as noted above, does have to approve and join in making most important legislation, so it has at least a blocking power and can suggest amendments. The Parliament must also approve the Community budget and also the members of the Commission. It may also remove the whole Commission, and although it has never voted to do so, the likelihood of this occurring led to the resignation of the Commission in 1999 as a result of allegations of financial irregularities against one of them.

The Commission is the administrative, arm of the Community. It implements policies and proposes legislation, and can itself make detailed regulations, particularly in relation to the Common Agricultural Policy. It also makes decisions on alleged infringements of Community law, for example in relation to competition law. It is responsible as 'guardian of the treaties' for ensuring that member states comply with their Community obligations.

The European Court of Justice, assisted by the Court of First Instance, has the sole responsibility, to the exclusion of the national courts of the member states, for interpreting EC law; it does so by means of rulings on points of law referred by national courts (Article 234 of the Treaty), deciding cases brought against the member states for alleged failure to comply with their obligations under EC law by the Commission (Articles 226 and 228–9) and by judicial review of the validity of acts of the institutions (decisions on particular cases or secondary legislation) on the application of other institutions, the member states and others directly affected (Article 230).

There are two forms of Act that amount to secondary legislation. These are Regulations and Directives; both are governed by Article 249 of the Treaty. Regulations, which may be made by the Council, with or without the Parliament, or by the Commission, are directly effective rules of Community law that must be obeyed by all persons and companies within the EC and will be enforced by national courts. Directives, which are normally made by the Council and Parliament, are used where the EC wishes to ensure that national law in all member states achieves the same results, but it is not appropriate to do this by way of regulation. One example is in relation to company law, where the law of the states is very variable in its form and terminology, so regulations would be meaningless.

Community law applies not only to states but also to individuals. This was not clear from the beginning, but the Court of Justice ruled in *van Gend & Loos* (1962) that an individual could rely on a treaty provision which was clear and complete and capable of conferring direct rights (in this case a prohibition on new customs duties) to defeat a claim by a state based on its own incompatible legislation. In *Defrenne* v. *Sabena* (1976) it was held that a treaty provision meeting these requirements (in this case the right to equal pay for women) could be relied on against a person or company, notwithstanding incompatible national legislation.

The position with regard to directives is more complex. They normally provide for an implementation period; while this is running they have no legal effect (*Pubblico Ministero* v. *Ratti* (1979)).

After the implementation date they are binding on the state,[13] so the state is prevented from relying on its own incompatible law. In addition, the state can be obliged to act in accordance with them (*Marshall* v. *Southampton and SW Hants AHA* (1986)).

This binding effect applies to the courts, which must interpret national legislation 'as far as possible' in accordance with the directive, even in cases involving two private litigants with no state involvement (*Marleasing* (1992)). This applies particularly to rules relating to remedies, which must be effective (*von Colson* (1986)). However, where the two cannot be reconciled, national law will prevail (*Wagner Miret* (1993)).

A directive cannot be relied on as such against a private individual or company (*Faccini-Dori* v. *Recreb* (1995)), although the court can be asked to interpret national law as above.

Where an individual or company suffers loss as the result of the failure of the state to implement a directive properly or at all, as a last resort the state may be held liable in damages (*Francovich* (1993)) provided that the breach is sufficiently grave (*Brasserie du Pêcheur/Factortame* (No. 3) (1996)). In principle this liability extends to a court decision that fails to apply community law (*Köbler* (2004)). Note also that this remedy may be available where the state fails to comply with EC law in other ways, as was the case in Factortame.

English courts have been willing to apply very radical interpretative methods to English legislation introduced specifically to give effect to EC requirements, even 'reading them down' to the extent of reversing the apparent meaning of the English legislation. The reasoning behind this is that it was the primary intention of Parliament to comply with the EC requirement, and the words used were believed to achieve this, so any reinterpretation meets that underlying purpose, even if it is not the obvious interpretation of the particular passage (*Pickstone* v. *Freemans* (1989); *Litster* v. *Forth Dry Dock* (1990)). After considerable uncertainty it seems that the same will apply to other legislation not passed specifically to meet EC requirements (*R* v. *Secretary of State for Employment ex p Equal Opportunities Commission* (1994); *Webb* v. *EMO Air Cargo* (No. 2) (1995)) although there is some suggestion that the English courts are happier to see damages claims for non-implementation, rather than radical interpretation (*Kirklees MBC* v. *Wickes* (1993)).

1.2 The English legal system

The English legal system has developed over many centuries, and although there have been piecemeal reforms, many old procedures and systems remain in place. This applies particularly to titles. Why should the principal judge of the civil side of the Court of Appeal be called the Master of the Rolls? He has nothing to do with either baking or gymnastics. What actually happened was that an official responsible for keeping the official records, or rolls, of the Chancery was gradually given a judicial role and by the nineteenth century, when the Court of Appeal in its modern form was established, he had become a senior judge and was therefore the right person to be appointed to preside over the Court of Appeal. Effectively there are two court systems in England. The criminal courts concentrate on crime, and the civil courts deal with everything else. There are some exceptions, where specialised tribunals have been set up. The most important of these are probably the Employment Tribunals[14] and the Employment Appeal Tribunal, which deal with most employment-related issues, including equal opportunities, although the various tribunals within the social security system deal with more cases. There are also separate tribunals for income tax and VAT.

1.2.1 Criminal justice system

All cases start with an appearance in the magistrates' court. Usually the case will have been investigated by the police and will be prosecuted by the Crown

Prosecution Service, but other government departments and agencies, local authorities and bodies such as the RSPCA also prosecute cases. Private individuals may prosecute, but rarely do. There are a total of some 2,000,000 cases each year[15] of which 75% are purely summary offences (motoring offences such as speeding, careless driving and defective vehicles, and other minor offences of drunkenness, vandalism, assault, etc.). These must be dealt with in the magistrates' court. The great majority of defendants plead guilty or do not contest the case. The remaining more serious offences fall into two groups. The most serious offences, such as murder, rape and robbery, can only be tried at the Crown court, 'on indictment'. The magistrates' court only deals with bail and legal aid. These are actually a small proportion of the total. The others are the middle range of offences (e.g. most assaults, theft, fraud and burglary). These are said to be triable 'either way'. This means that if the defendant admits the charge when it is put to him in the magistrates' court he is convicted there, although he may be committed to the Crown court for sentence if the magistrates' powers of sentence[16] are inadequate. If he does not admit the offence the magistrates must decide whether they have power to hear the case, having regard to its seriousness and complexity. If they decline to hear it the case must go to the Crown court. If they agree to hear the case the defendant may still elect trial at the Crown court.

Where a case is heard by the magistrates the defendant may appeal against sentence (and, if he pleaded not guilty, conviction) to the Crown court. These appeals are heard by a judge sitting with magistrates. Although an appeal against conviction is a full rehearing, it will not be before a jury. Both prosecution and defence may appeal to the Queen's Bench Division of the High Court[17] where they consider that the final decision is wrong on a point of law (as opposed to being a wrong decision on the facts). They may also apply to the same court for judicial review of any preliminary decision (e.g. on bail or legal aid).

The Crown court deals with about 80,000 cases a year, of which about 20,000 are contested trials. About 40% of these result in acquittals. These trials are before a judge and jury, with the judge responsible for decisions on matters of law, evidence and procedure, and the jury responsible for matters of fact and the final verdict.

The defendant may appeal to the Court of Appeal (Criminal Division) on the ground that the verdict is unsafe. The Court considers whether the defendant was prejudiced by irregularities at the trial such as rulings of the judge on law, or the admissibility of evidence, or errors in the judge's summing up. In effect the Court is asking, 'Can we rely on the jury's verdict, or do we feel that they would have decided otherwise if the irregularity had not occurred?'. The prosecution may not appeal against an acquittal, although they may ask the Court of Appeal to consider the point of law involved in an acquittal on a hypothetical basis by an Attorney General's reference. The defendant may, with leave, appeal against sentence, and the prosecution may appeal against an unduly lenient sentence. There is an appeal to the House of Lords for both prosecutor and defendant from the Court of Appeal where the case raises a point of law of public importance.

Although nurses may commit crimes, there is usually no direct connection with their professional activities. The availability of controlled drugs in a hospital environment may lead nurses into temptation, and there may be cases of delib-erate harm to patients, which will be prosecuted as assaults under the Offences Against the Person Act 1861, or in extreme cases as murder, as in the notorious case of Beverley Allitt, a children's nurse at Grantham hospital, who in the 1990s mur-dered or seriously harmed a number of children in her care. Nurses have no general privileges in relation to the physical management of patients, but most actions undertaken reasonably and in good faith will be protected by the ordinary law of self-defence, actions taken to prevent crime (restraining one patient to prevent an attack on another) and necessity. Restraint is also specifically authorised in some circumstances under the Mental Health Act. Prosecutions usually result from actions that go well beyond normal practice, for which there is no apparent explanation, and that are clear abuses of the nurse's professional responsibil-ities. In extreme cases health professionals may find themselves facing criminal charges arising from decisions made and actions taken within normal profes-sional parameters:

- Manslaughter by gross negligence. Where one person owes another a duty of care (and a nurse owes this duty to a patient), there may be criminal liability where there is a clear and obvious breach of this duty that obviously exposes the victim to a specific risk of death, and the victim dies (*R* v. *Adomako* (1994)). In *R* v. *Misra and Srivastava* (2005) this principle was applied in a case where junior doctors failed to recognise that a post-operative patient was suffering from an iatrogenic infection. Arguments that the offence was incompatible with the ECHR were rejected, as were arguments that negligence, even gross negligence, was inappropriate as a basis for criminal liability.
- 'Mercy killing' or active euthanasia. Any action that results in the shortening of life, and that is undertaken with that intent, is murder. It is irrelevant that the victim is terminally ill and in acute distress or severely disabled, and whether or not the victim or the next of kin consents. Juries are notoriously unwilling to convict,[18] and reliance is often placed on 'double effect', which legitimises the use of strong pain control, even if life is incidentally shortened.

1.2.2 Civil justice system

The general system was, in the late 1990s, significantly reformed by the intro-duction of new Civil Procedure Rules.[19] These create a new overriding objective of dealing with cases justly, having regard to ensuring that the parties are on an equal footing, expense and proportionality to the importance and complexity of the case. In practice this means that all cases are allocated either to the 'small claims track' for speedy and informal disposal of small-scale disputes, to the 'fast track' for routine cases requiring limited court time or to a 'multi-track' which allows for more complex cases to be handled as they deserve. Procedural judges take charge of the timetable of the case and the parties have to comply with the standard timetable of the fast track, or the agreed timetable in the multi-track. In the process the distinction between the county court and the High Court has been blurred. Most cases will actually be tried in the county court, including many high-value claims, but High Court judges will continue to hear the most complex cases. A decision of a procedural judge may be appealed to a circuit judge, and an appeal from the decision at a trial may be made to the Court of Appeal. There are special arrangements for family law cases.

Much of the work of the High Court is now judicial review. This is, in effect, a review of the legality and propriety of decisions by government departments and other public bodies while exercising statutory powers. The main grounds of review are illegality, where the decision is outside the powers given; procedural impropriety, such as a failure to give the applicant notice of the allegations against him; and irrationality, or reaching a decision that no reasonable body, carefully considering all relevant considerations, could have reached.

There is an appeal from the county court or High Court to the Court of Appeal, provided that the leave of either court is obtained. There is an appeal from the Court of Appeal to the House of Lords, but as in criminal cases there must be an issue of public importance.

One aspect of civil law that impinges directly on the health care profession is negligence. This is dealt with in depth in Chapter 6. At this stage it is important to note that liability for negligence is essentially liability for failure to reach a proper standard of care in dealing with someone to whom a legal duty is owed. In many cases this duty is imposed by the law in general terms, but in others it arises from a prior contractual agreement.

Since the eighteenth century it has been established that a physician or surgeon (and by extension any health care professional who takes responsibility for a patient) owes a duty to that patient. This general duty covers all NHS patients. It does not extend to practitioners who are 'off duty' and may be required to intervene if, for example, they come upon an accident victim in the street. In private medicine there is a contract between the practitioner and the patient. Ordinarily, this contract will merely require the practitioner to use reasonable care and skill[20] and this is the same standard as under the general law. However, in some circumstances the patient may have greater rights under the contract. The contract may specify a particular model of artificial hip, and failure to provide this is a breach. There would be liability to an NHS patient only if the device fitted was one that was not regarded as suitable by a responsible body of opinion. Normally a practitioner undertakes to use proper care and skill, but does not guarantee a cure. However, a contract may include a warranty of a cure, although this would be unusual (*Thake* v. *Maurice* (1986)).

Another important function is the inherent jurisdiction of the court to protect the interests of the incompetent. This is particularly relevant to 'end of life decisions' but also occurs in relation to consent to treatment. These cases often take the form of an application for a declaration. However, often the issues at stake are essentially questions of trespass to the person. Touching or restraining a person is normally a wrong, but if it is in the best interests of an incompetent person it may be justified by necessity. Examples include the PVS cases of *Bland* v. *Airedale* (1993) and the 'informal detention' case of *L* v. *Bournewood* (1998) which we have already met. These issues are dealt with in depth in Chapter 7.

1.3 Legal method

Judges have two roles. First, they are responsible for ensuring that the facts of the particular case are ascertained. They do this directly in civil cases, and supervise the jury in criminal cases. This is an important task, and vital for the parties to the case. It is not, however, the more legally significant of the two roles. The crucial role is in ascertaining the law, so that it can be applied to the facts of the case. The facts are usually quite specific, and affect only the parties,[21] but the legal principle is of general application. As indicated above, ascertaining the law may involve a review of existing common law rules or an interpretation of statute, Community law or the European Convention on Human Rights.

In English law, judges have the power to state the law. In this they differ from judges in most Continental European systems, who have no status to declare the law but merely a duty to interpret and apply the law that is to be found in the national legal codes. Of course these interpretations are entitled to respect and are usually followed for the sake of consistency and because they reflect a learned opinion on the meaning of the texts. However, if judges can state the law, it is necessary to have rules as to which statements are authoritative and must be followed (whether later judges agree with them or not).

1.3.1 Binding authority

The following statements of law, forming the basis of legal principle on which a case was decided, are binding on later judges:

Decisions of the European Court of Justice bind all English courts. Subject to the above, decisions of the House of Lords bind all other English courts. The House itself may, if it is persuaded that there is good reason to do so (either because there is a strong case that the earlier decision was wrong, or because the earlier decision is no longer appropriate to modern social and economic conditions) depart from an earlier decision and restate the law. Decisions of the Court of Appeal bind the Court of Appeal and all lower courts. Decisions of the Divisional Court bind magistrates' courts.

Judges may consider any other material; this will, however, merely be persuasive. It can include obiter dicta or comments in a judgment that do not form part of the basis of the decision,[22] statements in dissenting judgments,[23] statements by more junior judges,[24] decisions in other jurisdictions and academic comments. Decisions of the European Court[25] of Human Rights come into this category.[26]

An earlier statement of law will only be binding if the present case raises the same legal issue. It is possible to distinguish cases by explaining how, while similar, they do not raise the same legal issues. It is also possible to cheat by claiming to distinguish cases where the judge does not want to follow the earlier ruling, or vice versa, and it is often difficult to be sure whether judges are using this technique properly or not. Applying the law is an art, not a mechanical process.

In practice judges need to go beyond earlier statements of the law. New issues arise and new social and economic conditions arise. In the past judges were very coy about admitting that they did make new rules rather than reinterpreting old ones, but they now accept that they do. They are usually very conservative, preferring to go no further than strictly necessary. When in *Airedale NHS Trust* v. *Bland* (1993) the House of Lords was asked to rule on whether treatment could be withheld from a patient in an irreversible persistent vegetative state, they did so on the narrow basis that there was no justification for intrusive treatment as it did not serve the patient's best interests, and expressly stated that they could not consider general arguments based on the legality or desirability of general rules on euthanasia. That was a matter for Parliament.

1.3.2 Interpreting statutes (and Community law)

The law has been laid down here by Parliament (or the Community institutions). The judges may or may not approve, but in principle they must apply the law as passed. Unfortunately not all law is clear. There may be inconsistencies or ambiguities, or there may be situations that Parliament did not foresee and therefore did not cover.

Over the years the judges have worked out an approach to interpretation which allows some flexibility but stays as close as possible to the words actually enacted by Parliament. The approach will depend to some extent on the type of legislation. Criminal and tax legislation is always interpreted against the state in cases of doubt, while legislation intended to meet a Community law requirement will be interpreted to achieve that purpose.

The priority is to give effect to the words of the statute if they have a plain and unambiguous meaning. This will be applied even if it is not what Parliament 'meant', as in the case of *Fisher* v. *Bell* (1961), where Parliament had clearly introduced legislation designed to prohibit trading in flick knives. However, it created an offence of 'offering' such a knife for sale, and when a shopkeeper was prosecuted because she had one on display in the window the court ruled that since it had already been decided that it was the customer who made an offer for goods on display, she was not guilty of the offence. The words used were clear, and it was wrong to look back at what the underlying intention was as this was a criminal case and the statute had to be interpreted in favour of the defendant anyway. Where wording is ambiguous various approaches may be used:

- Preferring a sensible meaning to an absurd meaning. So the word 'marry' in the definition of the crime of bigamy was interpreted in *R* v. *Allen* (1872) as 'go through a form of marriage' rather than 'contract a [valid] marriage' which would have made the offence impossible to commit, as someone already married cannot validly marry again.
- Consideration of the underlying intention of the statute. In *Kruhlak* v. *Kruhlak* (1958) the expression 'single woman' in the context of affiliation proceedings was interpreted to mean any woman not living with her husband or supported by him; that is, it could include a divorcee or widow. The mischief was the need to ensure financial support for illegitimate children, whatever the marital status of the mother. Similarly in *Knowles* v. *Liverpool Council* (1993) a broad interpretation was given to the expression 'equipment' in the Employers'

Liability (Defective Equipment) Act 1969, in order to give effect to the broad aims of the legislation in the light of the known mischief.
- Refer to any authoritative statement in Hansard by the sponsoring minister on the meaning of the particular provision (*Pepper* v. *Hart* (1993)).

The main danger in interpretation is that the greater the leeway the judges allow themselves, the more likely it is that they will be accused of interpreting to suit their own notions of what is right and proper. As most such cases either involve issues of political controversy or raise contentious ethical issues, and this will increasingly be the case under the Human Rights Act, there is increasing concentration on the judges, and questions are increasingly being asked about their qualifications to adjudicate on these controversial issues as opposed to technical legal matters, where their expertise is acknowledged.

1.4 The legal context of nursing

Nurses are governed by three separate sets of legal rules,[27] quite apart from the law that establishes the framework of the NHS and the general law of the land. There are legal obligations to patients, normally arising in the context of allegations of negligence. There are professional obligations, imposed in the case of nurses by the NMC, which is responsible for education, registration, professional standards and discipline. The essence of the professional standards[28] established by the NMC in its Code of Practice are that each nurse must:

- safeguard and promote the interests of individual patients and clients
- serve the interests of society; justify public trust and confidence
- uphold and enhance the good standing and reputation of the professions.

Specific obligations in the Code of Practice require the nurse to respect the right of the patient to be involved in the planning of care, to work cooperatively with colleagues and to report anything that adversely affects the standard of care being provided.

The large majority of nurses work as employees in the NHS or the private health sector and thus have a legal employment relationship. Despite the reforms of the 1980s which were intended to create an internal market of independent NHS Trusts, each establishing its own terms and conditions of employment to replace the earlier national Whitley Council arrangements, in practice terms and conditions have remained relatively uniform. The employer is entitled to a professional standard of performance of the duties assigned, and the employee is entitled to be treated properly. Three aspects of employment law appear to be particularly relevant to the nursing profession:

1.4.1 Equal opportunity

Equal opportunity, both between the sexes and in relation to ethnicity, has been a major issue for many years. The latter is a purely English matter, regulated by the Race Relations Acts, while the former is regulated by the Equal Pay Act and the Sex Discrimination Act, both supplemented by Community law. Direct discrimination is rare, and most difficulties concern disguised discrimination.

Disadvantageous treatment of part-time workers may amount to indirect discrimination because these part-time workers are predominantly female (*R* v. *Secretary of State for Employment ex parte EOC* (1995)). The salary scale for a particular group may be depressed because the profession or group is largely female, and this may constitute indirect discrimination (*Enderby* v. *Frenchay Health Authority* (1993)) although it is important that the two groups are actually comparable, and where one is objectively rated as more demanding, the case will fail.[29] The law will seek to deal with historical anomalies based on gender-specific recruitment, but cannot resolve complaints about the relative valuation of different jobs.

1.4.2 Psychological and stress-related industrial illness

Employers are increasingly being held liable for psychological and stress-related industrial illness where it arises from the way in which work is organised and allocated. In *Lancaster* v. *Birmingham City Council* (1999) the employer transferred an administrative employee to a new post in a significantly different area with a promise of training and support that did not materialise. The employer admitted liability for the resultant disabling stress. In *Walker* v. *Northumberland CC* (1995) the employee, a social work manager, became ill with work-related stress. On his return to work he received no support and his workload increased. The employer was held liable when he suffered a recurrence. In *Johnstone* v. *Bloomsbury Health Authority* (1990) the Court of Appeal held that a junior doctor had an arguable case that the conditions under which he was obliged to work constituted a reasonably foreseeable risk to his health. Since much of the work in some areas of the NHS, in particular A&E departments and ICUs, is inherently highly stressful, and other work can easily become so if poorly managed or short-staffed, this is clearly a significant area. The House of Lords has now confirmed that there may be liability in such cases provided that the employer is aware that there is a risk of such harm: *Barber* v. *Somerset CC* (2004).

1.4.3 'Whistle blowing'

'Whistle blowing' has been problematic. Nurses are under a professional duty to report circumstances that may adversely affect patient care. They may also be under a duty to the patient. Some employers, including NHS Trusts, place greater weight on the management of information and resent adverse publicity, whether or not it is justified. Nurses who have publicised matters of concern have in the past attracted considerable attention and suffered serious consequences, like Graham Pink, a nurse at Stepping Hill Hospital, who became frustrated at what he considered to be managerial indifference to his complaints over staffing levels and in the early 1990s drew these to public notice, attracting disciplinary action from his employers as a result. Some protection is now given by the Public

Interest Disclosure Act 1998. This protects an employee from dismissal or other retaliatory action if he discloses information relating to circumstances which disclose an apparent breach of legal duties or a threat to the health and safety of any person. The disclosure must be to the employer, to the Secretary of State if the employee is in the public sector (including NHS Trusts, but not GP practices) or to the press or public where the employer has not taken action on an earlier report to him.

Most of the time these three duties do not cut across each other. Most of the time employers and employees have a common interest in promoting the welfare of patients in an efficient and professional manner. There are problems, however. The employee may feel professionally obligated to report deficiencies in the employer's services to patients or may feel that other professionals are not respecting the patient's autonomy, or allowing the nurse to act as an effective patient advocate.[30] In these circumstances the law is, at best, an imperfect instrument. Balancing the three duties is difficult, and a legal process that focuses on which of two cases has the better basis in law and in fact is not well adapted to weigh more complex issues.

1.5 Notes

1. We only have time for a brief consideration of these matters; for a more detailed treatment see either Terence Ingman, *The English Legal Process* (London, Blackstone Press, 2000) or Michael Zander, *The Law-Making Process* (London, Butterworths, 1999).
2. A bill may be voted down. This often happens to bills proposed by individuals (private members' bills) but rarely to government bills because the government can usually guarantee that its MPs will support it. The Lords is less predictable even after the recent reforms, but cannot block financial and tax bills, will not block bills that are part of the manifesto on which the government was elected and can in any event only delay bills for one year.
3. There are over 1400 references to 'medical practitioner' in statutes ranging from obvious ones such as the Mental Health Act to others such as the Deregulation and Contracting Out Act and the House of Commons (Disqualification) Act.
4. The position in Scotland is different. The Scottish Parliament can pass primary legislation on a large range of issues, including the health service.
5. As occurred in the *Factortame (No. 2)* case [1991] 1 AC 603.
6. See *Ghaidin* v. *Godin-Mendoza* [2004] UKHL 3007.
7. The European Court of Human Rights (ECtHR) case of *X* v. *UK* (Case 7215/75, judgment 5.11.81) established that the original advisory role of the Mental Health Review Tribunal did not meet this requirement. As a result the MHRT now makes the decision itself.
8. Measures to provide a review procedure for these patients will be introduced as amendments to the Mental Capacity Act 2005.
9. There may be a positive obligation on the police authorities where an individual is under specific threat: *Osman* v. *United Kingdom* (1998) ECtHR Reports 1998-VIII. In *LCB* v. *United Kingdom* (1998) ECtHR Reports 1998-III, the court considered 'that the first sentence of Article 2, section 1, enjoins the State not only to refrain from the intentional and unlawful taking of life, but also to take appropriate steps to safeguard the lives of

those within its jurisdiction', but this was again in the context of non-health-related government action (exposure to radiation during nuclear tests).

10. *N* v. *Home Office* [2005] UKHL 31.
11. *Pretty* v. *DPP* [2001] UKHL 61; *Pretty* v. *UK* 2346/02.
12. These are, essentially, that the decision was illegal because it was made without power to act, was irrational or was in breach of procedural fairness.
13. Which includes state agencies such as the NHS.
14. Formerly Industrial Tribunals.
15. This excludes some 7,000,000 fixed penalties for motoring and parking offences. Source: *Home Office Digest* 4: http://www.homeoffice.gov.uk/rds/digest4/digest4.pdf
16. Up to 12 months' (or in some cases two years') custody and usually fines of £5000 per offence.
17. Additionally, this may be done after the defendant has exercised his right of appeal to the Crown court.
18. *R* v. *Arthur*, *The Times* 5.11.81, was a case where nutrition was withheld from a severely disabled neonate, who died. There was some evidence of acute ailments other than those initially identified, and which might have led to death. The doctor appeared to have decided, with the parents, that they did not want the child to survive, but was nevertheless acquitted by the jury. In *R* v. *Cox* [1993] 2 All ER 19 the jury were in tears as they convicted of attempted murder relating to an elderly terminally ill patient who had repeatedly asked for release from her intractable pain.
19. The so-called 'Woolf Reforms', following a report by Lord Woolf.
20. Section 13, Supply of Goods and Services Act 1982.
21. There are of course important cases where the facts affect many different people, such as industrial disease and drug defect claims, but these are in the minority.
22. The so-called 'neighbour principle' expounded by Lord Atkin in *Donoghue* v. *Stevenson* in 1932 has been extremely influential in the development of liability for negligence over the past 30 years.
23. A dissent by Lord Justice Denning in *Candler* v. *Crane Christmas* in 1949 ([1951] 2 KB 164) formed the basis of the decision of the House of Lords in *Hedley Byrne* v. *Heller* in 1964 ([1964] AC 465).
24. The so-called *Bolam* test for medical negligence was laid down by Mr Justice McNair, but has been endorsed by many senior judges in the Court of Appeal and House of Lords.
25. Also decisions of the European Commission on Human Rights and of the Council of Ministers of the Council of Europe, both of which formerly had a role in the application of the European convention.
26. Human Rights Act 1998, section 2.
27. Those working in mental health are also governed by the Mental Health Act, making four in all.
28. See http://www.nmc-uk.org/aFramedisplay.aspx?documentID=201
29. As in *Southampton & District HA* v. *Worsfold* (1999) LTL 15.9.99, where a female speech therapist's work was rated at 55 and a male clinical psychologist's at 56.5.
30. UKCC Guidelines for Professional Practice 1996, pp. 9–11.

2 The Ethical Dimension: Nursing Practice, Nursing Philosophy and Nursing Ethics

Alan Cribb

What are the values that shape nursing practice? This is a much debated question. In fact most of the debate that takes place in nursing and in the academic nursing literature is about values. The only exception is debate about purely factual or technical matters. Value debates take place about the nature of professional–patient relationships, and about ideas like empowerment, partnership and advocacy. More specifically there are a host of particular debates about such things as how midwives can best protect the interests of pregnant women, or how far the work of health visitors should be dictated by public health targets. Set alongside these are discussions about the professional standards of nursing, the framework of which is reviewed in the next chapter. All these debates should be seen as continuous with nursing ethics, because they all involve making value judgements about the means or ends of nursing care; in short, they all ask: 'What is good nursing?' Anyone who has an interest in, and some grasp of, these issues is already 'inside' nursing ethics although they may not have thought about their concerns in these terms.

This is not meant to imply that nursing ethics is easy – far from it: all of these issues are complex. In any case even if someone was very good at debating the nature of 'good nursing' this would not make them 'a good nurse'. If nursing ethics is to be of more than academic interest it should have something to say about how people might become good nurses. I will return to this question later, but notice that there is some apparent ambiguity in it. If we talk about a nurse being 'a good nurse' are we talking about her professional or technical skills or are we making an ethical judgement about her character, or perhaps both? It would certainly seem odd to call someone a good nurse if she could demonstrate many 'competences' but lacked any concern for or commitment to her clients or colleagues. In this respect it seems very different from calling someone a good mathematician – having a set of skills that is, on the face of it, compatible with being lazy, insensitive, and self-centred!

All nursing practice is necessarily informed, partly implicitly, by some nursing philosophy. Such a philosophy embodies answers to a range of questions that are faced by any nurse. These include questions about the aims of care, professional–client relationships, working in teams and with colleagues, and wider questions about institutional, local or national policies. Although nursing involves activities other than patient or client care, such as health care research and management, it seems reasonable to view care as central, and to see the other activities as supporting this central one. But 'care' is too broad a notion to be of much help in clarifying the aims of nursing; care is the focus, but what are the aims of care?

One example of the debate about nursing philosophy and the aims of nursing is represented in what has been called the shift 'from sick nursing to health nursing'.[1] This shift – which is dramatic in some areas of practice and incremental in others – is from doing things to patients towards working with them; from an approach that is 'disease based' and expert centred to one that is 'health based' and patient centred. Such a shift follows from and reflects many things including changing patterns of ill health, emerging professional roles, an increase in consumerism, and developing ideas about health promotion. But at its heart is what might be called an ethical shift, a shift in values which has two interrelated components. First, and rather crudely put, there is a move from treating people as passive towards treating them with respect as equals. This is not only because individuals have an important role to play in their own care, but also because individuals 'deserve' to be treated with respect, whether or not to do so is useful to professionals. Secondly, there is a move from equating the best interests of patients with being 'disease free' towards an acceptance that there is much more to well-being. Quality of life, peace of mind, and self respect, for example, are legitimate concerns for a nurse, as well as disease management. These two components are closely related because one aspect of well-being, an aspect that many see as fundamental, is being able to make choices and have them treated with respect. These issues will be discussed more fully in the next section.

This example of a cultural shift shows the importance of what can be called 'habitual ethics':[2,3] the ethical judgements that individuals make as a matter of course; the values that are built into ways of working. Any shift in the philosophy or culture of nursing which entails that normal practice and expectations are changed, has enormous impact. Practice can be enhanced (or made worse) for literally thousands of people. Generally speaking much less rests upon the prolonged agonising about particular cases, however difficult they are. Of course these sorts of shifts in normal practice are difficult to implement: they involve reform of policies, institutions and so on. To reformers they might seem an overwhelming task, like trying to get the earth to spin on a different axis, yet they are the bedrock for any practical ethic.

2.1 Promoting welfare and well-being

Let us say, to use a piece of shorthand, that nursing is about the promotion of well-being. This seems a useful phrase yet, at the same time, it throws up a lot of questions. Many of the key ethical issues faced by nurses and other health care workers can be identified and clarified by working through some of these questions.

Is this formulation of the nurse's role not too broad? There are many aspects of well-being; someone's well-being may be increased by a tour of the Mediterranean, by acquiring a new friend, or by learning Latin. None of these things, nor many others like them, seem to be the function of nursing. So perhaps it would be better to say that nursing is about the promotion of certain elements of well-being. One version of this, for example, is to equate nursing with the promotion of health. This is only an improvement if we can give a meaning to health that is less all-encompassing than well-being, and yet less narrow than the idea of absence of disease, which fails to capture all of the work of nurses. A number of authors have advocated a 'middle-order' conception of health, with the intention that such a conception would help clarify the central objectives and priorities of health workers.[4,5] Broadly speaking this conception identifies health with what others would call 'welfare': that is, someone is healthy to the extent that they have the resources to pursue and achieve well-being or fulfilment. In practical terms this would mean that nursing is about helping to ensure that individuals are in a position to travel, or to learn languages and so forth. This is not the place to review all of the discussions that have taken place on the theme. But it is possible to make a few comments on the central issues.

Although it is useful to try to clarify the aims of nursing, there is no reason to suppose that a single phrase or formula will capture everything that nurses aim at. It is reasonable to assert that the central or overall aim of nursing is to contribute to welfare, but this simple formula needs to be qualified, otherwise it is arguably both too broad and too narrow. First, the way in which welfare is promoted is, in the main, based around the management (including prevention) of suffering or risk rather than wider aspects of welfare promotion such as financial assistance or education, although there is a place for these within health care. That is to say that nurses rightly do not regard the promotion of all aspects of all people's welfare as within their remit. They respond to the suffering of individuals, or to the risks faced by certain populations. Secondly, once in a relationship with a client they need to have regard to all aspects of well-being that might be relevant to caring for that person. This is part of what is meant by holistic care, but it also follows from a concern with the promotion of welfare, for how can you know whether you are contributing to someone's welfare if you do not see what you do in the context of their whole life? Only by having regard to the whole can nurses ensure that their work is in the interests of their clients.

It is not possible to promote welfare, for example, without having regard to both the costs and the benefits of proposed interventions. Any intervention is likely to have some 'cost' or risk for the client which has to be weighed against the expected benefit; and there will be wider costs and benefits for others affected directly or indirectly. (We will return to this below.) Neither can welfare be promoted without having regard to the wishes or preferences of clients. This is because an important part of my welfare consists in having my wishes respected. So even if a nurse is clear about her aims, and has a clear view of what is in the interest of her client, she faces a number of potential problems of fundamental importance. What if the client disagrees about what is in his or her interest? What if the client agrees that in some respects the nurse's preferred intervention is in his or her interest but for some reason does not wish the intervention to take place? What if the client is not in a position to express an opinion? Under all of these sets of circumstances an appeal to 'promoting welfare' is not sufficient. A well-intentioned intervention is not necessarily in the best interest of clients, and even in those cases where it is, that is not sufficient to justify unwanted 'interference' in people's lives.

The possible tension between 'welfare' and 'wishes' is one of the key issues in health care ethics. Many of the contributions in this book discuss it in one form or another. How should nurses balance promoting the welfare and respecting the wishes of their clients? This is, for example, the background against which the importance of informed consent is discussed. This issue is so important in health care contexts because these typically involve, on the one hand, a patient who is in some distress and in a relatively powerless state and, on the other hand, a group of health professionals in relatively powerful positions who are charged with looking after the patient. This creates a constant temptation to 'take over' in one way or another for the sake of the patient, without proper regard for the patient's wishes. The ideal circumstances are those in which a client is able to discuss and understand the options facing him, and able to negotiate care and freely assent to any intervention. This assumes that the client is conscious, of sufficient maturity, mentally well and in an open and non-pressurised environment. When one or another of these conditions is not met there is scope for ethical debate about how best to act. It is usually relevant to consider what the client would wish if they were able to express themselves freely. This might entail imaginatively 'putting ourselves in their shoes', or consulting their family and friends about their views. Sometimes health professionals or family members may be able to make an informed judgement based upon the wishes previously expressed by the client.

2.2 Respect for persons and respect for autonomy

Although it is certainly essential to take into account the views or wishes of clients, it should not be assumed that it is always right for these wishes to prevail. What is needed is an ethical account of why 'wishes' are of such importance, and when, if ever, they can be overridden. The intuitions that lie behind this judgement are so basic that it is difficult to produce an account. But the idea of 'respect for persons' helps to articulate it. In brief this is the idea that each of us has an intrinsic value which, if we are to recognise one another properly, cannot be ignored or 'traded off' for some other end. To treat someone only as an object, or only as a tool or resource, is to fail to treat them as a person. This way of expressing the value of persons is derived from part of Kant's moral philosophy, and for many people it expresses something close to the essence of ethics. One way in which respect can be exercised is by taking seriously the autonomous choices that people make and by not ignoring or overriding them. Hence the importance of consultation, partnership, and informed consent.

However, respect for persons does not only involve respecting autonomous choices. Parents may recognise the choices of their teenage children as autonomous,

and yet may choose to override some of their children's wishes without necessarily being guilty of treating them as 'objects'. Indeed they may be treating them
with great respect and love, and they may be motivated purely by concern for
their children's welfare. Acting in what you judge to be the best interests of
someone else, in a way that overrides or limits the exercise of their autonomy, is
called paternalism (or sometimes parentalism). As we have seen, paternalism is
a constant temptation in health care, and if we are to respect autonomy there
should be a presumption against it, but are there occasions on which it might be
justified?

There are two reasons why nurses may, from time to time, be justified in acting
paternalistically. First, autonomy is partly a matter of degree. How autonomous a
choice is depends upon a number of factors including the level of understanding
and reasoning of the chooser. A choice made by a client may be judged autonomous at a minimum level, and as worthy of respect and serious consideration. Yet
judged against a more demanding standard the same choice may not be seen as
sufficiently autonomous to decisively settle the matter. Secondly, it is often difficult
to assess the degree of autonomy of a choice. Sometimes we cannot be clear what
lies behind a decision or action, in particular how far it rests upon a mispercep-
tion, a whim, a disturbed temperament, or external pressure. Under these conditions it might be justified to postpone a decision, or even override an apparently
autonomous choice, in order to assess how far a choice is really autonomous. Both
of these reasons are more likely to come into play if the risk to welfare is great
(a suicide attempt is the paradigm case here).

Paternalism involves limiting a person's exercise of autonomy for his or her
own sake, but there are, of course, other reasons to limit the exercise of autonomy.
Respect for persons means taking into account the interests and wishes of all
those affected. Normally this means that the client concerned has the overriding
voice, but this is subject to important qualifications. A patient or client, even if
we assume they are 'fully' autonomous, cannot merely demand an intervention
whatever the cost to other people, or regardless of the views of health professionals. If we are to respect persons then nurses cannot merely be used as objects or
tools to meet the demands of other people – whether doctors or patients. This will
happen unless they are involved in appropriate decision-making, and allowed to
withdraw in a responsible fashion from involvement when they strongly object
to what is decided. Also there is sometimes more than one client. A nurse may, for
example, be supporting a bereaved family. Here respect for autonomy necessarily
entails balancing the wishes of different individuals together, and having regard
for the well-being of the family as a whole. Finally a nurse acting as a budget
holder or policy maker has to consider the overall implications of decisions for
the general population.

2.3 Utilitarianism and the public interest

This takes us on to a second cluster of problems concerning the promotion of
welfare. How are nurses supposed to balance together the interests of different
individuals, and how are they to consider both the needs of their immediate

clients and a commitment to the general welfare or the public interest? A large number of practical dilemmas turn upon these two questions. Dramatic examples of the first kind include those cases where individuals donate organs to others, or cases in which the interests of pregnant women and fetuses can come into conflict. Dramatic examples of the second kind arise when clients are a potential danger to the health or safety of others. If someone has a highly infectious and serious condition, or is seriously mentally disturbed, under what circumstances should they be able to determine their own lifestyle in the community?

One way of thinking about these dilemmas is to see them as about considering the expected costs and benefits of alternative courses of action in order to see which course produces the best overall outcome. This way of thinking is described as utilitarian, and there is a tradition of moral philosophy called utilitarianism in which it is defended as the basis of ethics. There are many debates about utilitarianism, and within utilitarianism, which cannot be summarised here. But it is possible to indicate both the plausibility and some of the difficulties of the central idea.

Its plausibility arises because it seems odd to see ethics as simply about following rules for their own sake. Surely what we are interested in is bringing about better, rather than worse, states of affairs. A nurse who is asked to adopt 'ethical standards' will expect to see how they are connected to protecting or promoting welfare, how they make the world 'a better place'. Yet a rule or guideline that seems to work well most of the time may, on occasion, seem to do more harm than good. For example, it seems important to have rules to protect the confidentiality of clients, but it also seems that there are circumstances where the risks or costs of silence may be so grave that confidentiality could justifiably be broken. It appears that in this kind of example a more fundamental, and utilitarian, ethic is being appealed to.

However, there are some problems with this way of thinking. There is no exact ethical accountancy by which the different sorts of costs and benefits can be optimised, and different individuals are likely to disagree about when a guideline is unhelpful and can be broken. At the extreme this could lead not only to a climate of uncertainty about policy, but to a nurse's idiosyncratic conception of what counts as a cost or benefit having undue influence.

More generally a concern about utilitarian thinking is that it can involve sacrificing some people's interests for the sake of others, and that this could amount to treating people merely as objects or resources. There is, on the face of it, a tension between certain examples of utilitarian thinking and the idea of respect for persons.

For example, consider resource allocation as an ethical issue that, on the face of things, lends itself to utilitarian thinking. A nurse manager might have to decide how to divide a budget between a number of patients and the professionals who work with them. It is plausible to suppose that she should use her experience, and research evidence, to determine which pattern of distribution would 'do the most good' (although note the complexity and uncertainty inherent in this), and opt for this pattern. This sounds fine in the abstract, but in the real world it would probably involve overriding the views and wishes of many of the patients and professionals involved. Certainly any decision that entailed not treating certain sick individuals at all because money 'wasted' on them might be better spent elsewhere would appear to treat the former with less than respect. For this reason many people react against utilitarian thinking, seeing it as amoral or even 'immoral'. Yet health professionals, including nurses, have some responsibility to the general welfare or the public interest, as well as to the individuals in front of them, and need to explore ways of balancing these responsibilities. This is merely one illustration of the way in which our basic approach to ethical thinking shapes the day-to-day practical decisions we might make.

2.4 Principles of health care ethics

One approach to health care ethics that has gained widespread currency is to set out fundamental principles, each of which needs to be taken into account when we make ethical judgements. This approach, and the so-called 'four principles', have been made famous by the work of Beauchamp and Childress[6] and Raanon Gillon.[7,8] The four principles are:

(1) the principle of respect for autonomy
(2) the principle of nonmaleficence
(3) the principle of beneficence
(4) the principle of justice.

In short, these principles mean that in deciding how to act health professionals ought to respect autonomy, avoid harming, where possible benefit, and consider (fairly) the interests of all those affected. This is not a formula for ethical decision-making, but rather a broad framework that can be used as a basis for organising ethical deliberation and discussion.

There is no substitute for reading about this approach in the source texts referred to above. These make quite clear the difficulties in interpreting and applying these principles, and the ways in which they tend to conflict with one another in practice. We have already seen that the idea of autonomy, and the ideas of costs and benefits, are open to different interpretations, and the idea of justice is, if anything, even more controversial. For example, some people would argue that a health care system in which health care is distributed by an open market, in which everyone has an opportunity to buy care, is perfectly just, whereas others would see this as profoundly unjust, arguing perhaps that health care ought to be distributed according to need.

This 'four principles' approach has come under criticism for being too superficial or too limited. Some of this criticism can be dismissed because it is based on misconceptions about what the proponents of this approach are advocating. They are not arguing that all ethical thinking can be reduced to a few key words, or that the four principles provide a quick and easy method for solving ethical dilemmas. Rather they are arguing that the principles provide a reminder of the key dimensions of ethical thinking, and that they can provide a common vocabulary and framework for individuals with different outlooks or philosophies. This approach is, in part, designed to avoid the paralysis of endless theoretical debate, and to be of practical help in real cases.

Leaving aside the question of its ultimate validity, the practice of applying the principles to cases provides important lessons for nursing ethics. Although the principles supply 'rules of thumb', we cannot assess what we ought to do in a specific case without considering the particular circumstances of the case. Ethical judgement depends crucially on questions of fact as well as questions of principle, and it is worth noting in passing that a good deal of apparent ethical disagreement stems from disagreements about the facts. Also, because so much ethical thinking involves weighing together the conflicting demands of different principles, it is possible for a small difference between two similar cases to result in apparently contradictory conclusions. We have already seen, for instance, how a decision to act paternalistically can rest upon very fine judgements about a client's degree of autonomy. Hence not only abstract reasoning but also sensitivity and attention to detail are essential parts of ethical thinking.

2.5 Philosophical ethics: its value and limitations

Philosophy students study 'Ethics' as an academic subject, albeit one that is normally seen to have an applied element. The questions typically considered in this context vary in their level of abstraction. The most abstract or general ones include, for example: What is the basis of ethics? Is it possible to have ethical knowledge? What are the meaning and the uses of the concept 'good'? Then there are middle-order questions that raise matters of practical substance but at a considerable level of generality, for example: What are the various conceptions of a fair society? Under what circumstances is it permissible to break promises? Finally there are the most applied questions in which philosophers analyse the 'rights and wrongs' of specific policies or actions. In relation to health care these might include consideration of specific cases in which it is asked if nurse X was right to Y (e.g. breach confidentiality) in circumstances Z (where these could be spelled out in some detail). Nurses who are also philosophers, or nurses who are interested in philosophy – and there are increasing numbers of both – will be interested in all of these questions, but what is their relevance to nurses with other interests?

Philosophers who wanted to 'sell' their subject could offer the following argument: every nurse has to answer the applied or practical questions, and it is impossible to avoid answering them even if only by default (i.e. faced with circumstances Z, you either do or do not breach confidentiality; you cannot fail to 'answer' the question merely by not thinking about it). But, it could be argued, answers to the applied questions lower down the list depend upon having or assuming answers to the sort of questions higher up the list. Therefore, if you want to answer the practical questions responsibly you must address the more philosophical questions. This is a very plausible argument. It takes the same form as all sales talk: 'You cannot do what you want to, or have to, without my product.' For this reason we should be suspicious of it; however, I would suggest that in essence it conveys a truth. The only way in which we can appraise specific circumstances is by standing back and comparing them with others. In so doing we will also find ourselves asking what kind of yardsticks, if any, we have. Are there some general standards we can apply, or do these vary from case to case, or from person to person?

Philosophical ethics is a discipline that is committed to this process of 'standing back' and systematic reflection and argument. There are a number of competing theoretical traditions that attempt to organise ethical reflection into systems of thought. At their most ambitious they attempt to produce a single theory (or a unified set of theories) to account for all our ethical judgements. Given such an overarching theory we could identify any particular decision, action, policy or person to be right or wrong, or good or bad, in specified respects. Philosophers disagree about the extent to which it is possible or desirable to aim for such general accounts, and whether they should be satisfied with the 'untidyness' of competing or complementary accounts. They also disagree about the extent to which ethics lends itself to rational analysis, and the extent to which it is rooted in conventional codes and customs (note that these two things are not necessarily incompatible). However, anyone with an interest in applied ethics is interested in seeing how far systematic thinking can be of help in making or evaluating ethical decisions.

Hence one of the benefits of philosophical ethics is that it allows us to reflect in more depth about such things as utilitarianism, the idea of respect for persons, and the idea of principles of health care ethics. What are the different versions of utilitarianism? How far are utilitarian ways of thinking inevitable, how far are they useful? And so on. We can ask this sort of question in the hope that we might arrive at a definitive overview of the basis and nature of ethics, or merely in the hope that we will illuminate some of the complexity of the subject. Although there is a danger that health professionals may see these philosophical questions as irrelevant traps (and something like the four principles approach may be pre-ferred as a 'working model'), it is important for everyone to recognise that these basic questions are hotly disputed – that is, there is no definitive 'knowledge base' in nursing ethics.

For example, in the health care ethics literature there is frequent mention of the value of 'autonomy', and there are many references to 'informed consent'. It would not be unreasonable for someone coming to the subject for the first time to assume that, in relation to such basic building blocks, there was a clear consensus as to their meaning and role. Thus it might easily be supposed that each time an author uses such an expression he or she is making use of a shared technical vocabulary; that, for example, 'autonomy' always means precisely the same thing, that it is always valued for the same reason, and that its relative importance to other values is agreed. In reality there are both commonalities and differences in the way these terms are used, and this is not a product of poor 'coordination' but a function of the inherent contestability of ethics. (Incidentally some of these com-monalities and differences are illustrated by the ethical perspectives in Part Two of this book, and some disagreements about the meaning and value of autonomy are discussed explicitly in the ethical discussions of consent.)

There are a number of other things that the philosophical tradition can offer to nursing ethics. First, there is a considerable literature in which the terms and issues of ethics are clarified and debated. So much has been written over centuries, and over recent years, about well-being and justice and so on. Secondly, there are conventions for debate, based upon ideals such as disinterested and reasoned discussion, which can serve as useful models for people entering the subject. Thirdly, there are many issues of health care ethics that have philosophical problems built into them. For example, questions about abortion and euthanasia do not turn only upon factual matters but also upon intrinsically philosophical matters to do with the nature and value of life. In these cases it is impossible to treat these issues seriously without some consideration of philosophical questions.

Finally, and paradoxically, one of the benefits of philosophical ethics is that it generates an awareness of its own limitations. Being philosophically skilled is not the same as being a good person. There may be some philosophers who believe that a full ethical theory would be sufficient to determine what should be done in every set of circumstances, but no one could think that this would be enough to make it happen. How would this perfect knowledge become embodied in practice? We all know that it is possible, sometimes all too easy, not to do what we regard as the right thing. For these reasons philosophers have to take an interest in character as well as in actions. What is it that makes people more or less likely to understand ethical demands, and to be inclined or disposed to meet them?

2.6 Being a good nurse

One tradition of philosophical ethics, which is concerned with 'the virtues', sees these questions about character as being at the heart of ethics. The tradition is usually associated with Aristotle's ethical writings but it is a thread that runs through all of ethics. The idea of 'virtues' may seem old-fashioned but it is a useful name for good qualities of character, in particular for admirable or desirable dispositions. To encourage children to do 'the right thing' we need not only to help them know what the right thing is but also to enable them to want to do it, preferably for it to become a habit or 'second nature'. The same goes for all of us.

It would be no exaggeration to say that nurse education and development are about the cultivation of desirable dispositions as well as the transmission of clinical skills. Some of these dispositions relate to professional attitudes and behaviour – such as research awareness – but underpinning them all is a disposition to care for patients or clients, including the habit of paying attention to and responding to needs. Unless a nurse has this quality she cannot be, except in very restricted circumstances, a good nurse. And this 'skill' of caring is intrinsic to ethics: it is not like other skills which may be used in good or bad ways. In fact caring is viewed by some as the pivotal concept of feminist ethics.[9] Caring does not necessarily mean a self-conscious emotional empathy or identification; there may be many instances where nurses are too tired or stressed to feel caring. The whole point of talking about a desirable disposition is to make clear that an attitude that is rooted in feelings will persist even when the requisite feelings are absent.

It would be an interesting, and perhaps useful, exercise to ask a group of experienced nurses to list the virtues necessary for nursing. At one time the Christian virtues of faith, hope and charity might have headed the list. Nowadays most people are likely to think of ideas such as honesty or integrity, whereas more 'old-fashioned' ideas such as patience or loyalty might be seen as more controversial. One thing is clear – as the conditions of nursing change a different balance of virtues is called for. No doubt humility is a good quality but as the pressures of individual accountability increase it needs to be tempered by courage and resolution. We all have some conception of what it is to be a good nurse. We can look at role models and try to identify which aspects of their character we admire. In this way we can set ourselves standards.

It is essential to note the difference between 'setting standards' for ourselves as individuals and the public kinds of standard-setting that have become increasingly important in health care – in the form of evidence-based guidelines, clinical governance, performance management and so on. Certainly the good nurse must take the latter into account and will, by and large, be happy to work towards publicly defined standards. But a nurse who has not only a sense of his or her personal accountability as a professional but also a strong sense of ethical integrity, and embodies nursing virtues such as courage, will want to 'aim above' public standards and – where necessary – critique, challenge or expose them. A number of the ethics authors in Part Two of this book point to ways in which ethics can be personally more demanding than the requirements of the law or of professional norms.

Hence, in the end, a serious engagement with ethics highlights some of the tensions between nursing as an ethical role and nursing as a professional or legal or institutional role – between the individual nurse and the nurse as part of the system. It is plausible to suggest that in the few years since the first edition of this book was published there has been a substantial increase in these kinds of tensions, and hence a heightening of importance for nursing ethics. On the one hand more and more emphasis is given to personal accountability in an ever growing range of health care agendas and settings. On the other hand there is a development and consolidation of both national and institutional policies, frameworks and guidelines. In many respects nurses are expected to 'do everything' – including being both personally responsible and jumping through other people's hoops!

This suggests that as well as cultivating courage nurses increasingly need to cultivate a form of constructive scepticism. They need, for example, to engage constructively with the systems of clinical governance that are put in place within their institution. Many things depend upon institutional systems and standards being in place. However, if nurses see aspects of these systems as misguided or ineffective – or if they find that they seem to be expressed only in apparently meaningless and self-referential jargon – they ought to explore means of saying so. In the health service the emperor is often quite naked and real standards sometimes depend upon people pointing this out!

So developing one's own personal standards is essential, but it is not a sufficient basis for establishing good nursing. Individual nurses cannot be expected to pull themselves up by their own boot straps. Only the exceptional few could achieve high ethical standards in an unethical environment. It is essential that the cultures and institutions of nursing foster the virtues of nursing. This is why it is important to continue the shift towards a philosophy of nursing founded upon ethical commitments. This is why it is important to have professional values and standards articulated in public documents and policies. This is why it is important for nurses to be able to debate the underlying principles and the particulars of ethics.

2.7 References

1. J. Macleod Clark, From sick nursing to health nursing: evolution or revolution? in J. Wilson-Barnett & J. Macleod Clark (eds), *Research in Health Promotion and Nursing* (Basingstoke, Macmillan, 1993).
2. M. Oakeshott, The Tower of Babel, in *Rationalism in Politics* (London, Methuen, 1962).
3. R.S. Peters, Reason and habit: the paradox of moral education, in *Moral Development and Moral Education* (London, Allen and Unwin, 1981).
4. D. Seedhouse, *Health: The Foundations for Achievement* (Chichester, John Wiley and Sons, 2001).
5. L. Nordenfelt, *On the Nature of Health* (Dordrecht, Reidal, 1987).
6. T.L. Beauchamp & J.F. Childress, *Principles of Biomedical Ethics* (New York, Oxford University Press, 2001).
7. R. Gillon, *Philosophical Medical Ethics* (Chichester, John Wiley and Sons, 1986).
8. R. Gillon, *Principles of Health Care Ethics* (Chichester, John Wiley and Sons, 1994).
9. C. Gilligan, *In a Different Voice* (Cambridge, MA, Harvard University Press, 1982).

3

The Professional Dimension: Professional Regulation in Nursing and Midwifery

Fiona Culley

Professional regulation in health care is not a new concept. The 1858 Medical Act established registration of qualified medical practitioners, and paved the way for other occupational groups, including nurses and midwives, to demand similar status. Registration of midwives began with the Midwives Act 1902, while nurse registration dates back to 1919, when the Nurses Act established the General Nursing Councils for England and Wales, and for Scotland. More recently, the Health Act 1999 stated that the common purpose of regulation among health care professionals is:

> to establish a country wide, professionally set, independent standard of training, conduct and competence for each profession for the protection of the public and the guidance of employers.[1]

It offers a contract between the profession, the public and employers. Despite its long history, the statutory self-regulation of the professions has been described as a shadowy subject that is not well understood.[2] This assertion appears reasonable, given that regulatory processes have to adjust to social and political circumstances. Much attention has been focused on increased personal and professional accountability of all health care professionals and their employers, through the introduction of a statutory duty of quality in health care (clinical governance[3]), and other initiatives such as *Standards for Better Health*.[4] Additionally Fitness to Practise decisions and orders of the regulatory bodies, and the reasons for them, now have to be published,[5] and regulators have a statutory duty to consult with the public and the professions. Study of this subject must therefore be neither underestimated nor abandoned in the wake of public and professional reaction to cases relating to poorly performing practitioners.

The Nursing and Midwifery Council (NMC) is the current regulatory body for nurses and midwives, established by the Nursing and Midwifery Order 2001 ('The Order').[6] It replaced its predecessor body, the United Kingdom Central Council for Nurses, Midwives and Health Visitors, on 1 April 2002. During 2006 the NMC handed over to a new Council, having completed its first term of office. The author of this chapter had the opportunity of working in the Fitness to Practise Directorate at the NMC during that first term, which helped inform this writing.

Revision of this text is now justified, as the previous edition was written at a point when The Order was in its draft form, and the NMC had yet to be appointed. Since then a number of changes have been implemented, which are summarised below. They include changes to the Council itself, to the NMC register, and to Fitness to Practise procedures. The first Fitness to Practise case considered under The Order was heard in January 2006,[7] which means that the 'new' procedures remain in their infancy. Nevertheless, early implications of these rules are now beginning to be realised.

As nurses and midwives remain the largest occupational group employed by the health service, and the majority (around 60%) of complaints at the NMC about fitness to practise come from employers,[8] the particular importance of understanding the role and powers of their statutory regulator, as well as considering their specific contribution to public protection, is self-evident. This chapter aims to develop that understanding, and will focus upon the NMC's role in professional regulation, explaining the approaches introduced by:

- the Health Act 1999
- the Nursing and Midwifery Order 2001
- the Nursing and Midwifery (Fitness to Practise) Rules 2004.

Fitness to practise is chiefly concerned with satisfying the regulator, and others, that those on the professional register are not only appropriately qualified, but are also of good character, and physically and mentally fit to practise. The NMC has to prescribe what is required of nurses and midwives up to and at the point of registration, and beyond.[9] The confines of this text do not allow examination of education and training or standards for admission to the register. Its aim is to outline information about some of the issues that commonly arise in Fitness to Practise cases, and the measures taken. It will also consider some of the challenges to the current system. This discussion is therefore by no means exhaustive and does not seek to replace the wide range of standards and guidance published by the NMC (www.nmc-uk.org), or the NMC Fitness to Practise Annual Report[10] which has, by law, to 'indicate the efficiency and effectiveness of the arrangements it has put in place to protect the public from persons whose fitness to practise is impaired'.[11]

An overview of the existing system now follows. However, it must be stressed that this reflects the time of writing and, as will become apparent, the system is set to alter.

3.1 Summary of the current nursing and midwifery regulatory system

Within health care, professional regulation remains a shared responsibility between Parliament, the statutory regulatory bodies, employers, registered practitioners, other health care workers and complainants. Between them, they must legislate, implement, monitor, review and report on standards of professional conduct, performance and ethics. The current system of nursing and midwifery regulation, and that of doctors and all other health care professionals in the UK, is state sanctioned self-regulation. This means that although the regulatory bodies work with the support of government to implement rules, and are accountable to Parliament through the Privy Council, they maintain a degree of independence in exercising their regulatory role.

Alternatives to this approach are independent regulation, where regulation is entirely independent of the state, or at the other end of the scale direct state regulation, where power to regulate rests entirely on legislation, and is led by government departments rather than the professions themselves.[12]

3.1.1 Challenges to the current system

Self-regulation is regarded by some as a privilege, and has, periodically, been criticised for promoting the self-interest of the profession, rather than protection of the public. For example, after the Kennedy Report into events at Bristol Royal Infirmary[13] the British Medical Association passed an overwhelming vote of no confidence in the GMC's regulatory processes, an opinion repeated more recently in the Shipman Inquiry.[14] These public reports serve as a reminder that the entire system of professional regulation in health care remains under close scrutiny, and is subject, at any time, to political reform. Although about half of the recommendations in the Fifth Report from the Shipman Inquiry relate to the GMC, there are implications for all regulators and their Fitness to Practise procedures.[15] The recommendations support the government's objectives within the NHS Plan,[16] and a separate report from the Cabinet Office,[17] that each regulatory body should become smaller, with more transparent procedures and greater accountability to the public and the health service, should offer consistency of approach and proportionality, and should be able to accommodate changing situations.

Following those recommendations, in 2005 the Department of Health[18] announced a review by the Chief Medical Officer (the Donaldson Review) into revalidation and regulation of doctors, and a separate review (the Foster Review) looking at the regulation of dentists, pharmacists, nurses, midwives, opticians, osteopaths, chiropractors and the 13 professions covered by the Health Professions Council. These led to further consultation, following which, in February 2007, the government published its White Paper (*Trust, Assurance and Safety: The Regulation of Health Professionals in the 21st Century*) outlining further proposals for change.

While the potential for reform appears increasingly evident, there is a clear statement in Chapter 27 of the Shipman Inquiry[19] that the recommendations should 'extend and improve the existing framework of protective systems' – not replace them. The report also calls for further independent review of the new Fitness to Practise procedures in three to four years' time (from 2004), upon the instructions of the Council for Healthcare Regulatory Excellence (CRHE), whose role is discussed further at 3.12 below.

3.2 The legal framework

The legal framework governing self-regulation of health care professionals rests in a number of Parliamentary Acts (primary legislation), and rules enacted through Statutory Instruments (secondary legislation). The legislation most relevant to the regulation of nurses and midwives is shown in Box 3.1.

The current regulatory system for nurses and midwives lies within a transition period, as allegations received by the NMC after 1 August 2004 are managed under the new legislation and procedures.[20] Cases received prior to that date are still dealt with under the Nurses, Midwives and Health Visitors Act 1997 and the Nurses, Midwives and Health Visitors (Professional Conduct) Rules 1993. There are also some transitional provisions relating to outstanding cases, in particular, where a committee wishes to postpone judgment, or where the applicant is applying for restoration to the register, or for the termination of a suspension.[21]

The Health Act 1999 moved the issue of professional regulation from the primary to the secondary legislative agenda, meaning the government can now amend regulation of the medical and health care professions by ministerial Order rather than an Act, if it is 'necessary or expedient' to do so.[22] While this points towards the likelihood of more timely reform, which might otherwise be precluded by a busy Parliamentary agenda, it may suggest a changed level of accountability as it will no longer necessarily be an issue openly debated in Parliament. The Health Act does, however, provide some protection for the current arrangements, as an Order, although amending regulation, cannot abolish the existence of any regulatory body.[23] In addition, the National Health Service Reform and Health Professions Act 2002 states that the independence of health care regulators should

---

Box 3.1   Legislation relevant to professional regulation of nurses and midwives.

1902 Midwives Act
1919 Nurses Act
1949 Nurses Act
1957 Nurses Act
1979 Nurses, Midwives and Health Visitors Act
1992 Nurses, Midwives and Health Visitors Act
Nurses, Midwives and Health Visitors (Professional Conduct) Rules 1993
1997 Nurses, Midwives and Health Visitors Act
Human Rights Act 1998
The Health Act 1999
The Nursing and Midwifery Order 2001 Statutory Instrument 253
The Nursing and Midwifery (Fitness to Practise) Rules 2004 Statutory Instrument 1761
The Nursing and Midwifery Order 2001 (Transitional Provisions) Order of Council 2004 Statutory Instrument 1762

be protected by their being made finally accountable to Parliament, not to any other body.

On a number of occasions since 1999 changes affecting the NMC, the General Medical Council (GMC), the General Dental Council (GDC) and the Health Professions Council (HPC) have been introduced by Order. The Health Act 1999 sets out what such an Order may provide for:

(a) the establishment and continuance of a regulatory body
(b) keeping a register of members admitted to practice
(c) education and training before and after admission to practice
(d) privileges of members admitted to practice
(e) standards of conduct and performance
(f) discipline and fitness to practise
(g) investigation and enforcement by or on behalf of the regulatory body
(h) appeals
(i) default powers exercisable by a person other than a regulatory body.

Other legislation relevant to professional regulation is the Human Rights Act 1998, which makes it unlawful for public authorities to act in a way that is incompatible with the rights expressed in the European Convention of Human Rights. In particular Article 6(1) states:

[E]veryone is entitled to a fair and public hearing within a reasonable time by an independent and impartial tribunal established by law.

The notion of being fair and being seen to be fair underpins the Fitness to Practise proceedings of all regulators.[24] There is an expectation that measures taken will balance protection of the public with fairness to the profession.

3.2.1 The Nursing and Midwifery Order 2001 ('The Order')

After the Health Act 1999, The Order established the NMC and set out its functions, constitution, statutory committees, procedures and election scheme (Box 3.2). It built upon the foundations of previous legislation laid out in the 1979, 1992 and 1997 Nurses, Midwives and Health Visitors Acts. Changes mainly arose as a result of a Department of Health commissioned review of the 1997 Nurses, Midwives and Health Visitors Act and the UKCC, which was carried out by JM Consulting in 1999 and which recommended a smaller, more accountable Council, and greater lay representation, all of which was accepted by the government and subsequently legislated for.[25]

Part V of the Nursing and Midwifery Order 2001 sets out the NMC's Fitness to Practise functions, with an explicit requirement to keep under review standards of conduct, performance and ethics expected of registrants and prospective registrants.[26] This is reflected in the rewording of the title of its most recent version of the professional code (discussed further at 3.5 below).[27]

A new concept introduced by The Order is the emphasis, within Part II, on the need for consultation with registrants, employers, service users and education providers. The NMC duly consulted upon Fitness to Practise during 2003, before

---

Box 3.2   Components of The Nursing and Midwifery Order 2001.

Part I General
Part II The Council and its Committees
Part III Registration
Part IV Education and Training
Part V Fitness to Practise
Part VI Appeals
Part VII EEA provisions
Part VIII Midwifery
Part IX Offences
Part X Miscellaneous
Schedules 1–5

---

finalising its new rules and procedures. These are provided by the Nursing and Midwifery Council (Fitness to Practise) Rules Order of Council 2004 (the Rules), which came into force on 1 August 2004 with the opening of the new three-part NMC register, determined by statutory instrument,[28] and further explained in 3.4 below.

3.2.2 Summary of Fitness to Practise procedures

In summary, the 'new' legislation allows the NMC to consider more categories of allegations relating to impairment of fitness to practise (see 3.7 below) and impose a wider range of sanctions than before (see 3.8 below and Table 3.1). With the additional categories of allegation there is a wider threshold for the referral of cases to the Fitness to Practise committees, from 'likely to lead to removal from the register' to 'case [of impairment] to answer'. This has resulted in a 100% increase in cases considered by the NMC from April to September 2005, compared with

Table 3.1   NMC sanctions for impairment of fitness to practise.

Previous rules	New rules (2004 onwards)
No action	As previous, plus
Caution	'Striking off' order
Removal from register	Suspension*
Interim suspension	Conditions of practice order**
	Interim order

* suspension cannot exceed one year in first instance, ** conditions of practice order has to be for a specified period of no more than three years. Under the new rules caution is for between one and five years.

the same period in 2004.[29] Other changes relate to the membership of the panels of the Fitness to Practise committees, and rules relating to the appeal period.

3.3 The Nursing and Midwifery Council and its committees

Like other regulators, the NMC is legally bound by The Order to maintain a professional register and to determine standards of professional conduct, performance and ethics, and manage allegations of unfitness to practise through the functions of its statutory committees (see below). The NMC is accountable to Parliament through the Privy Council, whose role is to advise the Queen on the approval of Orders in Council. Like its predecessor bodies, its prime objective is to:

> safeguard the health and well-being of persons using or needing the services of registrants.[30]

The NMC meets about four times a year to:

- consider and set policy and standards for nurses, midwives and health visitors
- consider issues of professional practice and implications for public protection
- monitor the work of the Council, for example performance in registration processes, professional conduct and financial management.

The Council is currently made up of 12 registrant members, 12 alternate registrant members and 11 lay members. The NMC is considerably smaller than the UKCC, which comprised 66 members, and aims to embrace greater public involvement. This is reflected in the larger proportion (around 30%) of lay members than previously appointed. It is recommended in the latest White Paper (see above) that the make-up of the NMC will become smaller and more board-like, with appointed members, and that at the least there will be parity between the number of registrant and the number of lay members.

The NMC has a number of statutory practice committees to carry out its strategic functions. Its Fitness to Practise responsibilities are undertaken by:

- the Investigating Committee (IC)
- the Conduct and Competence Committee (CCC)
- the Health Committee (HC).

Each committee has a strategic and an operational role, and deals with case work through its appointed panels at venues within the four countries of the UK. The fourth statutory committee is the Midwifery Committee, whose role is to advise the Council on any matters affecting midwifery,[31] including the circumstances in which, and the procedure by means of which, a midwife may be suspended from practice.

3.3.1 Fitness to Practise panels

The Order[32] allows the Council to appoint Committee members who are not Council members. Fitness to Practise panel members are appointed in this way to carry out the operational work of the three Practice committees. As well as imposing sanctions to restrict or prevent practice, panels of the CCC and HC also consider applications for restoration to the register from individuals who have been previously removed.

Panel members are expected to apply the same standards as Council members, including working within a competency framework, to guide their knowledge, skills and performance. The Order demands that panels comprise at least one member who is registered in the same part of the register as the person under consideration, and that the lay members may not be outnumbered by registrant members by more than one. If only one lay member is present, that person cannot be a registered medical practitioner.[33] The Council's current policy is that, for the time being, there will normally be a Council member present at each panel meeting. This is, however, not a legal requirement. It has recently been announced that the NMC is moving towards disqualifying Council members from taking part in Fitness to Practise panels from September 2007 in line with other regulators such as the GMC.[34] The Shipman Inquiry Fifth Report[35] recommends that the adjudication of the FTP procedures must be undertaken by a body independent of the GMC, with a call that 'consideration should be given to appointing a body of full-time, or nearly full-time, panellists who could sit on the FTP panels of all the healthcare regulatory bodies'. This has yet to be consulted upon, with arguments remaining for and against separation of functions.

3.3.2 The Investigating Committee (IC)

The first role of the NMC's IC is to consider documentary evidence in relation to any fitness to practise allegation, and decide whether there is a case to answer. The panels meet in private. Where the allegations are considered serious enough to warrant investigation, the panel will instruct solicitors to investigate and report on the strength of the evidence, which must meet the criminal standard of proof – in other words, that a panel is satisfied 'so that it is sure' of the facts alleged. The IC then has to decide, based upon the evidence before it, whether the allegation could be proved (to the criminal standard), and whether the facts could lead to finding that fitness to practise is impaired.

If the panel decides there is no case to answer, it will close the case. When closing a case, the panel can decide to keep a record of the allegation for three years. If a similar allegation is made within that period, the panel can reopen the original allegation or take it into account when considering the new one.

If the panel decides that there is a case to answer, it will refer it to the next stage of investigation, or consider mediation,[36] and subsequently refer to the CCC or the HC to decide the grounds on which fitness to practise is impaired.

If the IC refers a case to the CCC or HC, the NMC must notify the registrant's employer, LSA, any other body the individual is registered with and the Secretary of State/Minister for Health.[37]

During the course of these proceedings the panel will inform the registrant and complainant accordingly. All the evidence that is put before the committee panel is sent to the registrant who has been reported, inviting them to submit a written response to the panel at this stage. It is recommended that professional advice is sought in preparing any written response.

Another function of the IC is to directly consider allegations of fraudulent or incorrect entry to the register. These cases can be dealt with at a public hearing or at a private meeting. If a hearing is held, the registrant has the right to attend and to be represented, to cross-examine the Council's witnesses, and to give evidence and call witnesses. The hearings are generally held in public and are similar to hearings held by the CCC. If a panel decides an allegation is proved, it will order the Registrar to make the appropriate amendment to or deletion from the register. The Investigating Committee panel's decisions can be appealed at the county court or, in Scotland, to a sheriff.[38]

Any case that involves a health matter must be considered by a panel that includes a registered medical practitioner. They, like other members of the panel, are there to consider fitness to practise, not to diagnose, or act as medical examiner.

During 2004/2005 around 43% of cases were closed by the preliminary proceedings committee (PPC) (the predecessor committee to the IC).[39] The IC have a similar role to the PPC, but unlike the PPC they may no longer issue a caution under the new rules.

3.3.3 The Conduct and Competence Committee (CCC)

The Order requires the CCC to advise the Council on Fitness to Practise issues including:

- the performance of the Council's functions in relation to standards of conduct, performance and ethics
- requirements of good health and good character, and
- protection of the public from people whose fitness to practise is impaired.[40]

Through appointed panels, they consider allegations referred to them by the Council and its committees, as well as applications for restoration. Once a case has been referred to the CCC it must first decide whether to deal with the matter at a hearing. The Order does not require there to be a hearing unless the registrant asks for one or the panel decides a hearing is desirable. Hearings are often attended by the press, as well as observers. The majority of observers are registrants, who can learn about the importance of robust evidence, and will be able to reflect on the implications for practice of the decisions and reasons that have been presented by the panel. A list of hearings is published by the NMC on its website as a matter of public information. Additionally, the decisions of the Fitness to Practise Committee panels, and the reasons for them, are published. This is a requirement of The Order. The question of how much detail should be included in the reasons is a troubled one. In *Stefan* v. *General Medical Council* 1999[41] it was held that:

[t]he extent and substance of the reasons must depend on the circumstances. They need not be elaborate or lengthy. But they should be such as to tell the parties in broad terms why the decision was reached.

Registrants are entitled to attend and be represented at the hearing, normally by their professional body or trade union, or a solicitor or barrister. They do, however, have the right to be represented by any other person, and may choose to represent themselves on occasion. The Rules allow the Committee panel to proceed in the absence of the respondent, as long as they can prove that all reasonable efforts have been made to notify them.[42]

3.3.4 The Health Committee (HC)

The IC or CCC refers individuals to the Health Committee (HC), if it appears that their fitness to practise is impaired by their physical or mental health. The HC largely follows the same procedures as the CCC. The main difference is that the HC normally meets in private because of the confidential and often sensitive nature of the evidence involved. This may be submitted from the respondent, witnesses, the individual's own doctor and a medical examiner appointed by the NMC. If the individual does not agree to medical examination, the reasons for the absence of a medical report must be presented to the panel.

The Order has introduced a number of changes to the way in which health-related cases are handled and disposed of. Under the Professional Conduct Rules 1993 the HC (and the PCC) were allowed to postpone judgment, meaning that the case could be reviewed after a period of supported practice. That is no longer possible under the new legislation. However, the panel may opt to impose a conditions of practice order, placing specific restrictions upon registration. A conditions of practice order can be made at the same time as granting an application for restoration.

Another change under the new Fitness to Practise legislation is that there has to be a doctor (registered medical practitioner) on each of the Practice Committees, and on any Fitness to Practise panel where the health of the person is relevant to the case.[43]

Before considering the categories of allegation where fitness to practise may affect registration status, it is worth considering what the register stands for and how its composition has changed since 2004, as well as the standards the NMC expects of its registrants.

3.4 The register

A single professional register for nurses, midwives and health visitors was introduced in 1983 by the Nurses, Midwives and Health Visitors Act 1979. All nurses and midwives wishing to practise within the UK work within a jurisdiction that means it would be illegal to practise without effective registration.

In 1983, 11 parts to the register were established; these were later extended to 15 parts to identify the extra entry routes established by Project 2000. Those 15 parts distinguished between first- and second-level nurses, midwives and health visitors, and further separated the specialities of general, mental and learning disabilities, adult and children's nursing. The rules relating to the new NMC register are set out in Part III, article 5 of The Order, and through a statutory instrument[44] which gives an option for three parts. It states that it has to be accessible to the public at all times, and must include a part or parts for specialists in community and public health. Since 1 August 2004 the register has been divided into three parts only:

(1) nursing
(2) midwifery
(3) specialist community public health nursing.

The nursing part of the register is subdivided for first-level and second-level nurses and for adult, children's, mental health, learning disabilities and fever nurses. The midwifery part is open to all those with a midwifery qualification. The specialist community public health nursing part of the register includes health visitors on part 11 of the previous register, school nurses, occupational health nurses and family health nurses (in Scotland).

Registration processes are explained in Part IV of The Order, and allow names to be entered onto one or more parts of the register on completion of approved courses of education and training, and declaration of good health and good character. Renewal of registration also depends upon nurses and midwives signing a statement that they have fulfilled education and practice standards set by the NMC as part of their re-registration process, including maintenance of competence through professional development. As the PREP standards for nurses and midwives have recently been reviewed,[45] further details from the NMC on modernising revalidation will continue to emerge over time.[46]

3.5 Standards for conduct, performance and ethics

Section 2(1) of the Nurses, Midwives and Health Visitors Act 1979 states:

> The Principal functions of the Central Council shall be to establish and improve standards of training and professional conduct for nurses, midwives and health visitors.

Much of that statement is emulated by The Order, with some slight amendments. These include that in addition to standards of training and professional conduct, the Council is charged with establishing the standards for education and performance and ethics expected of registrants and prospective registrants.[47] The most recent version of the NMC professional code of conduct was updated in 2004 to take account of those changes, as is reflected in its title: *The NMC Code of Professional Conduct: Standards for Conduct, Performance and Ethics* (The Code).

There have been a series of revisions since the first edition of the code of conduct was published by the UKCC in 1983.[48] At the time of going to press the NMC are consulting on further revisions. Despite the changes, The Code's purpose remains constant and is summarised in its introduction. It stresses individual accountability, highlighting the need for registrants to accept responsibility relating to their particular knowledge, skills and competence. It also serves as the benchmark against which allegations of unfitness to practise would be measured.

However, a breach of any of those standards will not necessarily establish an impairment of fitness to practise.

The Code draws attention to the values shared among all the UK health care regulatory bodies. These are presented in an opening statement, which also reminds registrants of their individual responsibility and accountability, and informs the public, professions and employers of what may be expected of registered nurses and midwives:

> As a registered nurse, midwife or specialist community public health nurse, you are personally accountable for your practice. In caring for patients and clients, you must:
>
> - respect the patient or client as an individual
> - obtain consent before you give any treatment or care
> - protect confidential information
> - co-operate with others in the team
> - maintain your professional knowledge and competence
> - be trustworthy
> - act to identify and minimise risk to patients and clients.[49]

The Code is underpinned by the four ethical principles upheld by Beauchamp and Childress,[50] which encompass ideals commonly used as a basis to help decide the acceptability of practice in health care. They are autonomy, nonmaleficence, beneficence and justice.

3.6 Nursing and Midwifery Council Fitness to Practise proceedings

The NMC has published guidance for employers and managers to help them consider whether or not a registrant should be reported to the NMC, and the evidence that is needed in support of a complaint.[51] This states that one of the chief functions of the NMC is to protect the public from registrants whose fitness to practise is impaired and, in particular, those whose situation cannot be managed locally.

Anyone can complain to the NMC about an individual practitioner's conduct. The complaint should be made in writing, and should identify a named registrant by name, PIN and address. It should detail their job at the time of the allegations and key aspects of the post that may be relevant in considering the complaint. It should also detail any previous action undertaken through disciplinary, capability or health procedures. Documentary evidence such as patient care plans, adverse incident forms, medicine administration records, financial records and work diaries are normally required, as well as copies of notes of any investigative or disciplinary meetings.

A complaint is initially received by staff within the Fitness to Practise Directorate, who confirm that it concerns an NMC registrant, and fits the categories of allegation relating to fraudulent/incorrect entry or impairment of fitness to practise. If it concerns someone not on the NMC register, the staff will suggest the appropriate body to contact. If the allegation is not in the required form, staff will also advise. If the allegation meets the required form, it will be referred to the Investigating Committee (see 3.3.2 above).

3.7 Categories of allegation

The Order[52] identifies the following categories of allegation of impairment of fitness to practise:

- misconduct
- lack of competence
- a conviction or caution in the UK or a conviction elsewhere for an offence that if committed in England or Wales would constitute a criminal offence
- the registrant's physical or mental health
- a determination by another regulatory or licensing body that the registrant's fitness to practise is impaired.

The Order introduces a new power allowing the Council to handle allegations concerning actions alleged to have occurred outside the UK or when the person was not registered with the NMC.

The legislation also allows the NMC to deal with fraudulent or incorrect entries to the register. These categories of allegation provide a wider scope than previous arrangements, which charged the UKCC (and subsequently NMC), with considering allegations that fitness to practise was impaired by reason of misconduct or unfitness to practise due to ill health reasons only. The new powers led to the renaming of the Professional Conduct Department at the NMC as the Fitness to Practise Directorate, to reflect its broader remit. There is no further definition of these categories in The Order itself; however, following consultation in 2003 the NMC published their agreed definition in their guidance:

> Fitness to Practise means a registrant's suitability to remain on the register without restrictions.[53]

3.7.1 Misconduct

Defining professional misconduct can be testing, as it is a dynamic concept which not only is shaped by ethical and legal principles but also reflects social attitudes. For example, in 1934 one nurse was reported to have been removed from the register for 'staying in a hotel with a married man (who was not her husband)', and a second, a Matron, for having a child (out of wedlock) with a man employed on her staff.[54] Nowadays issues such as downloading illegal material from the internet have brought different challenges to the panels that consider fitness to practise.

Misconduct may relate to practice or non-practice-related issues, if public confidence in the profession is compromised. In 2003, the NMC revised its definition of misconduct to mean 'conduct which falls short of that which can reasonably be

---

Box 3.3   Issues arising from professional misconduct cases.

- Maladministration of drugs
- Neglect of basic care and unsafe clinical practice
- Failure to report incidents and failing to take appropriate action in an emergency
- Sexual, physical and verbal abuse of patients or clients
- Dishonesty, such as theft from patients or employers or claiming falsely to have qualifications
- Poor management practices and bullying
- Failing to collaborate with colleagues
- Miscellaneous: breach of confidentiality, failure to obtain consent, sleeping on duty, unfit for duty through alcohol or drugs
- Deliberate failure to deliver adequate care
- Deliberate failure to keep proper records
- Criminal convictions or cautions

Source: Nursing and Midwifery Council, *Fitness to Practise Annual Report, 2004–2005* (London, NMC, 2005).

---

expected of a registrant'. This means that a nurse or midwife would be judged against their professional code as any reasonable practitioner would be.

Examples of some contemporary issues commonly arising from misconduct cases are detailed in the NMC *Fitness to Practise Annual Report 2004–5*,[55] and shown in Box 3.3. There is no reliance on precedent with misconduct; however, decisions of the regulators, as well as the courts, can shape guidance and help determine and update standards.

3.7.2 Lack of competence

The Council's position on lack of competence is clearly stated in clauses 6–6.5 and 8.5 of the NMC *Code of Professional Conduct: Standards for Conduct, Performance and Ethics*, and within NMC guidance.[56]

Lack of competence means a lack of knowledge, skill or judgement of such a nature that the registrant is unfit to practise safely and effectively in any field in which the registrant claims to be qualified or seeks to practise.[57] This is a new category of impairment of fitness to practise for the NMC. The NMC lack of competence procedures are designed to deal with intractable incompetence, after all other avenues have been exhausted at a local level.

The NMC guidance sets out a number of prerequisites for employers and managers when considering reporting lack of competence. They include evidence that the registrant was made aware of the concerns about their competence and given an opportunity to improve their performance. There should also be evidence that a further assessment of the registrant's progress confirmed continuing lack of competence. This reminds employers that although the Council must undertake its regulatory role, it does not replace their responsibilities in managing lack of competence. In cases where the registrant is no longer employed, an assessment from a third party is likely to be required by the NMC in an area as similar as possible to that which gave rise to the allegation.

Previously, lack of competence would have been dealt with under the category of misconduct. It may still constitute misconduct if it is found, for example, that the practitioner worked outside of their area or level of competence, or where there is continued lack of competence despite opportunities to improve.

3.7.3 Convictions or cautions

The police have a responsibility to inform the NMC when a registered practitioner is convicted of a crime,[58] and more serious convictions may result in suspension or removal from the register. In *Balamoody* v. *UKCC*[59] it was held that professional conduct rules covered all criminal convictions irrespective of the seriousness of the crime or whether it was related to practice. In 2004/2005 the NMC was notified of 276 convictions, many of which were minor and did not require any further action; however, some involved serious convictions for rape, other violent crimes, downloading pornography or other illegal material from the internet, and dishonesty.[60] Other types of conviction that could lead to a finding of unfitness to practise include theft, fraud, sexual offences, and illegally dealing or importing drugs.[61] It is not the NMC's role to retry the evidence, but rather to determine whether the conviction was proved and whether the respondent before them is the same person who was convicted. Not all criminal convictions will necessarily constitute impairment of fitness to practise.

3.7.4 Impairment of fitness to practise due to physical or mental health

Consideration of allegations surrounding unfitness to practise for reasons of ill health is another important aspect of public protection. The majority of health-related matters referred to the NMC are made by direct referral from employers. Occasionally complaints will be made by the practitioner themselves, or a concerned relative or colleague. The majority of complaints relate to alcohol or drug abuse, depressive illness or other mental illness, with only 1% of health allegations relating to physical illness in 2004/2005.[62] Allegations about health issues are related not so much to a diagnosis as to behaviour or incidents that show impairment of fitness to practise due to ill health. The Investigating Committee can ask a solicitor to investigate and/or a medical examiner to assess the person's health.

3.7.5 A determination by another regulatory or licensing body that the registrant's fitness to practise is impaired

This means that upon receipt of any report from a regulator or licensing body within or outside of the UK that a registrant's fitness to practise is impaired, the

NMC has the power to instruct an investigation. If the NMC receives such a notification it will investigate it in the usual way following confirmation of the finding from the Registrar by the body and evidence about the proceedings and evidence that led to the finding.

3.8 Sanctions and indicative sanctions

Although it may be a common perception that the role of the regulator is to punish practitioners, judgments held in the hearing of appeals from regulatory bodies demonstrate that the regulator's role is to protect the public and also to maintain public trust and confidence in the trustworthiness of the profession and all that the professional register stands for.[63] Nurses and midwives are only removed from the register if the allegations satisfy the criminal standard of proof and are so serious as to put the public or the reputation of the profession at risk should the respondent continue to practise. Since 2004 the NMC has had a wider range of sanctions from which the panels may select, if fitness to practise is found to be impaired (Table 3.1).

This wider range of sanctions is similar to those adopted by most other health care regulators. In order to ensure consistency of approach among the panels, indicative sanction guidance is available to all parties. The guidance describes general principles panels should take into account when considering the appropriate sanction, sets out the range of sanctions, and details suggested criteria to apply when considering the sanction. General principles applied in considering any sanction have regard to the public interest, protection of the public, and trust and confidence in the professions and the regulator.

The use of indicative sanctions among regulatory bodies has been encouraged by the CHRE (see 3.12 below), and recognised by the courts as a way to improve consistency and openness of decisions.[64]

3.9 Interim orders

As well as the sanctions listed above, the NMC can in exceptional circumstances impose an interim order. Under the 1993 Rules the NMC has the power to suspend an individual's registration once an investigation is under way (interim suspension). The Order allows for similar arrangements, but also introduces interim conditions of practice. Interim orders are used in cases where the 'panel is satisfied it is necessary for the protection of the public, or is otherwise in the public interest, or is in the interests of the person concerned'.[65] This may be at any time that an investigation is under way. As all criminal cases need to be concluded before a Fitness to Practise committee can investigate and hold a hearing, a practitioner under police investigation for a serious criminal offence would probably be subject to interim suspension in the meantime. On occasion interim suspension may also be imposed upon practitioners in their own interest, for example if they are unfit to practise for health reasons, particularly where there is little or no insight into how that may affect their practice. Another example is where they have been accused of stealing and self-administering drugs, thereby putting themselves as well as the patients for whom the drugs are intended at risk. In all cases, the legal assessor will provide advice. Under the (new) Rules the period of interim order may not exceed 18 months without a court order.

3.10 Restoration to the register

Once a person has been removed from the professional register, they have a right to apply for restoration.[66] Under the previous Rules (the Professional Conduct Rules 1993) there was no restriction on how long a person must wait following removal from the register before submitting an application for restoration. This has changed under the new Rules, which require that an application for restoration shall not be made before a period of five years has elapsed. Any subsequent application may not be made within a year. Consideration of any application for restoration to the register is treated with the same degree of care as removal from the register. The applicant must attend the hearing so that they can be questioned by the panel. As well as considering the attitude and insight of the individual practitioner into the circumstances that led to their removal from the register, the panel must consider the effect that restoring the individual to the register would have on public confidence.

On occasions, restoration decisions have cast doubt upon the efficacy of nurses' and midwives' self-regulation. For example, a decision by the UKCC in 1996 to restore a convicted rapist caused unrest among the profession and others, and led to an extensive review of the process by which restorations were handled.[67]

Some applicants for restoration maintain that they are innocent of the matters charged, even following removal from the register. The Fitness to Practise panels must not become involved in discussing this issue. They are not there to change the original panel's findings, but must concentrate on the current position.

3.11 Appeals by the respondent

The 1979 Nurses, Midwives and Health Visitors Act introduced the right of appeal against an adverse decision to remove an individual from the register.[68] Appeals under that legislation, and section 12 of the 1997 Act, had to be made within three months of the decision. The Order, Section 38 (Part V) requires that Fitness to Practise appeals must be made within 28 days of a decision being served on a registrant. Appeals are dealt with by lawyers instructed by the NMC, and are generally based upon arguments about procedure or the law.

The court may:

(a) dismiss the appeal
(b) allow the appeal and quash the decision appealed against
(c) substitute for the decision appealed against any other decision the Practice Committee or Council, as the case may be, could have made
(d) remit the case to the Practice Committee concerned or Council, as the case may be, to be disposed of in accordance with the directions of the court or

sheriff (in England and Wales appeals about any order or decision of the Health Committee or Conduct and Competence Committee are made to the High Court, in Northern Ireland the High Court of Justice, and in Scotland the Court of Session).[69]

One of the UKCC's most significant appeals (*Brabazon-Drenning* v. *UKCC* 2000 QBD unreported) led to a successful challenge against the Council, the main issue being that it was unfair to proceed in the absence of the respondent, who had submitted medical evidence that she was unfit to attend. Reasons for the decision to proceed despite the medical evidence were not offered, and it was held that an adjournment on the grounds of ill health should only be refused in exceptional circumstances:

> Save in very exceptional cases where the public interest points to the contrary, it must be wrong for a committee which has the livelihood and reputation of a professional individual in the palm of its hands, to go on to a hearing when there is unchallenged medical evidence that the individual is simply not fit to withstand the rigors of the disciplinary process.

This case also served as a reminder that as part of natural justice a committee (panel) must provide reasons for its decisions.

More recently, an appeal against the NMC stressed the importance of reasons being given for decisions made by the adjudicating panels, even where there is no statutory requirement.[70]

Historically, there was only an appeal mechanism for the aggrieved respondent and no one else. Following recommendations in the NHS Plan[71] and the Kennedy Report,[72] the National Health Service Reform and Health Care Professions Act 2002 section 25(2) established a new organisation, directly accountable to Parliament, to act as an overarching body to cover the nine regulators responsible for around 1.5 million health care professionals in the UK. Their role in relation to appeals by other parties and their other responsibilities will now be explained.

3.12 Council for Healthcare Regulatory Excellence

The legislation (above) requires that an 'overarching' body be established to:

(a) promote the interests of patients and other members of the public in relation to regulating health care professions
(b) promote best practice in the performance of those functions
(c) formulate principles relating to good professional self-regulation and encourage regulatory bodies to conform to them
(d) promote cooperation between regulatory bodies, and between them and other bodies performing corresponding functions.

This body, established in April 2003, was originally known as the Council for the Regulation of Healthcare Professionals (CRHP), but was renamed in 2004 as the Council for Healthcare Regulatory Excellence (CHRE), because its role is not, as the original title suggested, to regulate individual practitioners, but to work towards a coordinated and consistent approach among the regulators. They can do this by recommending changes to regulators' rules (section 27), refer cases of 'undue leniency' to court (section 29) and advise health ministers (section 26(7)).

The appeal must be lodged on the grounds that a previous decision was felt to be 'unduly lenient', or that a relevant decision should not have been made, and that it would be desirable for the protection of the public for the CHRE to take action. Referrals have to be made by the CHRE to the High Court within 28 days.

Within this context the court has four options (section 29(8)):

(a) to dismiss the appeal
(b) to allow the appeal and quash the relevant decision
(c) to substitute for the relevant decision any other decision which could have been made by the committee or other person concerned, or
(d) to remit the case to the committee or other person concerned to dispose of the case in accordance with the directions of the court.

Between 2004 and 2005, 170 of the 590 cases considered by the CRHP/CHRE were from the NMC. Only one was referred to the High Court, and went to further appeal where it was dismissed by the judge, who stressed the importance of the adjective 'undue' in the leniency test.[73]

In 2005, another appeal by the CHRE against the NMC involving a case of misconduct was successfully upheld,[74] quashing the original decision of the Professional Conduct Committee (PCC) to take no action, and ordering that the case be remitted to the PCC for it to reconsider the decision as to the penalty imposed. It was also held that the reasons given by the panel were inadequate in providing a basis for their decision.

Although the number of CHRE appeals directly involving the NMC are nominal to date, the CHRE regularly publishes 'learning points' based on cases they have become involved in to help regulators and their panels understand how to improve Fitness to Practise processes, the kind of information that should be included in reasons, and similar issues.

3.13 Conclusion

At the time of writing, a characteristic of any conclusion in a text of this kind is that there can be no firm predictions about the future of professional regulation. All that can be said for certain is that the current system among health care professionals is set to alter, in response to public and professional opinion.

Whatever changes lie ahead, the importance of understanding the legal framework that underpins nurses' and midwives' professional conduct and accountability remains. This chapter serves as a reminder that registrants have an individual responsibility to maintain safe and effective practice, and to take appropriate action to deal with individuals who present an unacceptable risk to patients, to the public or to the reputation of the profession. It also demonstrates that there are transparent legal and professional standards that govern practice. In so doing it highlights the point that all health professionals, and their employers, need to be conversant with NMC standards and guidance, which

must be applied within their own context. Without that knowledge and application, and the ability to appropriately challenge regulatory processes, public
trust and confidence in the professional register and what it represents will
undoubtedly be compromised.

Finally, while the number of nurses and midwives investigated for alleged
impairment of fitness to practise remains a very small percentage of the profession,
there will always be some risk to public protection that no amount of regulatory
processes can legislate for.

3.14 Acknowledgements

The author wishes to thank former colleagues at the NMC, in particular Sonja
Wolfskehl, Senior Case Manager, Fitness to Practise, and Liz McAnulty, formerly
Director of Fitness to Practise, for their encouragement and advice, and for kind
permission to reproduce excerpts of NMC Fitness to Practise training materials
within this chapter.

3.15 Notes and references

1. Para. 333, explanatory notes to the Health Act 1999.
2. C. Davies & A. Beach, *Interpreting Professional Self Regulation: A History of the United
   Kingdom Central Council for Nursing, Midwifery and Health Visiting* (London and New
   York, Routledge, 2000).
3. Section 18, Health Act 1999, since replaced by section 45, Health and Social Care
   (Community Health and Standards Act) 2003.
4. Section 46, Health and Social Care (Community Health and Standards) Act 2003 sets out
   the legislative basis for the Healthcare standards in Department of Health, *Standards for
   Better Health: The Launch of Quality Standards for all NHS Foundation Trusts and Private and
   Voluntary Providers of NHS Care* (2004; updated by Department of Health, April 2006).
5. Part V, 22(9) The Nursing and Midwifery Order 2001, SI 2002:253.
6. Part V, 22(9) The Nursing and Midwifery Order 2001, SI 2002:253.
7. Nursing and Midwifery Council, *NMC News*, No. 15 (London, NMC, 2006).
8. Nursing and Midwifery Council, *Fitness to Practise Annual Report, 2004–2005* (London,
   NMC, 2005).
9. Part III, The Order.
10. Nursing and Midwifery Council, *Fitness to Practise Annual Report, 2004–2005* (London,
    NMC, 2005).
11. Part X, 50, The Order.
12. M. Moran & B. Wood, *States, Regulation and the Medical Profession* (Buckingham, Open
    University Press, 1993).
13. Bristol Royal Infirmary Inquiry (Kennedy Report), *Learning from Bristol: The Report of
    the Public Inquiry into Children's Heart Surgery at the Bristol Royal Infirmary* (1984–1995),
    Command Paper Cm 5207 July 2001, http:www.bristol-inquiry.org.uk
14. The Shipman Inquiry, Fifth Report, *Safeguarding Patients: Lessons from the Past – Proposals
    for the Future* (2004), www.the-shipman-inquiry.org.uk
15. Nursing and Midwifery Council, *Fitness to Practise Annual Report, 2004–2005* (London,
    NMC, 2005).

16. Department of Health, *The NHS Plan: A Plan for Investment A Plan for Reform*, CM 4818 (London, The Stationery Office, 2000).
17. Better Regulation Task Force, *Alternatives to Self Regulation* (London, The Cabinet Office, 2000).
18. Department of Health, *Government Widens Review into Healthcare Regulation*, Press release 2005/0121 (2005).
19. The Shipman Inquiry, Fifth Report, *Safeguarding Patients: Lessons from the Past – Proposals for the Future* (2004), www.the-shipman-inquiry.org.uk
20. Nursing and Midwifery Order 2001 SI 253 and The Nursing and Midwifery Council (Fitness to Practise) Rules Order of Council 2004, SI 2004:1761.
21. Nursing and Midwifery Order 2001 (Transitional Provisions) Order of Council 2004 SI 2004 No. 1762.
22. Section 60, Health Act 1999.
23. Section 7(1), Health Act 1999.
24. Viscount Hewart in *Rex* v. *Sussex Justices Ex parte McCarthy* [1924] K.B. 256, 259.
25. JM Consulting Ltd, *The Regulation of Nurses, Midwives, and Health Visitors*, report on a review of the Nurses, Midwives and Health Visitors Act 1997 (JM Consulting Ltd, 1999).
26. Part V 21(a), The Order.
27. Nursing and Midwifery Council, *NMC Code of Professional Conduct: Standards for Conduct, Performance and Ethics* (London, NMC, 2004).
28. Nurses and Midwives (Parts of and Entries in the Register) Order of Council 2004, SI 2004:1765.
29. S. Thewlis, Government rules increased NMC costs, *Nursing Times* (letter), **102** (2006), pp. 13, 16.
30. Part II 2, The Order.
31. Part VIII, The Order.
32. Schedule 1, The Order.
33. Schedule 1, Part II, The Order.
34. Nursing and Midwifery Council, *NMC makes historic decision on fitness to practise hearings*, press release, 23/2006.
35. Shipman Inquiry, Fifth Report, *Safeguarding Patients: Lessons from the Past – Proposals for the Future* (2004), www.the-shipman-inquiry.org.uk
36. Part V, 24.
37. Part 4, The Nursing and Midwifery Council (Fitness to Practise) Rules Order of Council 2004.
38. Part VI, 381(b) The Order.
39. Nursing and Midwifery Council, *Fitness to Practise Annual Report, 2004–2005* (London, NMC, 2005).
40. Part V, 27, The Order.
41. *Stefan* v. *General Medical Council* [1999] 1 WLR 1293.
42. Part 5, 21.
43. Schedule 1, 18, The Order.
44. Nurses and Midwives (Parts of and Entries in the Register) Order of Council 2004, SI 2004:1765.
45. Nursing and Midwifery Council, *The PREP Handbook* (London, NMC, 2006).
46. Nursing and Midwifery Council, Press Statement 24/2006, *NMC Position Statement re PREP* (2006).
47. Part II (2) and Part 1 (21), The Order.
48. UKCC, *Code of Professional Conduct for Nurses, Midwives and Health Visitors* (London, UKCC, 1983).

49. Nurses and Midwives (Parts of and Entries in the Register) Order of Council 2004, SI 2004:1765.
50. T.L. Beauchamp & J.F. Childress, *Principles of Biomedical Ethics*, 5th edn (New York, Oxford University Press, 2001).
51. Nursing and Midwifery Council, *Reporting Lack of Competence: A Guide for Employers and Managers* (London, NMC, 2004); NMC, *Reporting Unfitness to Practise: A Guide for Employers and Managers* (London, NMC, 2004).
52. Part V, 22.
53. Nursing and Midwifery Council, *Reporting Lack of Competence: A Guide for Employers and Managers* (London, NMC, 2004); NMC, *Reporting Unfitness to Practise: A Guide for Employers and Managers* (London, NMC, 2004).
54. E. Bendall & E. Raybould, *A History of the General Nursing Council* (London, HK Lewis, 1969).
55. Nursing and Midwifery Council, *Fitness to Practise Annual Report, 2004–2005* (London, NMC, 2005).
56. T.L. Beauchamp & J.F. Childress, *Principles of Biomedical Ethics*, 5th edn (New York, Oxford University Press, 2001).
57. T.L. Beauchamp & J.F. Childress, *Principles of Biomedical Ethics*, 5th edn (New York, Oxford University Press, 2001).
58. Home Office Circular 6/2006, *The Notifiable Occupations Scheme: Revised Guidance for Police Forces*.
59. *Balamoody* v. *UKCC*, *The Independent*, 15 June 1998.
60. Nursing and Midwifery Council, *Fitness to Practise Annual Report, 2004–2005* (London, NMC, 2005).
61. Nursing and Midwifery Council, *Reporting Unfitness to Practise: A Guide for Employers and Managers* (London, NMC, 2004).
62. NMC, *Fitness to Practise Annual Report, 2004–2005* (London, NMC, 2005).
63. *Bolton* v. *The Law Society* 1 W.L.R. 512; [1994] 2 All E.R. 486.
64. CHRE, *Annual Report and Accounts 2004/5*.
65. Part V, 31 (7).
66. Part V, 33, The Order.
67. UKCC Council Paper CC/96/32.
68. Section 13.
69. Part V, 38.
70. *Needham* v. *Nursing and Midwifery Council* 2003 EWHC 1141.
71. Department of Health, *The NHS Plan: A Plan for Investment A Plan for Reform*, CM 4818 (London, The Stationery Office, 2000).
72. Bristol Royal Infirmary Inquiry (Kennedy Report), *Learning from Bristol: The Report of the Public Inquiry into Children's Heart Surgery at the Bristol Royal Infirmary* (1984–1995), Command Paper Cm 5207 July 2001, http:www.bristol-inquiry.org.uk
73. *CRHP* v. *NMC and Stephen Truscott* [2004] EWHC 585, and *CRHP* v. *GMC and Ruscillo, and NMC and Stephen Truscott* [2004] EWCA Civ 1356.
74. *CHRE* v. *NMC and Claire McDonnell*, QBD, WEAC5350.

4 The Complaints Dimension: Patient Complaints in Health Care Provision

Arnold Simanowitz

'*Plus ca change . . .*' or, as the English would have it, 'The more things change, the more they stay the same.'

Once again there have been innumerable changes in the various aspects of the complaints procedures since the last edition of this book, and once again the situation for patients has been made, if anything, harder rather than easier. Of course there have been improvements, some of them quite fundamental and far reaching, and the relationship between complaints and the law becomes ever closer. But what has not been achieved is to give patients or their representatives who believe that there has been a problem with their care one simple system by which to initiate a complaint.

It may be thought that, with the third edition of the book, it was time to remove much of the history of the complaints system from this chapter. While some of it may be unnecessary, it is not possible to form a view of what is really required for a patient-centred complaints system without knowing how we have got to the present position. I will therefore retain what I regard as essential while making appropriate alterations.

Since this chapter was written for the first edition of this book, there have been major developments, if not advances, on all fronts in the ethical and legal spheres of health care, as the other chapters of the book demonstrate – some of an extremely far-reaching nature. In so far as complaints are concerned, the changes have been of a fairly fundamental kind. Indeed, while the issue of complaints was quite properly included in a book about law and ethics when the first edition was written, at that time complaints were not really seen as an ethical matter at all and had very little impact on or involvement with the law. With regard to ethics, on the one hand complaints were simply regarded by health care providers as an attack on the institution or individual involved, to be rejected if possible or diverted if not; on the other hand, patients believed, partly because of that very attitude of the providers, that if they complained they were doing something somewhat frowned upon by society and possibly harmful to the NHS. As a result, complaints were not seen as an ethical issue at all.

It was because of this that the original steps taken to introduce procedures to enable patients to complain satisfied neither patients nor health carers. On the providers' side, they were introduced grudgingly as a minimum that might satisfy the 'difficult' patient; on the patient's side, they did not begin to satisfy the first principle of a complaints procedure, which is to look at the problem from the patient's point of view. If someone of negative intent had sat down to create a system for patients to complain about health care, they would have been unlikely to have come up with anything as unhelpful as the system that operated before the changes brought in following the Wilson Inquiry in 1994.[1]

First, there was an entirely different procedure depending on where the treatment had taken place. If it had taken place in a hospital then the procedure under Health Circular (81)5 applied. This could lead to an 'independent' professional review by consultants from outside the region in which the care had taken place. While that procedure was described as independent, patients did not see it as such. Although the consultants carrying out the review were from outside the region, nevertheless they were seen as part of the health service and therefore likely to support their colleagues. A further problem was that if there was an allegation of negligence that might have been the subject of litigation then the complaint could not proceed.

Where the care complained of had taken place in a general practitioner's surgery, on the other hand, the complaint had to be made to the Family Health Services Authority, where the procedure was totally different. Even if the complaint involved an allegation of negligence it would, unlike hospital complaints, still be dealt with here.

Secondly, there was yet another distinction between types of complaint. If the complaint was about administration it could be made to the Health Service Commissioner (the Ombudsman) – but not if it related to primary care services in respect of which the Ombudsman had no jurisdiction.

Thirdly, if the complaint related to the conduct of a clinician, it might amount to professional misconduct and would therefore have to be made to the General Medical Council (GMC) or the United Kingdom Central Council for Nursing, Midwifery and Health Visiting (UKCC) (now NMC), where the doctor or nurse could be disciplined. The burden of proof of professional misconduct and the interpretation of it by the GMC or UKCC was, however, so heavy for the complainant that the vast majority of such complaints were rejected out of hand. But that was not the only way in which a hospital doctor working in the NHS could be disciplined. His or her employer, the hospital Trust, could itself implement disciplinary proceedings, the result of which could lead to dismissal but not to removal from the register, which was the purview of the General Medical Council alone.

Finally, if the complaint concerned damage to the patient who consequently wished for compensation, the only recourse was to the courts. It can be seen, therefore, that a patient wishing to complain was faced with a bewildering array of procedures any or all of which were mutually exclusive. Any one of them could involve a process of such length and complication that patients often did not have the stamina either to commence it or, once they had commenced it, to last the course.

Now there is more awareness on the part of many providers that there are two ethical aspects to the question of complaints. First, there is a recognition that how a complaint is dealt with can have an important effect on a patient and his or her family. It can be seen as part of the care of a patient, and as such the obligation to deal with it properly comes within the duty of care of all health care providers. The Chief Medical Officer recognised this in his seminal report on learning from adverse events in the NHS, *An Organisation with a Memory*:

> The processes of dealing with adverse events which lead to litigation are often themselves perceived by patients as further elements of poor care.[2]

Although this recognition is not yet universal, the concept, if not its consequences, is, certainly among the leaders in the professions, a reality and is accepted as applying not only to those events that lead to litigation but to those that elicit a complaint as well.

Secondly, there is a recognition that complaints have a major role to play in the improvement of health care; that they are 'jewels to be treasured' – they show, more than anything else, the shortfalls in the system.

At the same time, patients, greatly encouraged by the government, have at last come to recognise that the provision of health care is a service which, if not exactly the same as any other service – for example, the provision of electricity – is nevertheless something they are entitled to receive at a reasonable standard. If that standard is not attained they are far more prepared to complain without feeling that they are undermining the NHS.

In so far as the law is concerned, the complaints procedure has started to become an integral part of the legal process. It features both in the pre-action protocol, where it is something that should be considered before a claimant is advised to take legal action,[3] and, strongly, in the Legal Service Commission's guidance in clinical negligence cases where public funding may not be granted if resort has not been made first to the NHS complaints procedure.

There is little doubt that between the first and second editions of this book complaints moved further onto centre stage in the National Health Service and even began to make an impact in the independent sector. It is not within the scope of this chapter to describe in detail all the reasons for this. Nevertheless, it would not be appropriate to ignore entirely the three main causes. The first is the approach of the government. It is government policy to insist that the citizen is entitled to expect a good service in all public areas and to complain if they do not get it. It is the government itself that has insisted that the health service should in this respect be treated like any other service. Pursuant to that attitude, the government has established the Independent Complaints and Advocacy Service (ICAS), which is discussed later in this chapter.

The second is the high-profile disasters that have received such prominent reporting in the media, above all the Bristol Royal Infirmary tragedy. That disaster involved the avoidable deaths of more than 20 children and led to a public inquiry that lasted more than two years. The *BMJ* editorial in June 1998, commenting on the tragedy, started with the words 'All changed, changed utterly . . .'.[4] To the extent that the tragedy and subsequent public inquiry brought realisation to the wider public that doctors could be challenged, that statement was absolutely correct, and this has influenced attitudes towards complaints ever since. It is an irony that while Action for Victims of Medical Accidents (AVMA), now known as Action against Medical Accidents (AvMA), had by then dealt with over 25,000 adverse events – some equally devastating for the families concerned and involving at least as bad behaviour on the part of the doctors concerned – it was only after Bristol, which involved only 24 incidents, albeit of the most distressing kind, that the public, the media, the health care providers and the government began to take the matter of adverse incidents really seriously. Nevertheless, the important thing was that it did then start to take them seriously, and this had a major spin-off onto complaints.

The third reason for the increased importance of complaints is the change in approach that was recommended by the Wilson Report. While fundamental problems remain with the way complaints are dealt with, nevertheless both the underlying principles for a proper complaints procedure proposed by Wilson[1] and the new procedure itself have led to changes in the way complaints are perceived. It will be seen below that the new procedures introduced as a result of the Wilson recommendations addressed a number of the complaints about the previous procedure, but many remained.

4.1 The 'new' complaints system

While there have been further changes in the system subsequently, at the heart of the mechanisms for patients to complain about the service they have received from health care providers within the NHS is the complaints procedure that came into effect on 1 April 1996 following the report of the Wilson Inquiry.[1] This replaced all existing hospital, community health service and family health service complaints procedures with a two-stage procedure: local resolution and independent review. With only one major change, this procedure remains in force despite many of its defects. These defects, and the major change, are referred to later in this chapter.

4.1.1 Local resolution

The whole idea behind the procedure is that complaints should be dealt with as close as possible to the point at which the service was provided. The majority of complaints are investigated by the Trust or the general practitioner's practice itself. One of the major complaints made by patients about the previous procedures was the interminable time complaints could take. The guidance to this procedure recommends specific timetables for dealing with the complaint in an attempt to ensure that the patient receives a full response within a reasonable time.[5]

The procedure should, as recommended by the Wilson Report, be:

- accessible for complainants
- simple
- separate from disciplinary procedures
- able to provide lessons about the quality of service delivery

- fair
- rapid and open
- honest and thorough with the prime aim of resolving problems and satisfying the concerns of the complainant.

While there remains considerable dissatisfaction on the part of many patients about the way local resolution is conducted, this revolves largely around implementation by many of the Trusts and GPs and their personnel rather than the procedure itself. By and large the procedure is an improvement on what took place before, mainly because it has concentrated the minds of those responsible for dealing with complaints on their responsibilities to patients. Unfortunately the same cannot be said for the second stage of the procedure, the so-called independent review.

4.1.2 Independent review

The major complaint by patients' organisations about the review procedure for hospital complaints that existed before the Wilson Inquiry was that, notwithstanding its title, the Independent Professional Review was not really independent. Two consultants from outside the region would be appointed by the Regional Medical Officer; there would be no input into the review by the patient, who would have no knowledge of what investigations were made and would not see the statements made by other parties. (See the evidence of AvMA to the inquiry and their comments on the recommendations made by the Review Committee.)

Furthermore, there was no opportunity for the complainant to hear the explanation of the clinician, let alone cross-examine him or her. The consultants were at liberty to obtain the information they required in whatsoever way they considered appropriate, and the complainant would have no way of testing or challenging that information. At the conclusion of the 'review' the patient would simply be told what had been decided. If the decision was unsatisfactory there was no appeal. While on the face of it the review might seem independent because clinicians from outside the hospital concerned were making the decision, to the complainant it could not appear to be anything other than the doctors, or the NHS itself, 'sticking together'. If the aim of a complaints procedure is to satisfy complainants, which it is self-evident that it should be, then it can clearly be seen that such a situation was unacceptable.

What is more, even if the complaint were upheld, the complainant would not necessarily be told what action had been taken to ensure that similar incidents would not be repeated for other patients. In particular, if the complaint was against an individual clinician or other employee of the Trust, no information would be given to the complainant as to what action, disciplinary or otherwise, had been taken against that individual.

It is the experience of all those involved in dealing with complaints on behalf of patients that few are motivated by feelings of revenge. It is widely recognised that one of the major considerations on the part of those complaining about care, particularly where that care led to considerable distress for the patient or their family, is to ensure that others do not have to suffer in the same way. In many complaints, therefore, failure to inform the complainant of what action had been taken remained a cause of great dissatisfaction and resulted in the complainant feeling that the complaint had been a waste of time.

It is recognised that this is not a straightforward issue as matters of employment law, and now human rights legislation, are involved. Nevertheless, the health care provider must provide the complainant with reassurance that appropriate action has been taken if the whole complaints procedure is not to be undermined.

As far as complaints against general practitioners were concerned, the problem with the old procedure was a different one. The actual procedure was far more open, with the patient able to confront the doctor and ask him or her questions before a tribunal. The basic flaw with that procedure, however, was that it was a system aimed at dealing not with dissatisfied patients but with the relationship between the doctor and the Family Health Services Authority as employee and employer. Patients were therefore misled into believing that their grievances were going to be addressed when in fact the inquiry was simply to establish whether there had been a breach of the doctor's terms of service. Sometimes these aims were co-terminus, but often they were not.

Nevertheless, there were major advantages to this procedure over that for hospital complaints. In the first place the tribunal included a number of lay people and a lay chair; secondly, the proceedings were open, with the doctor subject to cross-examination – although not by lawyers, as they were not allowed to represent either party – and often findings that a doctor had been in breach of terms of service did amount to a vindication of the patient's complaint. Most importantly, the patient had the opportunity of seeing the person whom they considered responsible for the problem, who was required to account for his or her actions.

How much of the dissatisfaction with the old procedure was satisfactorily dealt with by the Wilson reforms? Under the 'Wilson' system, if patients were not satisfied with the result of Local Resolution they made a written request for an Independent Review. There was no automatic right to such a review. The decision as to whether a review should take place was taken by the convenor, who was usually a non-executive director of the relevant health authority or Trust board. If the convenor agreed, a review panel would be convened. Membership of the panel would comprise:

- an independent lay chair
- the convenor
- in the case of a Trust, a representative of the purchaser
- in the case of a primary care complaint, for a health authority panel, another independent lay person.

The panel would, in the case of clinical complaints, be advised by at least two clinical assessors nominated by the regional office, from a list compiled on advice from relevant professional bodies. The procedure adopted by the panel was decided by the chair on an ad hoc basis and there was no obligation to hold a hearing. Indeed, the thrust of inquiries was to avoid a confrontation between the patient and those who might be the cause of the complaint.

It will be seen that, from the patient's point of view, he or she would be confronted by a panel that, apart from the chair, was not independent, comprising and being advised by representatives of the very discipline about which they were complaining. The problem of lack of independence was therefore, from the patient's point of view, not satisfactorily addressed; the patient was still left without the right to hear the evidence of the clinician or to test it. It was common for the chair to agree to a hearing of sorts, but no legal representation was allowed; there remained no right of appeal; and the patient would still never be informed as to what action had been taken with regard to any practitioner who might have been found to have acted inappropriately. Furthermore, the more open procedure that applied to general practitioners was subsumed into the new procedure, which was not as open.

A report published by the Public Law Project following extensive research into the working of the new procedure concluded:

> In the course of our analysis, certain key characteristics of panel hearings emerged which raised serious questions about their independence, fairness and ability to achieve satisfactory outcomes for complainants.[6]

It will be seen that the main objection to the operation of the new complaints procedure rested with the second stage, the review. While some improvements on the previous position had taken place, the essential problem remained that complaints were not being approached from a patient-centred perspective.

In 2000 the government published the NHS Plan, which proposed significant reforms to the NHS.[7] The vision of these reforms was that care of patients in the future would be patient-centred. This philosophy was naturally to be applied to the complaints procedure as well. Changes to the first stage were to await the outcome of the Shipman Inquiry,[8] but the more urgent problems relating to the second stage were addressed.

In accordance with the plan, the second stage was taken over by the Healthcare Commission in 2004. For the first time, complaints were to be addressed by a body entirely independent of the organisation or person complained about. Furthermore, if a complainant is unhappy about the outcome of the first stage, they have the right to ask the Healthcare Commission for an Independent Review. The Healthcare Commission can:

- refer the matter back to the NHS body where the complaint arose with recommendations for action to resolve the complaint
- refer the complaint to the General Medical Council or other health regulatory body
- refer the complaint to the health service Ombudsman
- carry out a further investigation of the complaint with or without a hearing before a panel
- take no further action.

Apart from the more obvious improvements that this represents, a major step forward is that if the complainant has gone down the wrong route, the Healthcare Commission has the power to correct this by referring the complaint to a health regulatory body. This goes some way towards addressing the multiple confusing routes confronting a complainant but it will be seen that it does not really resolve the problems in the way that a 'one-stop shop' for all complaints would do.

Unfortunately, as I said at the beginning of this chapter, the more things change, the more they stay the same. The Healthcare Commission is having great difficulty in dealing with the number of complaints it receives. In November 2005 it was reported that it had received over 8000 requests from people wanting their complaint independently reviewed in the 12 months to August 2005.[9] This compared with 3700 requests for independent review in 2003/04, when the NHS dealt with second-stage complaints.

Unless there has been a dramatic increase in the number of incidents giving cause for complaint, this suggests that the fact that there is finally a truly independent forum for dealing with complaints has encouraged dissatisfied patients to take some action. The Commission's Head of Operational Development said:

> The number of NHS complaints referred for independent review has gone up dramatically. We have been working as hard as we can to get as many complaints resolved as quickly as possible and those efforts are now bearing fruit. However, all Trusts must also play their part. Patients want complaints resolved quickly and locally so NHS Trusts need to be good at this. It is worrying that so many of the NHS complaints that come to us – over one in three – are having to go back to the NHS to be put right.

Two conclusions can be drawn form this. The first is that after all this time, and despite the government's urging of the NHS to become more patient-centred, many Trusts are still unable to deal with complaints satisfactorily. The second is more fundamental. The pressure both on Trusts and on the various systems for dealing with complaints will not be reduced, and as a result patients will not be satisfied, until the causes for complaint are substantially reduced. That is the ethical issue for the Health Service to address. Everything else is firefighting.

That is where the National Patient Safety Agency (NPSA) comes in. This body was established following the report by the Chief Medical Officer, *Organisation with a Memory*, in 2000.[2] The report proposed the introduction of a new system for identifying patient safety incidents in health care in order to gather information on causes and to learn and act to reduce risk and prevent similar events occurring in the future. The NPSA defines a patient safety incident as 'any unintended or unexpected incident which could have or did lead to harm for one or more patients receiving NHS-funded care'.

The NPSA set up a National Reporting and Learning System, enabling the health service and members of the public to report patient safety incidents directly to it. This system is already beginning to address the disgrace that existed whereby the same incidents were occurring time after time in different – or often the same – health care sites with no action taken to prevent this. In due course the system should make a major contribution to patient safety, and consequently the number of complaints will fall.

But it is not only the NPSA's reporting system that will have an effect on complaints: two other initiatives of the Agency should also have that effect. The first is their Please Ask campaign. This encourages patients, who are naturally wary of challenging health carers in hospital, to ask those carers – doctors as well as others – if they have any concerns. It is surprising how often a sensible question can remind a health carer to take some action that has been overlooked.

Even more important than the Please Ask campaign is the Being Open project. The purpose of this project is to encourage health carers to be open with patients when something has gone wrong or is suspected to have gone wrong. My experience at AvMA, and one that is shared by all those who are engaged in helping people who believe they have suffered a patient safety incident, was that it is often the way in which health carers react to such an incident that compounds the problem. If patients' questions are not properly answered, if health carers are defensive and if they fail to give an honest explanation and sincere apology, patients and their relatives or carers frequently feel that they have no option but to make a formal complaint and can even be driven to litigate.

The Being Open project seeks not only to ensure that patients are properly dealt with when something goes wrong but to demonstrate to health carers that it is in their own interests to be open, honest and empathic when that happens.

4.2 The Health Service Commissioner (Ombudsman)

The role of the Ombudsman, too, has changed considerably. Until 1996 the Ombudsman's remit extended only to complaints about administrative matters and did not include issues of clinical judgement. This often caused considerable frustration for both patients and the Ombudsman. Following the Health Service Commissioner (Amendment) Act 1996, the Ombudsman is able to look at the whole of a complaint, including clinical care. His remit is also extended to complaints about Family Health Services, from which he was previously excluded.

A particularly helpful aspect of the Ombudsman's role under the procedure prior to 2004 was that if the convenor refused or failed to set up an independent review the complainant could complain to the Ombudsman, who could then require that a review be implemented. Now the role is somewhat different, as the complaint will in most cases have been through a truly independent review. The Ombudsman will nevertheless reconsider the complaint and if necessary may carry out a formal investigation. Either before that investigation or as a result of it, the Ombudsman can request the NHS body to carry out action deemed necessary or appropriate.

Effectively this means that the Ombudsman can act as a form of appeal. If a complainant has been through all the steps of the complaints procedure but still remains dissatisfied, the Ombudsman can investigate the matter further. Indeed, the fact that the Ombudsman states quite clearly on the website 'Usually you should have already complained to the organisation or practitioner involved and to the Healthcare Commission before sending us your complaint...' demonstrates that the power to investigate even after consideration by the Healthcare Commission is there.

4.3 Complaints in the independent health care sector

All the procedures described already apply only to complaints with regard to NHS-funded health care. Until 2000, patients who were unhappy with any aspect of care within the independent sector had no recourse to any formal complaints procedure. They were left to take up their complaint with the hospital administration or the clinician direct. Furthermore, there was no support system available to them as the remit of the Community Health Councils did not extend to the independent sector. The attitude of successive governments appeared to be that as they were not responsible for treatment outside the National Health Service, problems within that sector were not their concern. This left patients who had problems with no redress, and often they were driven to litigation as the only way in which they could ensure that their complaint was taken seriously.

However, in 2000 the Independent Healthcare Association introduced a pilot complaints procedure for the sector. Although some consultation with interested parties had taken place before its introduction, the procedure was not in a form that was acceptable to a number of patients' organisations. Those organisations that were not members of the Independent Healthcare Association also introduced a form of complaints procedure.

The fact remains, however, that complaints in the independent sector are not subject to scrutiny by the Healthcare Commission or the Ombudsman. That means that complainants are at the mercy of whatever procedure a particular institution has decided to introduce. With the fragmentation of care taking place as a result of recent government legislation, great confusion will arise as to the rights of NHS patients in so far as complaints are concerned.

4.4 Disciplinary issues

For patients, the most disappointing aspect of the whole system for complaining about a doctor has in the past been the General Medical Council. Most people have little or no knowledge of the system for complaining about doctors generally and only learn about it when they come to have need of it. There is a vague awareness, however, that doctors are subject to some control and that if something goes wrong there is a body that will discipline the doctor. What they discovered when something did go wrong, however, was that that body was reluctant to address their problem, confining itself only to what appeared to be the most arcane complaints; that it was extremely difficult to persuade it to investigate a complaint; that the procedures were complex, lengthy and did not involve the patient to any meaningful degree; and that the entire system was heavily weighted in favour of the doctor.

In recent years the GMC has taken major steps to try to address these problems. It has extended its remit so that it can deal not only with complaints involving potential impairment of fitness to practise (formerly expressed as serious professional misconduct) but also with issues of poor performance. That has meant that it can consider a complaint by a patient that a doctor has treated him or her badly. It is far more prepared than in the past to investigate any complaint, not hiding behind difficult issues of definition; however, only if the complaint discloses a serious defect in the doctor's performance will the GMC deal with it. It is also far more helpful to individuals who wish to make a complaint, and patients are seen much more as part of the process and are given more support. By including many more lay people both on the Council and in the disciplinary process, it appears less biased in favour of the doctor.

Nevertheless, two facets of the GMC's procedures tend to leave patients unhappy with those procedures. First, the GMC remains in the position of both prosecutor and judge. It is the GMC, through its case examiners, that decides whether a complaint should go forward; it is then the GMC that collects the evidence and prosecutes the complaint against the doctor; and it is the GMC, through its Fitness to Practise panel, that decides whether the complaint has been proved and what sanction, if any, should be imposed. Dame Janet Smith, in her Fifth Report on the Shipman Inquiry, strongly supported this criticism and suggested how this should be addressed.[10]

The second area of major dissatisfaction is the standard of proof that the GMC demands in order to uphold a complaint. It is not that which applies in civil cases, where proof must be on a balance of probabilities, but rather is equivalent to that applied in criminal cases. The case must be proved beyond reasonable doubt, which makes it more difficult to prove complaints. Interestingly, the General Dental Council, which deals with disciplinary issues involving dentists, has introduced the civil standard of proof. Nevertheless, although the GMC has carefully reviewed this issue it has at present no proposals for change.

However, Dame Janet recommended a change on this issue as well. At the time of writing the Chief Medical Officer has an expert group considering the action to be taken in respect of her report, and the GMC could be compelled to change.

4.5 Help for complainants

Until September 2005, despite the difficulties facing patients who wished to make a complaint of any kind, there was no statutory body with the specific power to assist them. The only statutory bodies that did deal with complaints were the Community Health Councils (CHCs). As 'patients' watchdogs', many of them had taken on that role notwithstanding that statutorily it was not included in their remit. The lack of statutory authority meant, in the first place, that not all CHCs undertook complaints work, and secondly, that there was great discrepancy in the skills and effectiveness of those CHCs that were prepared to deal with complaints and no overarching body to maintain standards. Nevertheless, as independent bodies committed to the welfare of patients, they were able, although having limited resources and lacking statutory backing, to assist a large number of patients in achieving a just outcome to their complaint.

The government, in its NHS Plan published in 2000,[7] stated its intention to abolish Community Health Councils in England. (In Wales, which was now responsible for its own health service, CHCs would remain, as would their equivalent in the Scottish system.) In their place it planned to establish a Patient Advocacy and Liaison Service (PALS) situated within each Trust, among other things to assist patients with their complaints. Various bodies were to be established to deal with the other tasks previously undertaken by the CHCs.

The proposals attracted a great deal of criticism. First and foremost, the objection was to the lack of independence of the PALS given that they would be established within the hospitals, with their officers answerable to the chief executive.

In addition, it was argued that dealing with complaints was not something that could be isolated from CHCs' other work. Their vast knowledge of the operation of the Health Service in their area accumulated over 25 years gave them the background to deal far more effectively with the complaint of an individual patient about the service that had been provided.

As a result of these criticisms the government modified its proposals and, in so far as complaints were concerned, proposed an Independent Complaints Advocacy Service (ICAS) in addition to the PALS, which would be a Patient Advisory Liaison Service situated within the Trusts and simply giving advice to patients. This would leave complaints and advocacy to the ICAS. In addition, it agreed to set up Patients' Councils, which would be responsible for that service. The exact remit and powers of those Councils were unclear and seemed unsatisfactory.

This still left the public without a national patients' body, which had been a major demand from the time when the government had announced the abolition of the CHCs. It had long been clear that patients and public needed a statutory voice with clout to advise government on the health and service needs of the public, and it appeared essential that the new bodies to be created – the Councils, PALS and ICAS – had to be part of a national organisation able to coordinate the service as well as provide training and maintain standards. The campaigners argued that this could be achieved by maintaining the CHCs and strengthening their remit and governance, rather than by undoing a system which, notwithstanding acknowledged deficiencies, had credibility and had achieved so much.

After much controversy and challenge in Parliament, most notably in the House of Lords, the bill setting up the new system was finally enacted. A patient and public national organisation was established with the clumsy name of the Commission for Patient and Public Involvement in Health (CPPIH, immediately christened Chippy). Clumsy or not, the name indicates exactly what the remit of the organisation was to be – not involved in the health service alone but in health itself. It seemed that the campaign for a national body had been successful. From there, however, it was downhill. Rather than the CPPIH being wholly responsible for the bodies on the ground that would involve patients and the public in health, the health service and complaints, the system remained fragmented. PALS would remain as an advisory service within the Trusts, charged with dealing with the 'concerns' of patients within those Trusts. Complaints would be dealt with by a new service, ICAS, the responsibility of the CPPIH, and involvement in the remaining areas of health and health care would be dealt with by Patient & Public Involvement Forums – Acute, Primary Care, Mental Health and Ambulance – of which there would be one for each of the 512 Trusts in the country.

The possibilities for confusion for the public are obvious. Where did concerns end and complaints begin? How were the Forums to know about, so as to be able to address them, the issues that were raised by complainants with ICAS? To compound the problems, the CPPIH was given insufficient funds, either to set up the Forums directly serviced by the CPPIH or to manage ICAS. The first of these problems was dealt with by the CPPIH contracting with local voluntary bodies to service the Forums. These would be known as Forum Support Organisations. This solution was considered by many to be very unsatisfactory. The second problem was dealt with by the Department of Health taking direct responsibility for ICAS, thereby placing a question mark over its independence, by franchising different groups to run the service in different areas. It was not intended, at that stage at any event, that this arrangement for ICAS would be a permanent one. The legislation still provided for the CPPIH to be responsible for ICAS and it was believed that, once the CPPIH was functioning satisfactorily, ways would be found to enable it to take over responsibility for ICAS so as to make it truly independent and, just as important, to be perceived as such.

For a report on how the ICAS performed in those areas where the provider of the service was the Citizens Advice Bureau, see their report 'The pain of complaining', May 2005.[11]

A further cause of confusion is one aspect of the role of the NPSA. For patients and members of the public, this agency – by its very name, if nothing else – can appear to be a body that can help them in dealing with their complaint. As the NPSA does not in fact deal with individual cases but wants to record the experiences of patients and public in order to provide additional feedback to the NHS, this can cause confusion and distress for those who contact it hoping for assistance. The agency is making every effort, both in its publicity and in the way it handles callers, to try to ensure that this misconception does not arise or cause problems.

As far as it goes, the new system for complaints is nevertheless a major improvement on its predecessors. First, there is now a statutory body, albeit responsible to the Department of Health, charged with assisting patients and the public to complain. Secondly, the second stage of any complaint, whether against a hospital or a general practitioner, is now dealt with by the Healthcare Commission, a body in no way connected with those being complained about, and there is effectively a right of appeal to the Ombudsman.

4.6 Changes to the system

It was to be hoped that, having introduced major changes to the system for patient and public involvement, incorporating an improved system for patient complaints, the government would allow it a reasonable amount of time to prove itself. Unfortunately, that was not to be. In July 2004, following what was known as the Arm's Length Review of health bodies sponsored by the Department of Health, the Secretary of State for Health announced the abolition of the CPPIH in June 2006. Because the Department had no idea of how patient and public involvement would be organised after its abolition, that period had to be extended to June 2007. An assurance was given, however, that the Patient and Public Forums would remain, although it was not clear how they would be serviced or supported.

Following a form of consultation with all interested stakeholders, including patients and public, the Department of Health set up an Expert Panel to review the responses to the consultation and make recommendations to the Secretary of State on the future of patients and public involvement. That body issued its report in May 2006. Contrary to assurances given it recommended that the Forums should be abolished. The bill to give effect to this is now before parliament which provides for the abolition of the CPPIH and the replacement of Forums with new local networks called LINKs. One of the major effects in the Bill is the omission of any national patients' body with the independent authority that was originally given to the CPPH. How all this will impact on the handling of complaints is not at all clear. That in itself is an indictment of the government's attitude towards complaints, which have certainly not taken centre stage in the debate.

4.7 Complaints and litigation

One of the major defects in the system for dealing with complaints is the fact that these and claims for compensation are corralled into rigidly separate compartments. If a patient makes a complaint but has either instigated legal action or has notified in writing that he or she intends to do so, the complaints procedure should be stopped.[12] Some health care providers interpret this requirement very narrowly – an approach from a solicitor, a request for medical records with a possible claim in mind, a brief reference to compensation or legal remedy in a letter – and work on the complaint immediately stops. The Ombudsman will not deal with a complaint if the above circumstances apply.

But patients need incredible stamina to follow first the complaints procedure – and possibly all three stages of it – and then, if they want or need compensation, to go down the legal route. Both the Health Service Commissioner and the Health Select Committee have strongly criticised the system. The Ombudsman has referred to patients' 'complaint fatigue'[13] and the Committee noted that 'when people did complain, it appeared they often became even more dissatisfied with the process and the outcome of the complaint and confused by a regulatory system which gave them a number of options for taking action'.[14]

But most patients only know, or suspect, something has gone wrong. They may want compensation but often that is not in the forefront of their minds, and in any event it is only one part of what they are seeking. More commonly – and today this is generally recognised – what they seek is an opportunity to air their concerns; if appropriate, further treatment to resolve the medical problem; a full and open explanation of what has happened and why; and, if there has been a mistake or unacceptable service, an apology and assurances that lessons will be learned for the future. Compensation is often only an issue if the other remedies are not provided, or not quickly enough, or the damage suffered by the patient is very serious.

Most patients have no previous experience of making complaints or claims, and have little or no knowledge of the complaints or legal system, or of the cost, stress and difficulty of pursuing a legal claim in particular. Many of those who seek advice from a solicitor only do so out of frustration at the NHS body's seeming inability to understand and try to resolve the problem. Yet the system obliges dissatisfied patients to choose, often artificially and too soon, which route to follow. Pushing patients into litigation that they do not really want makes very little sense from any perspective.

Best practice in the NHS has given a strong pointer as to how complaints should be handled. Enlightened claims managers will identify quickly what the patient is after and will ensure not only that the complaint is adequately and expeditiously dealt with but also that if the patient is entitled to a small amount of compensation this is paid. The provision that all claims or complaints managers adopt a similar course, and that if the unresolved complaint proceeds to an independent review an award of limited compensation can be part of the remit of that review, would have a dramatic effect for patients and health service providers alike. Patients would be satisfied that all their grievances had been dealt with within a reasonable time; both patients and clinicians involved would be spared the distress of legal proceedings; and the NHS itself would save the considerable costs of litigation.

4.7.1 A hypothetical case study

After years during which the complaints system has been tinkered with, the position of a patient who has had a serious patient safety incident in a hospital and wants to complain could be as follows.

Naturally, the patient turns first to the institution where he or she believes the incident happened. The patient is referred to the PALS at the hospital. The kindly officer at PALS undertakes to speak to the consultant who operated on the patient. Having done so, the officer informs the patient that the consultant believes that the problem arose from the delay in the GP's referral to the hospital. Having no reason not to accept this, the patient makes a complaint to the GP. The GP is adamant that he or she acted quite properly and it is the error made by the consultant that caused the problem. The patient, now becoming somewhat bemused, decides to complain to the General Medical Council about the GP. The GMC quickly decides that, while the incident may be serious, it is not something that would affect the GP's registration. It therefore informs the patient that the complaint is not within its remit. The GMC does, however, suggest that the patient contacts ICAS, something that the PALS officer might have done save that he or she did not see the issue as a complaint and considered that the 'concern' had been satisfactorily dealt with.

ICAS assists the patient to launch a complaint against both the hospital and the general practitioner. After some time, the result that her complaint has not been upheld is communicated to the patient. Again, with the assistance of ICAS she asks the Healthcare Commission to reconsider it. The Commission upholds her complaint and advises both the hospital and the GP what action to take to avoid a similar problem in the future. (Hopefully it also ensures that the incident is reported to the NPSA.) Although the Commission has effectively decided that both the GP and the consultant were at fault, it cannot award the patient compensation. The patient must now embark on litigation if she wants to recover compensation.

4.8 The ethical aspect

As will have been seen, there have been many changes and not a few advances in the patient's situation with regard to complaints. We have seen that it is now recognised that a complaint can be dealt with as part of the care of a patient, and as such the obligation to deal with it properly comes within the duty of care of all health care providers. Indeed, the way Trusts deal with complaints could be the subject of examination by the Healthcare Commission. There remains, however, a fundamental flaw in the approach by the health service when there is a breach in that duty. It should not be an issue of complaint – blaming someone, some institution or even a system.

A complaint exposes a defect in care. That should be, and today often is, recognised by those providing the care when it happens, not when the patient draws attention to it. When that happens, the provider should deal with it under the NPSA's Being Open policy, as previously described. If the health care provider has not acted in accordance with that policy but, hoping for the best, has waited until the patient draws attention to it, then that is how it should be seen and categorised – not as a complaint, but as an issue of care to be dealt with.

At the time of writing, the proposals of the Department of Health for changes in the first stage of the complaints procedure are still awaited. Is it too much to hope that this approach will be enshrined in such proposals?

4.9 Latest Developments

4.9.1 Complaints

In June 2007 the Department of Health published for consultation its proposals for changes to the complaints system.[15] Although these proposals retain the concept of a complaint and do not enshrine a policy of 'being Open' the principles on which it is based could lead to a major improvement. The proposals state that the fundamental aim of a complaints process is to:

- respond promptly to complaints
- inspire user confidence
- facilitate effective handling at local level to the user's satisfaction
- encourage organisational learning to prevent similar occurrences in future; and
- provide a unified approach across all providers to the handling of peoples' complaints.

Who can quarrel with that? Unfortunately these principles may be undermined by the fact that the Healthcare Commission has been removed from the process leaving just two stages, Local Resolution and the Ombudsman. The paper justifies this move as follows: 'It is arguable that providing an independent stage through a separate organisation has worked against effective resolution of complaints at a local level because NHS organisations are aware that the Healthcare Commission will undertake the work.'

So because local organisations have not implemented the existing system sensibly, the independent safeguard against an inadequate local investigation is to be removed. Other arguments for this change are of course put forward and the proposed modernised role of the Ombudsman is meant to fill this gap.

An interesting aspect of the proposals, and one that demonstrates again the connection between complaints and the law, is the reference to the NHS Redress

Act 2006. The proposals suggest that the Redress Scheme under that Act will help local organisations respond better to their patients as it makes provision for investigation, explanation and, where appropriate, apologies.

It is the overall aim of the proposals to create a cultural shift within the NHS and social care, with the emphasis towards preventing harm, reducing risks and learning from complaints. It remains to be seen whether, after consultation on the proposals the new system will achieve these laudable aims.

4.10 The General Medical Council

In February 2007 the Department of Health finally published a White Paper[16] in response to Dame Janet Smith's Fifth Report.[17] It deals robustly with the two issues highlighted earlier in this chapter. It has required the GMC to give up its adjudication role which will now be undertaken by an independent body. This leaves the GMC as the investigator and prosecutor only. Insofar as the standard of proof is concerned the GMC had already become resigned to moving to the civil standard. The White paper has now confirmed that that will happen. The GMC is in discussions with the Department of Health as to exactly how these changes will be brought about.

4.11 Notes and references

1. *Being Heard*, report of the Review Committee on NHS complaints procedures, chaired by Professor Alan Wilson, May 1994.
2. Report of an expert group on learning from adverse events in the NHS, chaired by the Chief Medical Officer, May 2000, p. 58, para. 4.33.
3. Pre-action Protocol for the Resolution of Clinical Disputes, Civil Procedure Rules Practice Direction.
4. *British Medical Journal*, **316**, p. 1917.
5. *Guidance on Implementation of the NHS Complaints Procedure* (NHS Executive, March 1996).
6. *Cause for Complaint? An Evaluation of the Effectiveness of the NHS Complaints Procedure*, published by the Public Law Project.
7. The NHS Plan, published by the Department of Health on 1 July 2000.
8. Independent Inquiry by Dame Janet Smith into the issues arising from the case of Harold Shipman, published on 9 December 2004.
9. Parliamentary answer, House of Lords, column 1726, 24/11/05.
10. Fifth Report, published on 9 December 2004.
11. 'The pain of complaining', CAB ICAS evidence of the NHS complaints procedure, May 2005.
12. *Guidance to the NHS Complaints Procedure*, 2004 Regulations (Department of Health), sections 3.15–3.16.
13. In an address to the UKCC on 7 June 1999.
14. *Procedures Related to Adverse Clinical Incidents and Outcomes in Medical Care*, Health Committee Session 1998–99 Sixth Report.

5 The Policy Dimension: Moving Beyond the Rhetoric towards a Safer NHS

John Tingle

As the previous chapters have indicated, the legal and health policy contexts of nursing have changed significantly since the second edition of this book appeared in 2002. My chapter in the second edition discussed the NHS Plan and the concept of 'patient empowerment'. Writing in 2006, four years on, the tenets of the concept of patient empowerment still remain. There have, however, been major changes. Controls assurance has gone; clinical governance now comes under integrated governance. Patient choice is a new buzz word and we have a bill going through Parliament to bring in a new NHS Redress Scheme, which maintains the potential to provide a significant alternative to the courts for patients seeking compensation for injuries caused by clinical negligence in the NHS. The term 'compensation culture' is also being bandied about by various groups and the government is worried that the perception, rightly or wrongly held, of a 'compensation culture' may be inhibiting public services such as the NHS and schools from doing their jobs properly.[1] Stories have appeared in the media of schools banning conker matches or insisting that pupils wear goggles while playing conkers. Some schools ban the common style of pencil sharpeners because they have razor blades in them. The chief executive of the NHSLA (National Health Service Litigation Authority) has given an unequivocal 'no' to the question of whether a compensation culture exists in the NHS or not.[2] However, the reality or otherwise of the issue remains an issue to be hotly debated.

The government responded to the compensation culture debate by passing the Compensation Act 2006 on 25 July 2006.This Act does a number of things including giving a stronger public focus to the issue of suing for negligence. Judges are reminded that when they assess the standard of care to be exercised in a case, perfectly innocent activities like school trips and conker matches may suffer as a result. Putting the standard at too high a level may have the effect of cancelling out socially very useful activities. In a clinical context, Good Samaritan health professionals may be put off rendering assistance. For example, a renal dialysis nurse with no first-aid training may have done her reasonable best at a road traffic accident, but the patient feels that she should have done more and sues. Section 1 provides that when considering a claim in negligence or breach of statutory duty a court may, in determining whether the defendant should have taken particular steps to meet a standard of care (whether by taking precautions or otherwise), have regard to whether a requirement to take those steps might prevent an activity that is desirable from taking place (either at all, to a particular extent, or in a particular way), or might discourage persons from undertaking functions in connection with the activity. Section 2 provides that an apology, an offer of treatment or other redress shall not of itself amount to an admission of negligence or breach of statutory duty. This provision is intended to reflect the existing law, as section 1 does. No new law is created, but the courts are gently reminded of what the law is, and it reassures the public and our institutions. We do not want to lose socially useful activities because of an unfounded fear of litigation, or through a risk-obsessed culture. Thinking they might be sued for something naturally puts people off doing things, but proving negligence in reality is a very hard thing to do. Sadly, the media and some claims companies present a false picture of this reality. The Compensation Act 2006 will hopefully work to redress the balance.

A related issue for this edition of our book is whether the NHS has gone too far down the road of patient empowerment and has created in the minds of patients unrealistic expectations of what can be achieved. Stories abound in the press of Trusts making large job losses despite record government NHS funding. Is it time to try to introduce patients to the notion that the NHS cannot always guarantee a perfect outcome? In Michael Powers's terms,[3] to introduce them to 'the politics of uncertainty'?

Also notably different since the time of the last edition is that the government has realised it has duplicated, and confused somewhat, the regulatory infrastructure of the NHS. The clinical risk, clinical governance and performance management structure has overlapping sections, with too many agencies with competing agendas involved. This is being dealt with, and mechanisms have been put into place to try to cut bureaucracy and the number of regulatory inspections in the NHS by introducing a Concordat.[4] The Healthcare Commission – statutory name Commission for Healthcare Audit and Inspection (CHAI) – has emerged as the lead inspection body.

The most notable substantive development since the last edition in the litigation and clinical risk field, however, must be in the area of patient safety. The work of the National Patient Safety Agency (NPSA) has proved to be very significant in developing a sound infrastructure for reflective and safe clinical practice. The NPSA maintains an impressive armoury of tools to help Trusts develop and maintain an effective patient safety culture, including the NRLS (National Reporting and Learning System). The NRLS is the world's first comprehensive patient safety adverse incident reporting system. The NPSA has been the subject of some criticism for its delay in introducing the NRLS and in its feedback to Trusts. NHS Trusts generally perceive that the NPSA has failed to maximise learning because it has not provided feedback quickly and regularly. There is also a question mark over the value for money being achieved by the NPSA.[5] The NHSLA has also positively contributed to improving patient safety by the CNST (Clinical Negligence Scheme for Trusts) and its other schemes. The NHSLA is a Special Health Authority and part of the NHS. It has a number of functions, which include indemnifying English NHS bodies against claims for clinical negligence, NHS litigation management, and raising the standards of risk management in the NHS.

The NHS can now be seen to be developing, albeit slowly, an engrained patient safety culture. It has been a long time coming and there is a long way to go, but positive steps have been made. The NHS now seems to be a much safer place than it was when the second edition of our book was published. The difficulty remains, however, that there is at present no scientifically based outcome measurement to prove all this.

In this chapter there will be a discussion of some of the themes mentioned above, and conclusions will be drawn.

5.1 NHS litigation levels: still a problem

In 2004/2005, the NHSLA[6] paid out £503 million for all clinical negligence schemes (2003/2004: £422 million). However, there was a drop in the actual number of claims made, from 6251 in 2003/2004 to 5609 in 2004/2005. The NHS expects to make future payments totalling £6.9 billion (at today's prices) in respect of known or expected claims (2003/2004: £6.3 billion). Of this, £2.8 billion is expected to be paid within the next five years. An additional £3.1 billion of claims is possible, but unlikely.

Figure 5.1 shows the trend in provisions over the past five years.[7] According to the NAO, however:

> whilst the provisions have been increasing over recent years, the amounts paid out to settle claims have remained stable.[7]

The NHSLA provides some interesting statistics on clinical negligence claims:[8]

> In 2005–06, 5697 claims of clinical negligence and 3497 claims of non-clinical negligence against NHS bodies were received by the NHSLA. This compares with 5609 claims of clinical negligence and 3766 claims of non-clinical negligence in 2004–05.
>
> £560.3 million was paid out in connection with clinical negligence claims in 2005–06. This figure includes both damages paid to patients and the legal costs borne by the NHS. In 2004–05, the comparable figure was £502.9 million. The figures for non-clinical claims are £31.3 million for 2005–06 and £25.1 million for 2004–05.
>
> The average time taken to deal with a clinical claim under the Clinical Negligence Scheme for Trusts, from notification of the claim to the NHSLA to the date when damages are agreed (or the claim is discontinued), is 1.46 years.

Litigation in the NHS can still be seen to be a big and expensive problem, which is better avoided. The Chief Medical Officer summed up quite well the nature of the clinical negligence system:

£ billion

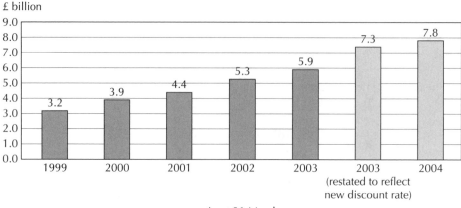

As at 31 March

Figure 5.1   Provisions for clinical negligence within the NHS.

Source: National Audit Office and the Audit Commission, *Financial Management in the NHS (England) Summarised Accounts 2003–04*, Report by the Comptroller and Auditor General, prepared jointly by the National Audit Office and the Audit Commission, HC 60 – Session 2005–2006 (London, NAO, The Stationery Office, London, 24 June 2005). © UK National Audit Office. Reprinted with permission.

> Legal proceedings for medical injury frequently progress in an atmosphere of confrontation, acrimony, misunderstanding and bitterness. The emphasis is on revealing as little as possible about what went wrong, defending clinical decisions that were taken and only reluctantly releasing information. In the past, cases have taken too long to settle. In smaller value claims the legal costs have been disproportionate to the damages awarded. In larger value claims there can be lengthy and expensive disputes about the component parts of any lump sum payment and the anticipated life span of the victim.[9]

The Bristol Royal Infirmary Inquiry Report expressed similar sentiments:

> The system is now out of alignment with other policy initiatives on quality and safety: in fact it serves to undermine those policies and inhibits improvements in the safety of the care received by patients. Ultimately, we take the view that it will not be possible to achieve an environment of full, open reporting within the NHS when, outside it, there exists a litigation system the incentives of which press in the opposite direction. We believe that the way forward lies in the abolition of clinical negligence litigation, taking clinical error out of the courts and the tort system.[10]

The clinical negligence tort-based system, however, has not been abolished and remains largely intact. When all the arguments are considered and balanced, it is hard to see why it should be abolished in regard to clinical errors. The courts provide a very useful mechanism of accountability in health care. Doctors and nurses are called to account for their actions or omissions, and reported court cases provide a rich source of education. The tort system also can be seen to act as a deterrence mechanism for poor conduct. To avoid going to court health carers need to practise safely. The tort system exists perfectly well for other professional disputes and the arguments used to support its abolition in respect of clinical negligence cases just do not measure up. The Woolf reforms discussed in the Department of Health's *Making Amends*[9] and in the second edition of our book have worked to improve the situation in regard to clinical negligence litigation, and the NHS Redress Scheme discussed below has the potential to offer a really good alternative.

5.2 Changing the clinical negligence compensation system

There has been since the second edition of this book a lot of soul-searching about our clinical negligence system.[9] The tort system has not fallen to any no-fault-based compensation schemes such as those that exist in New Zealand and Sweden. These and other no-fault systems were discussed in *Making Amends*[9] and rejected largely on grounds of their likely expense. The *Making Amends* report was very thorough and provides an excellent real-time account of the clinical negligence litigation system and its issues. Amongst the 19 recommendations of the report, the major one was for the establishment of an NHS Redress Scheme, described in Recommendation 1:

> An NHS Redress Scheme should be introduced to provide investigations when things go wrong; remedial treatment, rehabilitation and care where needed; explanations and apologies; and financial compensation in certain circumstances.

Recommendation 12 was also a key proposal:

> A duty of candour should be introduced together with exemption from disciplinary action when reporting incidents with a view to improving patient safety.

The CMO in *Making Amends* also invited views on whether the *Bolam* test should continue to be used for the NHS Redress Scheme:

> The NHS Redress Scheme
> - What should be the qualifying criteria: the 'Bolam' test currently used in assessing clinical negligence or a broader definition of sub-standard care?
> - If the latter, what would be the preferred formulation?[9]

5.2.1 Progress so far

The NHS Redress Bill was introduced into the House of Lords on 12 October 2005 and has been subject to major amendments. The government was defeated when the Lords voted by 157 to 144 to allow apologies and offers of treatment or redress to be made without admission of liability.[11] The bill provides for the establishment of a scheme to enable the settlement, without the need to commence court proceedings, of certain claims that arise in connection with hospital services provided to patients as part of the health service in England, wherever those services are provided. The applicable law to be applied will be the common law of tort, and the *Bolam* and *Bolitho* principles will apply.

5.2.2 *Bolam* and *Bolitho*

Unfortunately, the CMO and the government did not feel the need to depart from the traditional common law tort definitions of fault with its focus on peer-related reasonable practice, and this is a major criticism of the bill. AvMA have suggested that a different, 'avoidability' test should apply:

> An adverse event is compensatable except where it is the result of an unavoidable complication regardless of treatment or non-treatment . . . The onus would be on the NHS to demonstrate that it was an unavoidable complication, or offer redress . . . [12]

This AvMA proposal works in effect to switch the burden of proof from the claimant onto the defendant to disprove negligence. The test makes a lot of sense but it could and probably was viewed as too radical and perhaps too alien a construct to adopt in the context of a tort-based adversarial legal system. Lawyers and others are more comfortable and used to dealing with the *Bolam* and *Bolitho* framework for establishing fault. It is quite a bold step to say that as a Trust, unless you can prove otherwise, you have to compensate the patient because he or she was treated in your hospital.

The tort system is, by its very nature, adversarial, and justice surely dictates that both claimant and defendant should be treated from a basis of equality and fairness and should start off from a level playing field. The patient clearly is the weaker party in the care equation, but then they would be if suing a commercial company for breach of contract or for faulty goods or services. Why should suing for clinical negligence fundamentally alter their status? The fact that they can now access proper specialist professional legal advice corrects that power and knowledge imbalance as it does in the other suing instances mentioned. There was a discussion of legal services and the benefits of clinical negligence specialist solicitor accreditation in my chapter in the second edition of our book.

5.2.3 NHS Redress Bill

In order for the NHS Redress Bill to work properly, it is important that patients have proper access to legal advice when entering the scheme and progressing through it as well as when considering any offer made under it. The NHS Redress Bill[13] establishes the parameters of the cases to which any such scheme can apply, and which bodies can be members of a scheme, and gives the Secretary of State powers to set out in regulations the detailed rules that govern the scheme. It is envisaged that the scheme will cover people with claims in tort arising out of hospital treatment as part of the NHS wherever that hospital treatment may be provided.[14] Not all tort claims are covered, but only those that are 'qualifying liabilities in tort'. These are defined as:

liabilities in tort (a) in respect of personal injury or loss arising out of a breach of a duty of care in relation to the diagnosis of illness, or the care or treatment of any patient, and (b) arising as a consequence of any act or omission by a health-care professional.[13]

The intention is that the scheme will provide for financial compensation to be offered, and will specify an upper limit on the total amount of financial compensation that may be included in an offer under the scheme. It is currently intended that this limit will be set at £20,000 initially.[14] The DH states that the scheme will not cover systems negligence:

> A claim which alleges that a scheme member is directly liable in negligence for system failure or organisational error will not be within the scope of the scheme if the organisational error did not involve any act or omission by a health care professional. The reason for this is that the scheme is intended to cover low-level clinical negligence claims, which can be quickly investigated and resolved.[14]

The bill has not had an easy passage through Parliament and many believe it is fundamentally flawed. AvMA states:

> AvMA, like most patients' organisations, welcomes the stated intentions of the NHS Redress Scheme which the Bill creates, but believes that, as currently designed, the scheme is fundamentally flawed and would have the opposite of the desired effects.

Sixteen other patients' groups formally agree with AvMA that improvements are needed to the Bill and are signed up to the following statement:

> The NHS Redress Bill should be improved to address:
> - the need to have an independent means of deciding upon the merits of cases for redress under the scheme, rather than decisions being made by the NHS Trusts/the NHS Litigation Authority themselves
> - the need for the advice and assistance to be provided to patients/their families during the scheme to be sufficiently expert in medico-legal matters and clinical negligence
> - the need for more robust measures to ensure that lessons are learnt from medical errors identified through the scheme and action taken to improve patient safety.[15]

The bill is notably thin on detail and fundamentally, as *Bolam* and *Bolitho* remain the tests for deciding fault, the patient does need advice and assistance at the start, during and at the end of the claim. Clinical negligence litigation is generally notably complex and the NHS Redress Scheme must not just be seen as a financially driven short cut that compromises patient rights. The government to its credit does not see it that way, and the roots of its thinking can be seen in *Making Amends*[9] and in the words of the Bristol Inquiry report.[10] The key is to make the scheme 'robust, independent and fair'. The bill is improving, however, as it progresses through Parliament (at the time of writing, August 2006). The bill was amended significantly at the report stage debate in the House of Commons on Thursday, 13 July 2006, and changes made to make the scheme more independent, to give specialist advice and representation to patients, and for measures to ensure that patient safety lessons are learnt and implemented. At the time of writing, more amendments are possible.

As presently drafted, the NHS Redress Scheme seems as transparent and independent as the discredited NHS complaints system did until the Healthcare Commission became involved. The complaints system is far from right yet, as A. Simanowitz discusses in Chapter 4.

The statutory duty of candour was also missing from the bill when it was originally published. The softer option of leaving it to the NPSA to tell Trusts to develop candour policies into patient communication strategies has been adopted.[16]

5.2.4 Patient safety initiatives

Since the second edition of this book appeared, a number of significant developments have occurred in the patient safety area within the NHS. A developing and pro-active patient safety infrastructure can be seen slowly being moved into place. It is in this area that nurses and other health carers can make the most fundamental contribution to helping patients and securing their safety. There is a need for the individual nurse to be aware of the patient safety systems that exist, to understand why errors occur and then to guard against them. Participation in and promotion of the NPSA patient safety strategies is vitally important if an engrained patient safety culture is ever going to be developed in the NHS.

5.2.5 Tentative first steps

The DH set the scene for the development of an NHS patient safety structure with *An Organization with a Memory*.[17] This report examined the key factors at work in organisational failure and learning. Practical experience from other sectors was analysed and conclusions and recommendations drawn. One major recommendation was for the creation of a new national system for reporting and analysing adverse health incidents. The report noted that patient safety research and the knowledge of adverse incident rates in the UK was in its infancy:

> Yet the best research-based estimates we have reveal enough to suggest that in NHS hospitals alone adverse events in which harm is caused to patients:
>
> – occur in around 10 per cent of admissions – or at a rate in excess of 850,000 a year;
> – cost the service an estimated £2 billion a year in additional hospital stays alone, without taking any account of human or wider economic costs . . . Inquiries and incident investigations determine that 'the lessons must be learned', but the evidence suggests that the NHS as a whole is not good at doing so.[17]

The next stage was to take forward the recommendations made in *An Organization with a Memory*, and this was done in *Building a Safer NHS for Patients*.[18] This report focused on the implementation strategies for developing a patient safety culture in the NHS, to ensure that patient safety lessons are learnt across the whole NHS. The foundation stones of the NPSA were laid in this document. The report placed patient safety within the context of the government's NHS quality programme and highlighted linkages to other government initiatives. Central to the plan was the creation of a new national mandatory reporting scheme for adverse health care events and near misses within the NHS, now known as the NRLS (National Reporting and Learning System).

The NPSA was set up in July 2001. The first NHS organisations were connected to the NRLS in November 2003 and all NHS organisations have had the capacity to report incidents to the NRLS since December 2004.

5.2.6 The state of play on patient safety incidents

The NPSA published its first NHS patient safety data analysis, which gave some indication of how patient safety matters are proceeding in the NHS, in 2005.[19] Up until the end of March 2005, 85,342 patient safety incidents were reported. Most of these incidents (68% of the total) resulted in no harm to patients. Of the reported incidents, about one in 100 led to severe harm or death. In acute hospital settings, about three in every 1000 reported incidents resulted in death. Based on incidents and deaths reported over a three-month period by 18 Trusts, the NPSA has estimated that each year there would be approximately 840 deaths and 572,000 incidents reported in acute Trusts in England.

The most common types of incidents reported are patient accidents (in particular, falls) and incidents associated with treatment, procedures and medication. Reporting levels are, according to the report, 'increasing rapidly'. These data, which have not been available before, are important as they provide a useful picture of patient safety in NHS Trusts. The data can help inform the development of patient safety strategies at the individual health care, Trust and NPSA levels.

5.2.7 The NPSA patient safety tools: resources

The NPSA has developed, and is developing, training support resources that include e-learning training modules, the incident decision tree (IDT), video-based training workshops, a safety culture survey, Root Cause Analysis (RCA) training and workshops.[19] These can all help NHS health care staff and Trusts develop a safer patient care environment. Key NPSA publications include *Being Open: Communicating Patient Safety Incidents with Patients and Their Carers*,[16] the *Manchester Patient Safety Framework* (MaPSaF),[21] Patient Safety Bulletins[22] and *Seven Steps to Patient Safety*.[20] *Seven Steps to Patient Safety* is a simple checklist for NHS staff to follow and to measure their performance against so that they can ensure a safe health care environment (Box 5.1).

The above NPSA publications and tools are all well written and contain straightforward and well-considered advice. If the advice is followed, an engrained patient safety culture in the NHS may yet become a firm reality.

Box 5.1   The seven steps to patient safety.

Step 1   Build a safety culture
Create a culture that is open and fair
Step 2   Lead and support your staff
Establish a clear and strong focus on patient safety throughout your organisation
Step 3   Integrate your risk management activity
Develop systems and processes to manage your risks and identify and assess things that could go wrong
Step 4   Promote reporting
Ensure your staff can easily report incidents locally and nationally
Step 5   Involve and communicate with patients and the public
Develop ways to communicate openly with and listen to patients
Step 6   Learn and share safety lessons
Encourage staff to use root cause analysis to learn how and why incidents happen
Step 7   Implement solutions to prevent harm
Embed lessons through changes to practice, processes or systems

Source: National Patient Safety Agency, *Seven Steps to Patient Safety: An Overview Guide for NHS Staff*, 2nd Print (NPSA, London, April 2004). © NPSA. Reprinted with permission.

It is important to determine whether all this patient safety activity has worked. In order to find out, a number of possible performance indicators need to be considered. In considering these, it also needs to be accepted that in a complex health care environment such as the NHS, which treats over a million patients every day, some errors will be inevitable. In reality, the best we can hope to do is to try to minimise their occurrence as much as possible through adopting effective patient safety and clinical risk management strategies.

5.2.8 Some error statistics

The NHS 2005 staff survey (Table 5.1) shows that errors are still fairly endemic in the NHS:

Errors and incidents:

- 40 per cent reported seeing at least one potentially harmful error, near miss or incident that could have hurt either staff or patients in the previous month
- a fall in the number of staff witnessing at least one potentially harmful error, near miss or incident from 47 to 40 in 2003 to 2005
- generally employees feel that trusts are encouraging them to report errors, near misses or incidents and 83 per cent said that the last potentially harmful

Table 5.1   Statements about incident reporting.

	% agree or strongly agree	% disagree or strongly disagree
My trust treats fairly those staff who are involved in an error, near miss or incident	40%	7%
My trust encourages us to report errors, near misses or incidents	75%	4%
My trust treats reports of errors, near misses or incidents confidentially	52%	6%
My trust blames or punishes people who make errors, near misses or incidents	9%	39%
When errors, near misses or incidents are reported, my trust takes action to ensure that they do not happen again	50%	8%
We are informed about errors, near misses and incidents that happen in the trust	30%	31%
We are given feedback about changes made in response to reported errors, near misses and incidents	33%	28%

Source: Healthcare Commission, *National Survey of NHS Staff 2005*, Summary of key findings (London, Healthcare Commission, March 2006). Reprinted with permission.

> error, near miss or incident they witnessed was definitely reported by them or a colleague
> * but fewer staff are confident that their employer treats those involved fairly, handles reports confidentially and takes action to prevent recurrence.[23]

5.3 Some patient safety performance indicators

5.3.1 Clinical governance

The concept of clinical governance lies at the heart of government NHS quality improvement strategies. The concept incorporates clinical risk management and CNST (Clinical Negligence Scheme for Trusts) compliance. If Trusts have good clinical governance ratings then they must be taking some positive steps in relation to risk management and patient safety. The Healthcare Commission is responsible for performance rating and monitoring Trusts in regard to clinical governance compliance.

According to the NAO:

> The key principles of clinical governance . . . are: a coherent approach to quality improvement, clear lines of accountability for clinical quality systems and effective processes for identifying and managing risk and addressing poor performance. It involves putting in place the information, methods and systems to

ensure good quality so that problems are identified early, analysed and action taken to avoid any further repetition. The Department of Health (the Department) expects clinical governance to integrate the previously rather disparate and fragmented approaches to quality improvement, such as clinical audit, risk management, incident reporting and continuing professional development into a single system and to ally it to accountability for quality.[24]

The NAO conclude in their report that the government's clinical governance initiative has had many beneficial impacts. Clinical quality issues have been made more mainstream and there is a greater or more explicit accountability of both clinicians and managers for clinical performance.[24]

The report notes that there has been a change in professional cultures towards more open, transparent and collaborative ways of working. Evidence of improvements in practice and patient care was also noted, though it is stated that Trusts lack robust means of assessing this and overall progress:

> However, our research and the outcome of the Commission for Health Improvement's reviews indicate that progress in implementing clinical governance is patchy, varying between trusts, within trusts and between the components of clinical governance. There is, not surprisingly, scope for improvement in: the support provided to trusts; putting in place overall structures and processes; communications between boards and clinical teams; developing a coherent approach to quality; and improving processes for managing risk and poor performance. There is also a need to improve the way that lessons are learnt both within and between trusts; and to put those lessons into practice. Overall, the key features of those organisations that have been better at improving the quality of care are quality of leadership, commitment of staff and willingness to consider doing things differently.[24]

5.3.2 Patient safety initiatives

The NAO also looked more recently at the government's patient safety initiatives and found that progress is being made:

> The safety culture within trusts is improving, driven largely by the Department's clinical governance initiative and the development of more effective risk management systems in response to incentives under initiatives such as the NHS Litigation Authority's Clinical Negligence Scheme for Trusts . . . However, trusts are still predominantly reactive in their response to patient safety issues and parts of some organisations still operate a blame culture.[25]

It was stated in the report that all Trusts have established effective reporting systems at the local level, although under-reporting remains a problem within some groups of staff, types of incidents and near misses; also, most Trusts pointed to specific improvements derived from lessons learnt from their local incident reporting systems, but these are still not widely promulgated, either within or between Trusts. It was also found that the National Patient Safety Agency has provided only limited feedback to Trusts of evidence-based solutions or actions derived from the national reporting system – a point emphasised and developed by the House of Commons Committee of Public Accounts.[5]

Another performance indicator of how well Trusts are doing in patient safety and clinical risk management is the Trust CNST achieved compliance level.[26] If they have a low CNST rating then probably not much is happening with patient safety; conversely, a high rating indicates a firm Trust commitment to the concept.

5.3.3 The NHSLA and CNST

The NHSLA currently provide five sets of standards, reflecting the different organisational, clinical and non-clinical risks faced by different kinds of health care organisations:[27]

- NHSLA Risk Management Standard for Acute Trusts (including specialist hospital Trusts)
- CNST Maternity Standards
- CNST Mental Health and Learning Disability Standards
- NHSLA Standard for Primary Care Trusts
- NHSLA Ambulance Standard.

Trusts (including PCTs) that provide labour ward services are subject to assessment against both the NHSLA Acute (or PCT) Standards and CNST Maternity Standards.

5.4 How they work

NHS bodies pay the NHSLA a contribution, which goes into a mutual pool. In return the NHSLA take over the claim and will pay any compensation awarded by a court. The NHSLA may decide to defend or settle the claim without going to court. Discounts in contributions are available to those Trusts that comply with the programmes of clinical risk management standards and to those with a good claims history. Discount levels are Level 1: 10%, Level 2: 20%, Level 3: 30%.[26]

The PCT Standard is currently set at just two levels.[28] Level 1A is a review of key risk management documentation such as the PCT's risk management strategy and incident reporting policy. PCTs who are successful at level 1A receive a 5% discount and are then eligible to apply for level 1B. This takes the form of an on-site assessment, focusing on the risk management systems developed by the PCT, and leads to a total 10% discount in contributions.[28]

Although scheme membership is voluntary, all NHS Trusts (including Foundation Trusts) and Primary Care Trusts (PCTs) in England currently belong.

Figure 5.2 is taken from NHSLA and gives details of the CNST general levels achieved. The NHSLA states:

> It is pleasing to report that for the second consecutive year there are no level 0 acute or specialist hospital trusts, and the number of trusts at levels 2 and 3 has risen from 35% in 2004/05 to 49% at the end of March 2006.[29]

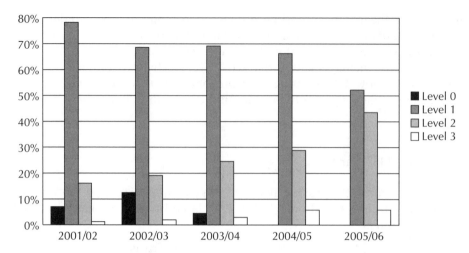

Figure 5.2   Comparison of levels achieved in the CNST general standards – acute and specialist hospitals.

Source: National Health Service Litigation Authority, *Report and Accounts 2006*, 11 July, HC 1179 (London, The Stationery Office). Reprinted with permission.

The NHSLA state that these standards are assessed progressively and that each criterion has been allocated to one of three levels:

> Level 1 criteria represent the basic elements of a clinical risk management framework. Levels 2 and 3 are more demanding. Many are concerned with the implementation and integration into practice of policies and procedures, monitoring them and acting on the results. These levels also require staff to have a good understanding of clinical risk issues.[30]

The new NHSLA Risk Management Standards state:

> The progression of organisations through the standards is logical and follows the development, implementation, monitoring and review of policies and procedures.
>
> Level 1 deals with establishing effective risk management systems and processes.
>
> Level 2 assesses whether the systems described at level 1 have been implemented.
>
> Level 3 concentrates on whether the organisation is monitoring its compliance with the systems and acting on the findings.[26]

5.4.1 Most Trusts are at level 1

The CNST is over ten years old, and while most Trusts are still at level 1, it is fair to say that there has been a drift upwards towards a generally higher compliance level. In 2005/06 the gap narrowed between those Trusts at level 1 and those at level 2. In assessing the success or otherwise of the CNST it is important to remember that level 1 shows that Trusts maintain the basic elements of a clinical risk management framework. Looking at the criteria again, level 1 Trusts have yet to implement, integrate and pro-actively work with the CNST standards, which is worrying.[26,30] The reasonable man or woman in the street or, to borrow from the law of tort, the man or woman on the 'Clapham omnibus', would surely assume that after ten years of the CNST most Trusts would be at level 2 if not 3. What have the Trusts being doing during these last ten years? How seriously have they taken clinical risk management and patient safety? According to the CNST levels, there has been only incremental developing interest over the period. The development of the NPSA patient safety infrastructure should bring about some more discernible improvements here. The basic underlying problem is that good patient safety practices have yet to filter down properly to Trusts and the workforce.

5.4.2 The CMO's view

In his annual report for 2004, the CMO (Chief Medical Officer) stated, in the section on compliance with patient safety alerts, particularly with intrathecal chemotherapy guidance:

> In spite of all this, and of the continuing risk of another tragic death in their hospitals, NHS Trusts took 19 months to comply with the original guidance and 18 months to comply with revised guidance and, worse still, after a first round of peer review visits, 47 per cent of trusts were still not fully compliant with the latest up-to-date guidance. This case study reveals much about the safety culture of the NHS, which is clearly not yet focused or organized enough to reduce a potentially fatal risk to patients rapidly enough.[31]

Fair comment by the CMO, which in a sense puts the less than satisfactory CNST Trust attainment levels in some perspective.

5.4.3 Government overkill and Trust financial austerity: a defence for Trusts?

Primary and secondary care in the NHS have been subject to many competing agendas over this last ten years – certainly since the second edition of this book – and they continue to be so. The NHS is in a constant state of reform or revolution as successive governments try to manage it effectively. It is a monolithic structure and by definition a high-risk and very technical enterprise. The NHS is also currently going through a period of financial austerity and it will be interesting to see whether the government patient safety and clinical governance agendas can survive in the new climate of thrift and financial austerity. Will the agendas remain at or near the top of Trust agendas as severe job losses take place and concentrate financial minds? There has been very little outcome measurement on whether risk management actually works and saves money. Our best guess is that it does. Common sense, however, would dictate that if you practise safely and more reflectively then the risk of adverse incidents occurring should be reduced.

Sadly, the government has been guilty of 'overkill' in its health quality reform agenda and has exposed Trusts to too much regulation in the field of health quality and patient safety. It has only recently started to consolidate overlapping arm's length agencies and policies that govern the area.

The Regulatory Impact Unit of the Cabinet Office in a joint report with the DH said:

> A multitude of organisations undertake some form of inspection, accreditation or audit in the NHS. The bulk are statutory organisations or professional bodies, but a significant number are voluntary. Front-line staff and management acknowledge the value added by inspection in driving up standards in health care, enhancing public accountability and ensuring patient safety. However, several recurring themes relating to review activity arose during the course of these interviews that were seen by staff to hamper effective delivery of health care. They were:
>
> - Multiplicity, overlap and lack of co-ordination between reviewing organisations and their functions
> - Duplication and inconsistency in requests for data and information
> - Proportionality and transparency of reviews
> - Burdens of preparation for reviews
> - Benefits of review outputs.[32]

This report led to a Concordat being published by the Healthcare Commission.[4] The concordat provides a code of objectives and practices for government and independent inspectorates to deliver more joined-up and appropriate inspection programmes that reduce the burden of inspection on health care staff.

5.5 Conclusion

The conclusion from this discussion must be that there have been major changes in the NHS as regards risk, litigation and the patient safety field since the last edition of this book.

Health care litigation and complaints are still with us, and perhaps always will be given the nature of what the NHS tries to do. Everybody seems to agree that health care is an inherently risky and complex business. There has been a general acknowledgement that the tort-based common-law system is not the best way to compensate patients but the government has left the system largely intact. We have the NHS Redress scheme, which in its draft bill form is regarded by some as being fundamentally flawed. Properly amended, it does maintain an important potential to change things for the better for the injured patient. We have also seen the development of a new patient safety infrastructure system with the NRLS, and the work of the NPSA is giving NHS staff the tools to deal with the patient safety problem. Nationally the NHSLA and CNST risk management standards do seem to have had a positive influence and Trusts can be seen to be moving, albeit slowly, towards higher levels of compliance. We have a developing NHS patient safety infrastructure and there is more joined-up thinking about what needs to be done in order to achieve an engrained patient safety culture in the NHS.

The NHS is probably a much safer place today than it was in 2002.

5.6 References

1. Better Regulation Taskforce, *Better Routes to Redress* (London, Cabinet Office Publications and Publicity Team, May 2004).
2. National Patient Safety Agency, Debate, 'Is there a growing litigation culture in the NHS?', NPSA Annual Review 2004–05 (London, NPSA), pp. 18–19.
3. M. Powers, *The Risk Management of Everything, Rethinking the Politics of Uncertainty* (London, Demos, 2004).
4. Healthcare Commission, Concordat, *Working in Partnership, Getting the Best from Inspection, Audit, Review and Regulation of Health and Social Care*, updated edition (London, Commission for Healthcare Audit and Inspection (Healthcare Commission), May 2006).
5. House of Commons, Committee of Public Accounts, *A Safer Place for Patients: Learning to Improve Patient Safety*, 51st Report of Session 2005–06, 6 July 2006 (London, The Stationery Office).
6. National Audit Office and the Audit Commission, *Financial Management in the NHS (England) Summarised Accounts 2004–05*, Report by the Comptroller and Auditor General, prepared jointly by the National Audit Office and the Audit Commission, HC 1092 – Session 2005–2006 (London, NAO, The Stationery Office, 7 June 2006).
7. National Audit Office and the Audit Commission, *Financial Management in the NHS (England) Summarised Accounts 2003–04*, Report by the Comptroller and Auditor General, prepared jointly by the National Audit Office and the Audit Commission, HC 60 – Session 2005–2006 (London, NAO, The Stationery Office, London, 24 June 2005).
8. National Health Service Litigation Authority, *About the NHS Litigation Authority* (NHSLA, London, 2006) http://www.nhsla.com/home.htm (accessed 22 August 2006).
9. Department of Health, *Making Amends: A Consultation Paper Setting Out Proposals for Reforming the Approach to Clinical Negligence in the* NHS, A Report by the Chief Medical Officer (London, Department of Health Publications, June 2003).
10. Final Report, *Learning from Bristol: The Report of the Public Inquiry into Children's Heart Surgery at the Bristol Royal Infirmary 1984–1995*, Command Paper: CM 5207 (London, The Stationery Office).
11. Guardian Unlimited, *Yesterday in Parliament*, Compensation Culture (Press Association, 8 March 2006) http://politics.guardian.co.uk/commons/story/0,1726124,00.html (accessed, 14 April 2006).
12. *Action against Medical Accidents*, Briefing on the NHS Redress Bill (Croydon, Surrey, 31 October 2005).
13. NHS Redress Bill [HL] Bill 137.
14. Department of Health, *NHS Redress: Statement of Policy* (Leeds, Department of Health, 2005).
15. *Action against Medical Accidents*, NHS Redress Bill, Briefing for Report Stage, House of Lords (Croydon, Surrey, AvMA, February 2006).
16. National Patient Safety Agency, *Being Open: Communicating Patient Safety Incidents with Patients and Their Carers* (London, NPSA, 2005).

17. Department of Health, *An Organization with a Memory*, Report of an expert group on learning from adverse events in the NHS chaired by the Chief Medical Officer (London, The Stationery Office, 2000).
18. Department of Health, *Building a Safer NHS for Patients: Implementing an Organization with a Memory* (London, Department of Health, May 2001).
19. National Patient Safety Agency, *Building a Memory: Preventing Harm, Reducing Risks and Improving Patient Safety*. The first report of the National Reporting and Learning System and the Patient Safety Observatory (London, NPSA, July 2005).
20. National Patient Safety Agency, *Manchester Patient Safety Framework (MaPSaF) Acute*, (London, NPSA, 2006).
21. National Patient Safety Agency, *Patient Safety Bulletin 1* (London, NPSA, July 2005).
22. National Patient Safety Agency, *Seven Steps to Patient Safety: An Overview Guide for NHS Staff*, 2nd Print (NPSA, London, April 2004).
23. Healthcare Commission, *National Survey of NHS Staff 2005*, Summary of key findings (London, Healthcare Commission, March 2006).
24. National Audit Office, *Achieving Improvements through Clinical Governance: A Progress Report on Implementation by NHS Trusts*, Report by the Comptroller and Auditor General, HC 1055, Session 2002–2003 (London, The Stationery Office, 17 September 2003).
25. National Audit Office, Department of Health, *A Safer Place for Patients: Learning to Improve Patient Safety*, Report by the Comptroller and Auditor General, HC 456 Session 2005–2006 3 November 2005 (London, The Stationery Office).
26. National Health Service Litigation Authority, *Risk Management Standards for Acute Trusts* (derived from the former CNST and RPST Standards), Pilot Version (London, NHSLA, April 2006).
27. *CNST Standards and Assessments* (London, NHSLA) http://www.nhsla.com/RiskManagement/CnstStandards/ (accessed 23 August 2006).
28. National Health Service Litigation Authority, *Primary Care Trusts Standards and Assessments* (London, NHSLA) http://www.nhsla.com/RiskManagement/PCTStandards/ (accessed 23 August 2006).
29. National Health Service Litigation Authority, *Report and Accounts 2006*, 11 July, HC 1179 (London, The Stationery Office).
30. National Health Service Litigation Authority, *Clinical Negligence Scheme for Trusts General Clinical Risk Management Standards* (London, NHSLA, April 2005).
31. Department of Health, 'Learning how to learn, compliance with patient safety alerts in the NHS', *On the State of the Public Health*, Annual Report of the Chief Medical Officer 2004 (London, DH, 19th July, 2005).
32. Regulatory Impact Unit, Public Sector Team, 'Making a difference, reducing burdens in health care inspection and monitoring' (London, Cabinet Office, July 2003).

Part Two: The Perspectives

6 Negligence

A The Legal Perspective

Charles Foster

Lawyers use the word 'negligence', confusingly, in two ways. First, they use it to describe a particular type of fault – a fault whose characteristics are defined by a statute or past legal decisions. Negligence in this respect can be either criminal (leading to prosecution) or civil (leading to an action in the civil courts for money). And secondly, they use it to describe that which must be proved in order for a claimant to succeed in recovering money ('damages') in respect of damage if caused by that fault. When used in this second sense, they are referring to the tort of negligence. A tort is simply a legal wrong that does not involve a breach of contract.

This chapter is concerned mostly with the tort of negligence. But criminal negligence is important too. Medical manslaughter features commonly in the newspapers. When a doctor is charged with killing a patient accidentally, he will be convicted by the Crown court of manslaughter if the jury finds that he has been grossly negligent – so negligent that his action or inaction deserves the penalty of criminal conviction.[1] This definition of gross negligence is of course circular: it comes down to saying someone should be convicted if he should be convicted. Precisely the same principles apply to the liability of a nurse for manslaughter, but as yet there are no reported English cases in which a nurse has been successfully prosecuted for manslaughter arising out of a breach of her professional duty to a patient.

The vast majority of medico-legal cases concern the civil law of negligence. They are tried in the county court or the High Court (depending on their value and/or their complexity) by a judge sitting alone, without a jury. Only a tiny proportion will ever get to court. Most are settled or abandoned long before trial.

Of those that do get to trial, many are decided in the defendant's favour. Clinical negligence cases are difficult for claimants to win. Some of the reasons for this will appear in this chapter.

It is very rare for nurses to be sued individually. If a nurse has been negligent, generally the employing health authority, NHS Trust, private hospital or clinic will be sued. This is a consequence of the doctrine of vicarious liability, which states that employers are liable for the torts of their employees when the act or omission that constitutes the tort occurred in the course of the employment. This doctrine does not absolve the employee from responsibility: the claimant can sue the employee instead of or as well as the employer, but generally it would be foolish for a claimant to do so when the claimant knows that the issues in the action against the employer will be identical to those in the action against the employee, and that the employer will certainly be able to pay damages, whereas the employee may well not be able to.

Where an employee has been negligent, and the employer is successfully sued in relation to that negligence, the employer can sue the employee for an indemnity (*Lister* v. *Romford Ice and Cold Storage Co Ltd* (1956)), but in practice this is almost unheard of in nursing cases. With the rapid expansion of private medicine, however, it may become a contractual requirement of employment at a private hospital that the nurse has a policy of professional indemnity insurance, which could pay an indemnity in the event of the hospital's liability. That fact, rather than any change in the substantive law of negligence, is likely in the future to lead to more actions against individual nurses.

6.1 The elements of the tort of negligence

To succeed in an action for clinical negligence, a claimant must show that:

(1) the defendant owed the claimant a duty of care (i.e. a duty to do something that should have been done, or a duty not to do something that has been done); and
(2) the defendant has breached the duty; and
(3) the breach of duty has caused some injury, loss or damage to the claimant of a type which the law acknowledges.

6.2 The existence of a duty of care

A duty of care between a claimant and a defendant will exist if the following three criteria are satisfied (*Caparo Industries plc* v. *Dickman* (1990)):

(1) the relevant damage was foreseeable; and
(2) the relationship between the claimant and the defendant is sufficiently 'proximate'; and
(3) it is 'fair, just and reasonable' to impose such a duty.

Foreseeability of damage is rarely an issue in clinical negligence cases, but the proximity of the relationship between the claimant and the defendant often is.

The courts have been reluctant, in cases involving doctors, to say that the necessary proximity exists beyond the confines of the ordinary doctor–patient relationship, and have defined that relationship fairly narrowly. A good example is *Kapfunde* v. *Abbey National* (1998). Here the claimant applied for a job with the first defendant. The first defendant employed a doctor, the second defendant, to take a medical view of applicants, based on completed medical questionnaires. The second defendant told the first defendant that the claimant was, because of her history of sickle cell anaemia, likely to have unusually long absences from work. The court held that there was no doctor–patient relationship between the claimant and the second defendant, and that accordingly no duty of care existed.

Another example is *Goodwill* v. *BPAS* (1996), in which the defendant performed a vasectomy on his patient, and then advised him that he was sterile. Three years later the patient met the claimant, and he told her that he was sterile. They had unprotected sexual intercourse, and the claimant became pregnant. She sued the defendant for the cost of upkeep of the child.[2] The court held that the action must fail. There was no sufficiently proximate relationship between the relevant doctor and the claimant because the doctor could not know that his advice would be passed on to and relied on by the claimant.

A number of the cases on proximity were decided alternatively on the grounds of 'just, fair and reasonable'. It may now be that the question 'is it just, fair and reasonable to impose a duty?' should be expanded to read 'is it just, fair and reasonable to impose a duty to pay damages as big as those claimed?', and that in order for damages to be recoverable there has to be reasonable proportion between the damages claimed and the duty assumed.

The Compensation Act 2006, section 1, provides that 'a court considering a claim in negligence or breach of statutory duty may, in determining whether the defendant should have taken particular steps to meet a standard of care (whether by taking precautions against a risk or otherwise), have regard to whether a requirement to take those steps might (a) prevent a desirable activity from being undertaken at all, to a particular extent or in a particular way, or (b) discourage persons from undertaking functions in connection with a desirable activity'.

6.3 Breach of duty

6.3.1 The general principles

A clinical professional will have discharged his duty to the patient if what that professional has done would be endorsed by a responsible body of practitioners in the relevant specialty at the material time. This is the famous and ubiquitous *Bolam* test.[3]

The *Bolam* test is a rule not only of substantive law (defining what amounts to adequate care), but also of evidence (indicating how a court determines whether adequate care has been given). Thus in *Maynard* v. *West Midlands RHA* (1985) Lord Scarman said:

> [A] judge's 'preference' for one body of distinguished professional opinion to another also professionally distinguished is not sufficient to establish

negligence in a practitioner whose actions have received the approval of those whose opinions, truthfully expressed, honestly held, were not preferred . . . In the realm of diagnosis and treatment, negligence is not established by preferring one respectable body of professional opinion to another. (p. 639)

In the past the *Bolam* test has been caricatured as asserting that a professional escapes liability if he can get someone who at some stage has qualified in the relevant specialty and avoided utter professional disgrace to stagger into the witness box and say that he or some of his (unspecified) friends would have acted as the defendant did. This was never the case in theory, although it may, in some more outlandish county courts, have worked like that.

That caricature was laid finally to rest in a case before the House of Lords called *Bolitho* v. *City & Hackney Health Authority* (1997). *Bolitho* underlined the word 'responsible' in the *Bolam* test. The central passage reads:

[I]n cases of diagnosis and treatment there are cases where, despite a body of professional opinion sanctioning the defendant's conduct, the defendant can properly be held liable for negligence . . . In my judgment that is because, in some cases, it cannot be demonstrated to the judge's satisfaction that the body of opinion relied upon is reasonable or responsible. In the vast majority of cases the fact that distinguished experts in the field are of a particular opinion will demonstrate the reasonableness of that opinion. In particular, where there are questions of assessment of the relative risks and benefits of adopting a particular medical practice, a reasonable view necessarily presupposes that the relative risks and benefits have been weighed by the experts in forming their opinions. But if, in a rare case, it can be demonstrated that the professional opinion is not capable of withstanding logical analysis, the judge is entitled to hold that the body of opinion is not reasonable or responsible. I emphasise that in my view it will very seldom be right for a judge to reach the conclusion that views genuinely held by a competent medical expert are unreasonable. The assessment of medical risks and benefits is a matter of clinical judgement which a judge would not normally be able to make without expert evidence . . . it would be wrong to allow such assessment to deteriorate into seeking to persuade the judge to prefer one of two views both of which are capable of being logically supported. It is only where a judge can be satisfied that the body of expert opinion cannot be logically supported at all that such opinion will not provide the bench mark by reference to which the defendant's conduct falls to be assessed . . . (p. 243)

Bolitho said nothing new, but caused a lot of unnecessary hysteria.[4] It was dubbed a 'claimant's charter'. It was feared that it would encourage medically illiterate judges to substitute their own uninformed views of what was medically reasonable for the views of distinguished practitioners. It is unlikely, as the cited passage clearly states, to have that effect in many cases. But it will have the effect of making experts look more critically at the practices they are defending. It will not lead to a proliferation of litigation, but it might lead to a proliferation of footnotes in expert reports.

The requirement that practice, to be defensible, has to be 'responsible' begs the question of whether, in a clinical world increasingly dominated by evidence-based medicine, a practice that the literature clearly shows leads to statistically worse results than another economically comparable practice can sensibly be said to be 'responsible'. It is likely to be found irresponsible not to adopt an evidence-based approach, and irresponsible not to adopt an intelligent strategy in deciding which evidence-based approach to use. The NMC's own code of professional conduct states: 'You have a responsibility to deliver care based on current evidence, best practice and, where applicable, validated research when it is available'.[5] It may be that the clinical negligence cases of the future will be battles between statisticians, with the issue to be decided by the judge being whether the published results that are said to justify a particular clinical approach really do justify it.

The standard that the law expects of practitioners is the standard that is appropriate to a person undertaking the relevant task. Thus a nurse undertaking the work that normally (and appropriately) a senior house officer would do undertakes to do it as well as a senior house officer would and cannot complain if she is judged by that standard.[6]

The standard of care expected is decided by reference to the post occupied by the person giving the care, rather than to the rank or status of that person or to the individual characteristics or training of that person. Thus, for instance, where the performance of work of a type reasonably done by staff nurses is criticised, the question of whether the work has been done negligently will be answered by reference to the standard expected of responsible staff nurses, not by reference to the standard that might normally be expected of that particular staff nurse with her particular experience.[7]

Liability for negligent prescribing by nurses is likely to be approached by the courts, at least for the next few years, by reference to the standard of prescribing expected of those doctors who originally performed the task that the nurse has taken on. Public policy considerations make it inconceivable that nurses will have less expected of them.

There is a legal duty to keep reasonably up to date,[8] but the courts do not expect practitioners to read every relevant article that appears in the professional press.[9] Of course the duty to keep up to date includes a duty to know about guidelines affecting the profession: it is far less excusable not to know of a relevant NICE guideline than it is not to have read an editorial in an immensely obscure specialist journal.

It is clear that one does not decide that a particular practice is or is not responsible by counting the number of practitioners who do or do not do it. This principle is important in cases involving super-specialists doing pioneering work (*De Freitas* v. *O'Brien* (1995)).

For some reason section 2 of the Compensation Act 2006 felt it necessary to declare that 'an apology, an offer of treatment or other redress, shall not of itself amount to an admission of negligence or breach of statutory duty'.

6.3.2 Obtaining properly informed consent

In the past the *Bolam* test has been held to apply to the issue of obtaining consent from patients. Thus a clinician would not be negligent if what he had told a patient about a procedure would be what a responsible body of practitioners in the relevant specialty would have told that patient (*Sidaway* v. *Board of Governors of the Bethlem Hospital and the Maudsley Hospital* (1985)).

This extension of *Bolam* to the realm of consent has recently been doubted by some commentators, although the *Sidaway* case, which asserted it (a House of Lords case), has certainly not been overruled. The doubts arise from an off-the-cuff comment in *Bolitho* to the effect that the remarks there about the *Bolam* principle were made in the context of 'cases of diagnosis and treatment',[10] not in the context of consent to treatment. In inserting this caveat the House of Lords might have had in mind the Senate of Surgery's document *The Surgeon's Duty of Care*,[11] which has subsequently been extended to all registered medical practitioners by the GMC's guidelines: *Seeking Patients' Consent: The Ethical Considerations*.[12] The details of these guidelines do not matter for present purposes. It is enough to say that they state categorically how consent must be obtained. If the ruling body of medical practitioners states that particular procedures must be followed, can it seriously be argued that there is a responsible body of medical practitioners that would not follow those procedures? The point is a moot one: it has yet to be tested in the courts.

The relevant guidelines on consent for nurses are in paragraph 3 of the NMC Code of Professional Practice (2004). They are much more sensible and general, and far less prescriptive than those imposed by the Senate of Surgery and the GMC, and nurses are unlikely to find that these guidelines deprive them of their *Sidaway* shield (*Sidaway* is discussed in Chapter 7).

6.3.3 The relevance of protocols to civil liability

The points above about guidelines raise the general question, important to nurse practitioners, of the relevance of protocols to issues of breach of duty. Clinicians from all medical and nursing specialities worry about protocols because they think that failure to follow them will necessarily connote negligence. In legal theory, of course, this is nonsense: *Bolam* does not cease to apply simply because a protocol has been drafted.

In the context of nurses failing to follow protocols, two situations have to be distinguished. The first is where a nurse has carelessly failed to do what the protocol says. An example might be failure to give the prescribed regime of post-operative antibiotics because of forgetfulness or ignorance of the regime. Here, *Bolam* will not protect, because *Bolam* never applied: there is no responsible body of nursing opinion that forgets or is ignorant of protocols. The second situation is where a nurse has failed to do what a protocol says because she exercised her own independent clinical judgement and decided to do something other than what the protocol says. Here, *Bolam* would excuse the nurse if there were a responsible body of nursing opinion that would, in the relevant circumstances, have acted in the way that the nurse did.

As a general rule, adherence to local or national protocols is likely to protect, because the courts are likely to find that those protocols represent responsible practice (if not embodying the only responsible practice).[13] Departure from local protocols may be *Bolam*-justifiable if the departure was made in the exercise of clinical judgement for responsible clinical reasons. Departure from national protocols, such as those imposed by NICE, may create problems, even if the departure is endorsed by other members of the same profession because the courts will tend to think that nationally endorsed protocols definitively circumscribe acceptable practice.

Note that *Bolitho*'s endorsement of the propriety of looking at the reasoning that leads to clinical decisions is likely to bring greater judicial readiness to look at the research and consultation that led to the formulation of the relevant guidelines. It is therefore important that the formulation process is well documented.

6.4 Causation

6.4.1 The conventional rule

The claimant has to show that but for the defendant's negligence he would probably have avoided the injury and loss claimed. Thus lawyers often talk about the '51% test' or 'proof on the balance of probabilities'. In the context of causation they simply mean that the claimant will succeed if he shows that it is more likely than not that the defendant's default caused the injury/loss.

Causation is an essential element of the tort of negligence. Beware of confusing questions about whether causation has been established with questions about how much the judgment should be for.

6.4.2 Loss of a chance

It is often asserted that damages for loss of a chance are not recoverable in the English law of tort. This is untrue. In some commercial fields such damages are regularly recovered.[14] But whether they can be or should be recoverable in clinical negligence cases is contentious. The authority generally cited for the proposition that such damages are not recoverable in tort is *Hotson* v. *East Berkshire Health Authority* (1987). But *Hotson* says nothing of the sort. The Court of Appeal in *Hotson* decided that loss of a chance was damage that the law recognised, and that accordingly to prove that one had lost a chance was to prove causation. The Court of Appeal was anxious to avoid treating claimants who sued in tort and in contract differently. Damages are uncontroversially recoverable for loss of a chance in contract.[15] Why, the Court of Appeal said, should an NHS patient who is deprived by a doctor's negligence of a chance of recovery be unable to recover damages, whereas the same patient, treated identically but privately (and therefore under a contract) by the same doctor, be successful? The court said that such an anomaly would be monstrous. The House of Lords never decided the question of recoverability of damages for loss of a chance: it merely decided that on the facts of that case it did not need to decide.

The question was considered again by the House of Lords, in the context of failure to diagnose cancer, in *Gregg* v. *Scott* (2005).[16] The House there rejected the loss of chance analysis in clinical negligence cases (at least those relating to failure to diagnose), adopting the straightforward balance of probabilities test. Lost chances have probably not left medical law completely, but the arguments that invoke them will have to be more complex than before.[17]

6.4.3 Causation: material contribution

Sometimes it will be impossible for the experts to say that the defendant's default has, on the balance of probabilities, caused the damage, but they may be able to say on the balance of probabilities that the default has materially contributed to the damage. Where this is the case, the claimant is entitled to succeed in full.

An example is *Bonnington Castings* v. *Wardlaw* (1956). The claimant there was a steel dresser. In the course of his work he was exposed to silica dust from two sources. The exposure to dust from one source was a consequence of the defendant's breach of statutory duty; the exposure to dust from the other was not. He developed pneumoconiosis. It was impossible to determine the contribution that the 'guilty dust' and the 'innocent dust' had made to his disease. All that could be said was that the contribution made by the 'guilty dust' was not de minimis. Those facts, said the House of Lords, meant that the claimant was entitled to judgment for damages representing all his illness and its financial consequences. Lord Reid said:

> I cannot agree that the question is: which was the most probable source of the [claimant's] disease, the ['innocent dust'] or the ['guilty dust']? It appears to me that the source of his disease was the dust from both sources, and the real question is whether the ['guilty dust'] materially contributed to the disease. What is a material contribution must be a question of degree. A contribution which comes within the exception de minimis non curat lex is not material, but I think that any contribution which does not fall within that exception must be material. I do not see how there can be something too large to come within the de minimis principle but yet too small to be material. (p. 621)

The House of Lords appeared to extend this principle in *McGhee* v. *National Coal Board* (1972). They said there that where the defendant's default had materially increased the risk of the injury that in fact occurred, the claimant succeeded in full. This case produced uproar among practitioners and academics. It was pointed out that if all you could do was to prove a material contribution to risk, you had failed to prove that there was anything causative about the defendant's default at all. Judges were extremely reluctant to follow *McGhee*, but it haunted the law of tort until it was exorcised by the House of Lords in *Wilsher* v. *Essex AHA* (1986). In *Wilsher* Lord Bridge said:

> *McGhee* . . . laid down no new principle of law whatever. On the contrary, it affirmed the principle that the onus of proving causation lies on the [claimant]. Adopting a robust and pragmatic approach to the undisputed primary facts of the case, the majority concluded that it was a legitimate inference of fact that the [defendant's] negligence had materially contributed to the [claimant's]

injury. The decision, in my opinion, is of no greater significance than that . . . (pp. 881–2)

Whenever the House of Lords describes the decision of a differently constituted House as 'robust and pragmatic' it is clear that there is deep intellectual embarrassment. The fact is that *McGhee* was plainly wrong.

It is surprising how seldom the *Bonnington Castings* principle is wielded in clinical negligence litigation. It is potentially extremely helpful to claimants in cases where experts cannot be pressed to agree with the artificial speculations about biological processes that lawyers love so much.[18]

6.4.4 Causation: multiple competing causes

Often in clinical negligence cases there will be a number of candidates for the post of 'cause' of the injury. That was the case in *Wilsher*. The claimant there suffered from retrolental fibroplasia. It was said that this was a result of the negligent administration of hyperbaric oxygen. But there were several alternative explanations, and it could not be said that the negligent explanation was probably correct. Accordingly the claimant failed to establish causation.

6.4.5 The requirement that the loss is legally recoverable

Not everything a claimant might justifiably complain of is recognised by the law as 'loss or damage' sufficient to ground liability. The most obvious examples relate to psychiatric harm. If the only harm suffered is psychiatric, the claimant will have to show, in order to obtain judgment, that a recognisable psychiatric illness has been suffered. Mere distress and shaking up are not enough.[19] A good example was *Reilly* v. *Merseyside RHA* (1994). The claimants were trapped in a hospital lift for 1 hour 20 minutes. They suffered fear and claustrophobia but no physical injury. They were not entitled to any damages.

6.5 The assessment of quantum

6.5.1 General

'Quantum' is simply the value of a case. There are a number of possible 'heads of claim' in clinical negligence cases. They are divided up as follows:

- pain, suffering and loss of amenity
- special damage
- future loss
- hybrid heads of claim.

Damages in negligence cases are almost always intended to be simply compensatory – to put the claimant into the position he would have been in had the defendant not been negligent in so far as money can do that. In rare circumstances damages can be awarded that are intended to represent the court's disapproval of the defendant's oppressive or otherwise immoral conduct. These are referred to as aggravated damages. A good example of aggravated damages in a clinical negligence case is *Appleton* v. *Garrett* (1995). There, a dentist who was sued in negligence and trespass for doing unnecessary dental work on patients in order to enrich himself, was ordered to pay aggravated damages, calculated as 15% of the compensatory damages for pain, suffering and loss of amenity that he also had to pay.

The claimant is under a duty to 'mitigate' his loss. That means that he has to take reasonable steps to reduce the total sum of damages payable. Thus he is not entitled to buy in extravagantly priced care, or go to his hospital appointments in a chauffeur-driven Rolls-Royce. If non-dangerous medical treatment would alleviate his condition, he may be obliged to have it: if he does not, he may forfeit that part of his claim that relates to the difference between the condition he is in fact in and the condition he would have been in had he had the treatment. All the comments below about damages have to be read subject to this caveat about mitigation.

6.5.2 Damages for pain, suffering and loss of amenity

These are exactly what they say. They are inevitably quantifications of the intrinsically unquantifiable. In trying to assess this head of claim, lawyers rely on guidelines that prescribe broad brackets of awards for particular types of injury and disability,[20] and on reported cases.

The Law Commission criticised awards of damages for pain, suffering and loss of amenity as being too low. That is a common complaint. Certainly the disparity between such awards and awards of damages in libel cases for injury to reputation can often be insulting to claimants who have suffered personal injuries. In *Heil* v. *Rankin and Others* (2000), the Court of Appeal decided that where the conventional award of damages for pain, suffering and loss of amenity was £10,000 or less there should be no change, and that above that there should be a gradual tapering up of awards so that the largest awards would be about one-third higher than they had previously been. Insurers were generally happy with this decision, since the vast number of cases they face attract awards of less than £10,000. The National Health Service will be hit particularly hard, since damages for pain, suffering and loss of amenity in clinical negligence cases are very often over the £10,000 threshold.

6.5.3 Special damages

These, broadly, are the financial losses that have accrued between the time of the negligence and the time of the trial. They can only be described broadly this way because they include heads of claim (for instance, the cost of care) that relate to work that has been done free for the claimant, and it is rather artificial to describe these as 'financial losses'.

They typically include the cost of travel (both of the claimant and of visiting relatives) to and from hospital, prescription and other medical expenses, the cost of care, lost earnings and the cost of equipment needed to cope with disability. In relation to each claim, the court will ask itself whether the claimant has proved that the loss has in fact occurred; whether the loss was caused by the negligence; and in relation to expenditure, whether it was reasonable in principle to spend money on whatever the head of claim is, and if so whether it was reasonable to spend the amount of money that is claimed.

If care has been given free by relatives or friends, the court values the cost of buying in that care and then reduces this sum by about 25% to 33% to take account of the fact that no tax or National Insurance has been paid, as it would have been had the care been bought.

In practice, special damages are often agreed. Judges rightly shout at barristers who ask them to decide whether the travelling expenses were £250 or £275.

6.5.4 Future loss

Because this involves speculation about future events, it is much more difficult to calculate. The basic system used is the multiplier–multiplicand system. The multiplier relates to the number of years over which the particular loss runs; the multiplicand represents the annual loss under that head.

Obviously the multiplier cannot simply be the number of years over which the loss runs. If a claimant will lose £1000 per year for ten years, he would be overcompensated if the court were to award him £10,000 because it has to be presumed that he will invest the award of damages. The amount of investment income has to be taken into account if the award is to represent the actual loss. The court in fact presumes that the award will be invested in index-linked government securities (*Wells* v. *Wells* (1998)). Exactly what the discount should be to take account of this presumption is controversial. Defendants said that it should be 3% per annum; claimants pointed out that the rate of return on these securities has fallen over the last couple of years, and often contended for a rate of around 2%. There is a statutory power to fix the discount rate.[21] Since 28 June 2001 it has been fixed at 2.5%.

The multiplier also needs to take into account future contingencies such as the possibility that the claimant would in any event have died, or (in the case of a future loss of earnings claim) have been unable to work in any event. The calculation of multipliers is becoming a sophisticated science in its own right – a science led by actuaries.

Significant heads of future loss often include future loss of earnings, future care, future accommodation requirements and the cost of equipment. Obviously in relation to equipment costs there needs to be expert evidence about the lifetime of each item of equipment. In the case of accommodation costs, claimants are given the costs of any necessary conversion and the costs associated with moving to the required accommodation, plus the court's valuation of the financial disadvantage resulting from the additional money tied up in the new property being unavailable. This is calculated, very roughly, in relation to the income that would have been earned had that sum been available for investment (*Roberts* v. *Johnstone* (1988)).

Sometimes it will be impossible to use the multiplier–multiplicand system to calculate future loss. It may be, for instance, that because of an injury a claimant would be at a disadvantage on the labour market were he to be made unemployed, but at the time of trial he is employed and that employment is expected to continue. Here, the court may make a (rather arbitrary) award to represent the disadvantage, and will assess in doing so the prospects of that claimant finding himself adrift on the labour market as well as the level of disadvantage once he is adrift (*Smith* v. *Manchester Corporation* (1974)).

6.5.5 Hybrid heads of claim

Some heads of claim do not fall neatly within the above categories. The best example is damages for loss of congenial employment – an award to compensate the claimant for not being able to continue doing a particularly satisfying job (*Hale* v. *London Underground Ltd* (1992)). Nursing is one of the classically cited examples of satisfying employment.

6.5.6 Structured settlements

The court most commonly awards, or the defendant agrees to pay, a lump sum of damages. That lump sum or part of it may then be invested in such a way that it produces an annuity that meets the claimant's assessed needs at various stages through his life. This form of investment is called a structured settlement. This may have tax advantages or be otherwise advantageous – for instance, if there are concerns that a claimant, or whoever would be managing the money, might fritter it away. The court now has power to order that the whole or part of the compensation due to a claimant should be paid by way of periodical payments.[22]

6.6 Proving the case

6.6.1 General

It is for the claimant to prove the case. Proof is on the balance of probabilities. The general rule is that things are proved by adducing evidence or by getting the other side to agree to them. If something is blindingly obvious and common knowledge the judge may 'take judicial notice' of it, thus dispensing with the formal requirement of proof or agreement. But this is an extremely limited and in practice unimportant exception to the general rule.

Evidence is a highly technical branch of the law in its own right, and cannot be dealt with in this chapter. It is important to remember that evidence includes evidence not only of fact but also of opinion from appropriately qualified experts.

6.6.2 The maxim *res ipsa loquitur*

Although Lord Woolf hated Latin tags, lawyers still use them because they are convenient shorthand. One of the most common is *res ipsa loquitur*: the thing speaks for itself. It refers to the situation where the mere facts of a case shout loudly and unequivocally 'negligence, and nothing but negligence'.

A lot of mystique has sprung up around this maxim. It has at various times been suggested that where the maxim applies the burden of proof shifts from the claimant to the defendant. It has now been established that this is wrong: the burden of proof never moves.[23]

6.7 Clinical negligence: the future

Clinical negligence claims are big business. The numbers of claims brought has increased very rapidly over the last few years. The loss of legal aid for clinical negligence claims might stop the trend. Such claims are now increasingly funded by 'no win, no fee' arrangements, and obviously such arrangements concentrate the mind of the claimant's lawyers harder on the merits than an unlimited legal aid certificate previously did.

Comparisons are often drawn between the rise in clinical negligence cases in England and the situation in the litigation-mad USA. The comparison is not a good one. In the USA juries generally assess damages, and are much less scientific, much more generous, and much less strictly compensatory about it than are the professional judges who assess damages in England. If irrationally large awards of damages are not going to become available, irrationally large numbers of clinical negligence actions are unlikely. In England, too, contingency fee arrangements for legal funding (whereby the lawyers get a percentage of the damages recovered – a clear incentive to push the damages as high as possible) are illegal. They should remain so. They are an invitation to sharp practice.

It is sometimes said that a lot of litigation is launched by litigants wanting an apology and an explanation rather than damages. This is true. Increasingly, procedures for investigation (and, if appropriate, compensation) that bypass the courts are available. These include informal mediation. Few clinical negligence cases have yet been arbitrated or mediated, but there seems to be no reason why these methods should not work in some cases.

It may seem unfair that a claimant's entitlement to damages should depend on his proving fault. The claimant's need for compensation is just as great whether or not fault can be proved. This consideration has led some to advocate no-fault liability schemes for clinical negligence. The basic problem is cost, and it seems highly unlikely that any British government in the foreseeable future will be prepared to finance such an initiative. In the case of National Health patients injured by National Health negligence, it is arguable that there is a de facto no-fault liability scheme in place anyway in relation to many of the costs claimed in clinical negligence actions. This is because much of the medical treatment and nursing care and many of the appliances that NHS negligence makes necessary are themselves provided by the NHS.

There have been some urgent calls for reform of the system of compensation for clinical negligence, notably in the Chief Medical Officer's paper *Making Amends*.[24] Many of the Chief Medical Officer's proposals have been embodied in the NHS Redress Act 2006. This may change radically the way that clinical negligence claims are handled. It allows for the establishment of redress schemes whereby certain categories of case were dealt with entirely outside the court system. It is too early to say what effect it will have. Many of its most significant effects will be through as yet undrafted secondary legislation. For the moment, the liability of NHS bodies and of individual practitioners will remain governed by the principles set out above.

6.8 Notes and references

1. See *R* v. *Adamako* [1994] 5 Med LR 277; *R* v. *Misra* (Amit) [2005] 1 Cr. App R. 21.
2. For actions in relation to the birth of an unwanted child now, see *Macfarlane* v. *Tayside Health Board* (HL) [2000] 1 Lloyds Rep. Med. 1.
3. Arising from Mr Justice MacNair's direction to the jury in *Bolam* v. *Friern Hospital Management Committee* [1957] 1 WLR 582.
4. For a discussion of this issue, see Charles Foster, Medical negligence: the new cornerstone (*Bolitho* v. *City & Hackney HA*), *Solicitors' Journal*, 5 December 1997, p. 1150; Charles Foster, *Bolam*: consolidation and clarification, *Health Care Risk Report*, **4**(5) (1998), p. 5.
5. Nursing and Midwifery Council, *NMC Code of Professional Conduct: Standards for Conduct, Performance and Ethics* (2004), para. 6.5.
6. See *Wilsher* v. *Essex Area Health Authority* [1986] 3 All ER 801; *Djemal* v. *Bexley Health Authority* [1995] 6 Med LR 269; and *Nettleship* v. *Weston* [1971] 2 QB 691. The *NMC Code of Professional Conduct: Standards for Conduct, Performance and Ethics* (2004) states, at para. 6.2: 'To practise competently, you must possess the knowledge, skills and abilities required for lawful, safe and effective practice without direct supervision. You must acknowledge the limits of your professional competence and only undertake practice and accept responsibilities for those activities in which you are competent.'
7. See *Wilsher* v. *Essex Area Health Authority* [1986] 3 All ER 801, per Lord Justice Mustill at pp. 810–13.
8. There is also an obligation in professional ethics: the *NMC Code of Professional Conduct: Standards for Conduct, Performance and Ethics* (2004) states: '6.1 You must keep your knowledge and skills up-to-date throughout your working life. In particular, you should take part regularly in learning activities that develop your competence and performance ... 6.5 You have a responsibility to deliver care based on current evidence, best practice and, where applicable, validated research when it is available.'
9. See *Crawford* v. *Charing Cross Hospital* (1953) *The Times*, 8 December; *Gascoine* v. *Ian Sheridan and Co.* [1994] 5 Med LR 437.
10. *Bolitho* v. *City & Hackney Health Authority* [1998] AC 232, per Lord Browne Wilkinson at p. 243.
11. The Senate of Surgery, October 1997.
12. General Medical Council, November 1998. Available on the GMC website at http://www.gmc uk.org/guidance/library/consent.asp
13. See *Re. C (a minor) (medical treatment)* [1998] Lloyds Rep Med 1; *Airedale NHS Trust* v. *Bland* [1993] 4 Med LR 39; *Early* v. *Newham HA* [1994] 5 Med LR 214; *Penney, Palmer and Cannon* v. *East Kent Health Authority* [2000] 1 Lloyds Rep. Med. 41.

14. See, for instance, *First Interstate Bank of California* v. *Cohen Arnold & Co.* [1996] 1 PNLR 17; *Allied Maples Group Ltd* v. *Simmons & Simmons (a firm)* [1995] 1 WLR 1602.
15. See, for instance, *Chaplin* v. *Hicks* [1911] 2 KB 786.
16. [2005] 2 WLR 268.
17. See the discussion in Charles Foster, Last chance for lost chances, *New Law Journal*, **155** (7164) (2005), pp. 248–9. Note, too, the curious and much criticised case of *Chester* v. *Afshar* [2005] 1 AC 134, in which it was held by the House of Lords that where (a) there has been a negligent failure to warn about an entirely randomly occurring risk; and (b) the patient would, if warned, have still undergone the procedure at the hands of the same operator and in identical circumstances, but at a different date; and (c) the randomly occurring risk in fact eventuates, without any intra-operative negligence at all on the part of the operator, the claimant succeeds in establishing causation.
18. Note, though, *Tahir* v. *Haringey* HA [1998] Lloyds Rep Med 105, in which the court laid down guidelines indicating when the *Bonnington Castings* analysis would be the correct one in a clinical negligence context.
19. See *Nicholls* v. *Rushton*, *The Times*, 19 June 1992.
20. *The Judicial Studies Board Guidelines for the Assessment of General Damages in Personal Injury Cases*, 4th edn (London, Blackstone Press, 1999).
21. Damages Act 1996, section 1.
22. See Damages Act 1996, section 2(1)(a), inserted by Courts Act 2003, section 100.
23. See *Ratcliffe* v. *Plymouth & Torbay HA and Exeter & North Devon HA* [1998] PIQR P170.
24. Department of Health, June 2003.

B   An Ethical Perspective – Negligence and Moral Obligations

Harry Lesser

It is fairly clear that in a broad sense the legal and ethical uses of the term 'negligence' are the same. Negligence is, roughly, failure to exercise the appropriate level of care. Nevertheless, there are a number of important differences between what is appropriate legally and what is appropriate ethically. These may be summed up briefly by saying that the ethical standard – the level of care required to be doing what one ought to do – is higher than the level required by the law. But there are a number of ways in which the ethical duty of care goes beyond the legal duty. To see what these are we need to examine closely section 8 of the NMC code of professional conduct (2004), and compare it with the requirements of the law.

6.9   Harm and risk

First – and this is made very clear in part A of this chapter – the courts come into operation only if harm has been done. There is a legal duty of care, as well as an ethical one, incumbent on nurses, midwives and specialist community public health nurses. But failure to meet this duty will concern the law only if some harm or damage results. The law has to decide such things as whether harm has been done, who is to be held responsible for the harm, how compensation for the harm should be calculated, and whether the negligence was criminal. But if no harm has been done, there is no place for the law. Ethics is different: a professional who exposes a patient or client to serious and unnecessary risk through failing to take standard precautions is still morally to blame even if by good fortune no harm is done. The law is concerned essentially with redressing, and sometimes with punishing, the harm done by negligence; ethics is concerned with the obligation to avoid negligence, whether harm in fact results or not. To make a very obvious point, a professional who has subjected a patient to unnecessary risk of this kind but without any harm resulting is in no danger of legal action, but ought nevertheless to have a 'bad conscience' and (more importantly) to resolve that this should not happen again.

6.10   The Code of Professional Conduct

It is therefore very appropriate that section 8 of the NMC Code has as its key concept not harm but risk. The general statement is: 'As a registered nurse, midwife or specialist community public health nurse, you must act to identify and minimise the risk to patients and clients.' Subsection 8.1 continues: 'You must work with other members of the team to promote health care environments that are conducive to safe, therapeutic and ethical practice.'

This goes beyond the law in three ways. First, as already mentioned, it requires the nurse not merely to do no harm, but not to risk doing harm. Secondly, it does not restrict 'harm' to certain types of harm, whereas for the law there is criminal negligence only if the injury, loss or damage is of a kind acknowledged by the law. Thirdly, the requirement is not simply to avoid subjecting patients and clients to risk, but to work positively to create as safe an environment as possible. More-over, environments are not only physical: the work must include appropriate training of the people involved, and, as a member of the team, helping to form the appropriate team ethos. And, as we shall see, still more is required by what is set out in subsections 8.2 to 8.5. But first, there is a problem to consider.

6.11 The problem of avoiding risk

The problem is this. Even in ordinary life it is impossible absolutely to avoid caus-ing some risk to oneself or others. One might try to deal with this by saying that risks should always be minimised. But if one literally tried to minimise risk, as the top priority, one would be able to do nothing worthwhile at all: after all, switching on the electric light, crossing the road, travelling in any vehicle, all involve some risk to oneself and others. This could be dealt with, it might be argued, by simple common sense in assessing which risks are so low, and which costs of not taking a risk so high, that the risk should obviously be taken. But in medical care the situation is still more complicated. At the very outset (1.2) the Code requires the nurse to 'protect and support the health of individual patients and clients', as well as the health of the 'wider community'; and at 2.2 there is a requirement to 'pro-mote and protect the interests and dignity of patients and clients'. At first glance this looks fully compatible with minimising the risk to their health, interests or dignity: one requirement is positive and one negative, but they involve the same purpose. But matters are not so simple. Not to care for a patient would very often result in harm or the risk of harm; but most, perhaps even all, forms of care them-selves involve some degree of discomfort, harm or risk. So there may be no way of absolutely safeguarding the interests of the patient, and it may be a matter of judging what is most likely to be in their long-term interests.

Often this may be straightforward. The likelihood of a cure may be very high, for example, and the side-effects of the medication a short-term discomfort clearly worth enduring for the sake of the cure; the nurse administering the medication is in this case fairly clearly acting in the patient's interest. But sometimes matters are much less simple, and it is by no means clear how to balance the risks and possible benefits of a particular type of treatment, and how to decide what is or is not in the patient's interest. Even if the spheres of authority of the doctor and the nurse can be distinguished (which is far from certain), these problems arise for the nurse as well as the doctor, and they can arise over both general and more specific decisions about treatment.

Ethically, three things seem to be required. One is always, if possible, to consult the patient, so that risks are run and discomfort or pain endured with their under-standing and consent; this is in any case required, and explained in detail, in section 3 of the Code. The other requirements are to avoid unnecessary risks not required for the sake of a likely benefit, and not to inflict harm greater than the benefit to the patient or client. All these arise essentially because of a difference between a legal and an ethical duty. Although, as the section on legal negligence makes clear, the legal obligations of a nurse are not something about which there is total clarity or precision, there is, rightly, an attempt to provide guidelines of such a nature that a nurse who acts according to those guidelines will not be guilty of legal negligence. But the Code of Professional Conduct is different. As the preceding discussion shows, one cannot simply 'act according to its provisions' or 'act within them', as one can at least try to do with the law. One is forced, whether or not one is conscious of this, to balance them against each other and to use intelligence and flexibility in translating them into action.

The reason for this complexity is one that lies at the base of many problems in health care ethics. Medicine – here taken to include the activities of nurses, doctors and other health care professionals – has three major aims: to cure or alleviate illness, disease and injury; to prolong life; and to relieve suffering. Very often these three aims coincide, and the same treatment will contribute to all three. But when they do not, problems arise about what should be done, and these problems are made worse by the fact that one is often dealing with probable or possible rather than certain consequences, so that it is not, for example, a matter of trading discomfort for cure, but of trading likely discomfort for a possible cure. Sometimes this can be dealt with by being left to the patient; sometimes it is not in the nurse's hands, but a matter for the doctor or the doctor and patient; sometimes the answer is obvious. But there is a residue of situations where the task of weighing up the pros and cons is going to fall on the nurse. And here the legal position is different from the ethical one. Legally, if things are balanced in this way, the nurse is probably covered whichever course of action he or she takes. Ethically, the nurse is still obliged to consider carefully (insofar as time permits) what is the best thing to do.

It is perhaps worth pointing out – though this is largely drawing attention to the obvious – that these problems cannot be solved by a demarcation of the duties of the nurse and the doctor. There has been a tradition of seeing medicine and nursing as clearly divided, with the functions of the nurse being, for example, to keep the patient as comfortable as possible and to carry out the doctor's instructions. It may be questioned whether this ever corresponded to what went on in practice; but it seems now to be agreed that no such exact demarcation of duties is either possible or desirable.

One may sum all this up by saying that ethics differs from law, in this field, by the fact that it operates all the time, and is concerned with working to avoid potential harm and not merely with redressing actual harm; by the fact that ethics is more complex than law, and may require not simply doing one's duty but working out the best thing to do; and by the fact that ethical standards are higher than legal ones, the Code being considerably more exacting than the law. This raises a further question: whether the personal ethics of the nurse ought to be even more exacting than the Code. For personal ethics, unlike formal codes, needs to be concerned not only with meeting standards but also with pursuing ideals. Professionals, such as nurses, need to be concerned to maintain a level of care above the minimum required by the law and the Code, and to remember that in one sense duty is never completely done.

However, as soon as one says this, one must at once use common sense to qualify it. On the one hand, one needs an ethics that goes beyond duty; on the other, one must remember that nurses, like other people, have been issued with one pair of hands and feet and live through days with 24 hours in them, that hospitals are under-staffed, and that even meeting the standards of the Code can take all the time available. Not only would it be unjust to nurses to expect more than is possible or reasonable: if the standards are set too high, the practical result will be worse rather than better. What seems to be required here is a combination of a resolution to maintain a standard of care at least a little above the minimum required by the law and the Code, with an aspiration to achieve still more when time, energy and opportunity permit. What is also required is a sensible use of one's personal feelings, so that they maintain the standard rather than weakening it. To recognise that one sometimes fails in one's duty and to resolve not to repeat those failures are both useful; but guilt feelings that are inappropriate (for example, at a failure of aspiration which is not an actual failure of duty) or excessive (for example, that persist after the resolution not to repeat the failure has been made) often have the effect, like setting excessively high standards, of making actual practice worse rather than better.

6.12 The ethical duty of care

We have now discussed, if sketchily, the concern of ethics with potential as well as actual consequences, the higher standard and greater complexity of the Code of Professional Conduct when compared with the law, and the way in which the personal ethics of individual nurses should, if possible, be a little higher and more complex than either and consider aspirations as well as duties. Much of this applies to other areas besides the avoidance of negligence, but this area affords a particularly clear example of the differences between legal and ethical obligation.

However, we now come to something that applies particularly to negligence: the extent to which there can be a specific ethical duty of care even when there is no legal duty. There are three cases where this may arise. The first is the case where a nurse happens to be on the scene of an accident. Legally, there is no obligation to help the victims; nurses, midwives and health visitors are under no obligation to stop and assist, unless they are already under a duty to help the person in question because of their contract of employment. But 8.5 of the Code says: 'In an emergency, in *or outside the work setting* [my italics], you have a professional duty to provide care. The care provided would be judged against what could reasonably be expected from someone with your knowledge, skills and abilities when placed in those particular circumstances.' This provision of the Code is very much in line with ordinary morality, which holds both that one ought to help those in need if one can, and that in the particular case of a medical emergency the obligation on health professionals to stop and help is greater than that on other people, because they have the relevant knowledge and skills. There is one problem here: although there is no legal obligation to offer care, once it is offered it is subject to legal obligations, and the victim has a legal claim if they suffer harm as a result. I would suggest that the existence of this legal paradox – that a nurse could not be sued for not offering care but could be sued for offering it negligently – is not a sufficient ground for saying there is no moral obligation to offer care. But it is to be hoped that the law of negligence will not develop, as it has in some countries, in such a way that the legal risk of offering help becomes so great that people become afraid to offer it.

Secondly, there are the moral and legal responsibilities of the manager, or the head of a team, or the named nurse given overall responsibility for a patient's care. The named nurse (or other practitioner) is legally responsible for the negligence of other members of the team only if that negligence is the result of their own acts or omissions – if, for example, they fail to give clear instructions, or to communicate properly information about the patient, or fail generally to make sure that all those to whom care of the patient has been delegated or entrusted were both adequately informed of their responsibilities and competent to carry them out.

This is the legal position. But the implications of section 8 of the Code go beyond this. Section 8.1, already quoted, requires working with the team to promote a safe environment; 8.2 requires quick action to protect patients or clients 'if you have good reason to believe that you or a colleague . . . may not be fit to practise'; 8.3 says that '[w]here you cannot remedy circumstances . . . that could jeopardise standards of practice, you must report them to a senior person with sufficient authority to manage them'; and 8.4 says in effect that managers have several duties – to patients, colleagues, the wider community and the organisation, but 'When facing professional dilemmas, your first consideration . . . must be the interests and safety of patients and clients'. These provisions of the Code can be carried out only if those in charge of a team, and indeed to some extent everyone in a team, accept an obligation (obviously only in ways consistent with good working relationships – on this see section 4 of the Code) not only to make sure that other members of the team are appropriately competent and fully and clearly informed and/or instructed, but also to maintain a constant check that standards of care are being maintained.

The third area where moral duty goes beyond legal duty concerns unborn children. Midwives and other health professionals have no legal duty to care for unborn children, and are not liable for pre-natal injuries to the child provided they have cared properly for the mother. But ethically it would seem that as long as the interests of mother and child are compatible the duty of nurse or midwife must be to both, so that whatever benefits the child should be done, even if it is of no direct benefit to the mother. (In any case, this would normally 'benefit' the mother by being strongly in accordance with her wishes.) There is a technical problem of ethical language and ethical concepts here: it is a disputed matter whether a fetus/unborn child is a kind of being to which duties can be owed. But this seems to be genuinely a purely linguistic problem with no practical effects (unlike many issues in ethics that seem linguistic but turn out to be substantive). One can simply rephrase by saying that the legal duty of the nurse or midwife is to care for the mother, but there is a moral duty also to care for the unborn child even if this goes beyond caring for the mother. For example, if doing, or refraining from doing, certain things will benefit the child but have no effect on the health of the mother, there seems to be no legal duty on the nurse or midwife either to inform the mother of this or to recommend it. But there is a moral duty to do both.

6.13 Conflicts between law and ethics

So far, we have been dealing with various ways in which the moral duty to 'promote and safeguard the interests and well-being of patients and clients' goes beyond the legal duty to avoid negligence, but is not incompatible with it. But there are two areas in which there may be an actual conflict between legal and ethical duty. One concerns the mother and unborn child: if the legal duty is to the mother, but the moral duty is to both, then a conflict is at least possible. Very often, of course, either the interests coincide or the mother strongly wants to put the child's interests first. In the main instance where they do not, that in which the mother is having an abortion, the law specifically allows a nurse with conscientious objections not to take part. The Code similarly, at 2.5, recognises in general the possibility of conscientious objections that may be relevant to professional practice and requires them to be reported 'at the earliest possible time', also requiring the nurse or midwife to 'provide care to the best of your ability until alternative arrangements are implemented'. One can conceive of a very determined opponent of abortion objecting even to this, and raising the question whether it could be the duty of a nurse or midwife not merely to refuse to take part but actually to try to sabotage the whole process. But, given that there seems to be no possible way of doing this successfully, and given how ethically dubious it would be, this is not a suggestion to be taken seriously.

Yet a problem remains. It seems clear that it is possible, though hopefully rare in practice, for a health care professional, faced with a situation in which the interests of the mother and the child are in conflict, to believe that the interests of the child ought ethically to prevail, and not be able simply to withdraw on grounds of conscience. For example, suppose, as sometimes happens, that a Caesarean section would be very advisable to prevent harm to the child, but the mother is refusing to have the operation. Legally, it seems, the midwife should support the mother's decision and not encourage her to expose herself to the risk of the operation; ethically, she might well feel that she should bring all reasonable pressure to bear in order to get the mother to agree. What she should do is a disputed matter; it might, for example, be argued that since the mother, however she feels now, does not want a brain-damaged child, the duty to both mother and child is to bring the pressure to bear. But it is important to point out that it is possible, though hopefully very rare in practice, for health professionals to decide that they have an ethical duty to the child which conflicts with their legal duty to the mother. What they should then do – and different courses of action may be appropriate in different circumstances, depending on the exact possibilities and likely consequences – is a matter for the person involved rather than the academic theorist.

The second case of conflict between law and ethics concerns a health care professional who is given instructions that they believe to be wrong or mistaken, by a person whose competence is not in doubt (so that 8.2 does not apply). Under such circumstances the nurse is legally required to question the orders. But if they are confirmed by the doctor or higher authority before being acted on, the nurse is not regarded as legally negligent. In contrast, 8.3, at least by implication, requires the nurse to report the matter to higher authority, rather than carry out the orders.

So the law will support a nurse who, under appropriate circumstances, questions an order or policy, or demands that a doctor carry it out personally, or for good clinical reasons exempts a particular patient from the established hospital policy. And the Code goes beyond this, and requires the matter to be reported. But ethically this may not be enough. If the consequences of, for example, administering a drug were sufficiently terrible, it would seem that there could be a moral duty not only to refuse to give the drug, and/or to report the matter, but also to prevent the doctor from administering it.

For while it is entirely reasonable that nurses, midwives and health visitors should comply with doctors' orders (if the orders relate to medical practice), nevertheless if in their professional judgement those orders are likely to result in harm to the patient or client, they have a clear moral and professional duty to question them, and even to refuse to carry them out or, if this is practicable, to prevent their being carried out. Section 1.3 of the Code says: 'You are personally accountable for your practice . . . regardless of advice or directions from another professional.' Benjamin and Curtis put the point very clearly some years ago:

> In so far as a nurse has an obligation to follow a doctor's orders, it is only a prima facie obligation, and may be overridden in certain circumstances by other factors. A nurse must be careful not to confuse a well-grounded prima facie obligation with blind faith.[1]

Similarly, hospital policy, or the policy of one's employer, whether in a private nursing agency, for example, or in industry, does not remove personal accountability. There is again a prima facie duty to comply with the rules and policies of one's employer or organisation, but this needs to be overridden if the policy does not meet agreed professional standards or fails to serve the best interests of the patient. Although this seems ethically clear, it is supported by the law only up to a point. Questioning the law or policy is positively required; refusing on professional grounds to carry out the policy has legal backing. But refusing on any other moral grounds is supported by the law only in the case of abortion; and trying to prevent an order being carried out has no support at all, as far as one can see. On the other hand, reporting to the appropriate authority what is going on – 'whistle-blowing' – though not required by the law, is required, as we have seen, by the Code, and is safeguarded by the law.

There is a real problem here. On the one hand, the running of any institution requires that individuals make some sacrifice of their personal judgement of what is best to the judgement of those in charge; life would be impossible if individuals constantly prevented decisions from being carried out, and even the questioning of orders – which is, up to a point, a good thing – has to be kept within very tight limits if activities are not to grind to a halt. It is also important to remember that anyone taking the drastic step of trying to prevent an order from being complied with may well face disciplinary action and find that, however morally right they may be, the law and the Code do not in practice adequately protect them. Even 'whistleblowers', who if they are reporting genuine instances of risk to patients are precisely obeying the Code, may find that, whatever the theory, they are in fact in serious trouble. But on the other hand, despite the need to keep the institution running, and despite the importance of not encouraging people to put themselves on the line when it is not necessary, one must always remember the harm, sometimes terrible, that can be done if people take no steps to prevent wicked, or even well-meant but mistaken, actions or policies.

In the end, each health professional must decide for himself or herself when the moment has come to put themselves on the line; one hopes most will be spared ever having to make such a decision. The only guideline one might suggest is that this should be considered only if the alternative is something widely agreed to be seriously harmful. It remains important to acknowledge that one's moral duty can conflict with one's legal duty. Which should be given precedence, in these unfortunate situations, has to be a matter of individual conscience, with awareness that there may be a price to pay.

6.14 Conclusion

A carer has both a legal and an ethical duty to avoid negligence. The ethical duty differs from the legal one primarily in the following ways:

(1) It operates whether or not any harm actually follows from the negligence, and whether or not the harm is of a kind acknowledged by the law.
(2) The NMC Code of Professional Conduct requires a higher standard than the law, and also has the consequence that the carer must on occasion be able to weigh up likely harms and benefits in order to decide what it is best to do.
(3) Time and energy permitting, the carer should have a personal ethical standard at least a little higher than that of the Code, and should also have an ethics of ideals as well as duties, again in line with what is reasonably possible.
(4) Ethics goes beyond the law in requiring a direct duty of care for unborn children; a duty towards accident victims if one can help them; a general duty to make sure that those whose work one is responsible for coordinating and supervising carry out their duties properly; and a duty to report circumstances in which care is endangered. (The first of these is not specifically in the Code but is a general moral duty, recognised even if one believes that abortion is sometimes right.)
(5) Ethics may occasionally require someone to actively prevent an order or policy from being carried out, even though this may conflict with their legal duty, or to uphold the claims of someone they are not legally obliged to care for in preference to the claims of someone for whom they are legally obliged to care. (These situations are rare but not impossible.)

6.15 Reference

1. M. Benjamin & J. Curtis, *Ethics in Nursing* (Oxford, Oxford University Press, 1992).

7 Consent and the Capable Adult Patient

A   The Legal Perspective

Jean McHale

Obtaining the consent of a patient to treatment is a crucial part of health care practice. It fosters the bond of trust between practitioner and patient by according the patient respect for her autonomy of decision-making. The Nursing and Midwifery Code provides that:

> 3.1 All patients and clients have a right to receive information about their condition. You must be sensitive to their needs and respect the wishes of those who refuse or are unable to receive information about their condition. Information should be accurate, truthful and presented in such a way as to make it easily understood. You may need to seek legal or professional advice or guidance from your employer in relation to the giving or withholding of consent.[1]

Obtaining consent before undertaking treatment is also part of the health professional's legal obligation.[2] If treatment is given without consent she runs the risk of being sued for damages in the civil law courts or prosecuted in criminal law.

The nurse has two main roles in the consent process. First, when she is acting as the primary carer, providing the patient with treatment, she has the task of obtaining the patient's consent. The expansion in the role of the nurse means increasingly that it is the nurse herself who will be taking on this role. Secondly, even if a doctor obtains the patient's consent, a patient may be confused or uncertain about her treatment choice and may turn to the nurse for clarification. When complying with her legal obligations in relation to consent to treatment the registered nurse needs also to be aware of her professional ethical obligations including her role as advocate for her patient. Here, as in other areas of her practice, the nurse may find herself torn between what she believes are the obligations required of her under the Nursing and Midwifery Council Professional Code and her obligations under the contract of employment.

Consent to treatment is one area of health care practice in which the courts may be invited to consider the application of the European Convention of Human Rights through the Human Rights Act 1998.[3] Issues that concern consent to treatment can be found in relation to the debates concerning many areas of health care and this is reflected in many of the other chapters of this book.[4] This chapter discusses consent to treatment and the competent adult patient. In section 7.1 the general nature of consent in law and capacity to consent to treatment is discussed. Section 7.2 considers the liability of the nurse in civil and in criminal law if she fails to provide the patient with information regarding her treatment. Section 7.3 examines the situation in which a nurse believes that the doctor has provided her patient with insufficient information with which to make a treatment decision. Some of the difficulties that can face the nurse in attempting to act as an advocate for her patient are examined, particularly in the context of inter-professional conflicts of disclosure.

It should be noted that while this chapter does give an introduction to the issues it is obviously not possible to explore the full breadth and range of complex issues that arise consequent upon consent to treatment; for a fuller exploration readers are referred to other sources.[5]

7.1 Consent to treatment: some general issues

7.1.1 The consent form

One of the most frequent cries to be heard in a hospital is: 'Have you got her consent form?' All nurses are familiar with the consent forms given to patients to sign before they go in for an operation. But the fact that the patient has signed a consent form does not necessarily mean that consent is valid. It depends upon the circumstances; simply signing a form does not by itself mean that the implications of that consent have been explained. Equally, consent given orally may be perfectly valid if the patient has been properly informed. However, while it is not strictly required, written consent has the advantage of drawing a patient's attention to the fact that she is consenting to a clinical procedure and it may provide some evidence of her consent should there be any future dispute as to whether consent was given.

7.1.2 Express and implied consent

While consent may be given expressly, whether in writing or orally, in some situations even express oral consent is not required. If a patient proffers her arm for a bandage to be applied, although she may say nothing her actions imply that she has consented to the procedure. But there are dangers in too readily assuming that a patient has given implied consent. For example, particular difficulties can arise in relation to blood tests. When blood samples are taken, a number of tests are usually performed on the samples. It can be argued that by giving general consent to a blood sample being taken a patient is consenting to all those tests being performed that the doctor considers to be necessary. But what if one of those tests is to determine a patient's HIV status? Is this a test of a different nature? It is clear that the implications for a patient if an HIV test is taken are considerable. For example, it may inhibit their ability to obtain insurance and employment. The precise legal position as to whether blood can be tested for HIV without consent remains uncertain.

Different legal opinions have been expressed on this point.[6] The General Medical Council stated in their 1997 guidance that consent must be obtained from patients before testing for a serious communicable disease.[7] This guidance goes on to state:

> Some conditions such as HIV, have serious social, financial, as well as medical implications. In such situations the nurse must make sure that the patient is given appropriate information about the implications of the test, and appropriate time to consider and discuss them.

It is submitted that this is the appropriate approach to take and that testing should not be undertaken without the patient being made clearly aware of the consequences.

7.1.3 Capacity to consent

In order for consent to be valid in law a patient must be capable of making that treatment decision. Adult patients are presumed to have capacity to consent or to refuse consent to a particular treatment, although this refusal can be rebutted.[8] But what is meant by 'capacity'?[9] Obviously the patient will require some understanding of the implications of the decision that he or she is to make, but how much? In Re C (adult: refusal of treatment) (1994) the court upheld the right of a 68-year-old paranoid schizophrenic who had developed gangrene in his foot to prevent his foot being amputated in the future without his express written consent. Mr Justice Thorpe suggested a three-part test to determine capacity:

> first, comprehending and retaining treatment information, secondly, believing it and thirdly, weighing it in the balance to arrive at a choice.

At the hearing it was claimed that C was not competent because of his delusions that he was a doctor and that whatever treatment was given to him was calculated to destroy his body. But despite these claims Mr Justice Thorpe held that he was satisfied that C was capable of giving or refusing consent because he understood and had retained the relevant treatment information, and believed it and had arrived at a clear choice. One potential problem with the test in Re C is that it makes capacity dependent on the information that the patient is actually given. If the nurse provides a patient with a great deal of complex information he or she may be unable to understand it and as a result lack capacity. In contrast, if a basic explanation is given the very same patient may possess the capacity to consent.[10]

This approach was followed in 1995 by the Law Commission in their report *Mental Incapacity* concerning the care and treatment of those patients with mental incapacity. They stated that the test should be decision-relative. They proposed that legislation should provide that a person should be deemed to lack capacity if at the material time he or she is:

(1) unable by reason of mental disability to make a decision on the matter in question
(2) unable to communicate a decision on the matter because he or she is unconscious or for any other reason.

The Law Commission defined 'mental disability' as being 'any disability or disorder of the mind or brain, whether permanent or temporary which results in an impairment or disturbance of mental functioning'. They proposed that a person should be unable to make a decision on the basis of mental disability 'if the disability is such that, at the time when the decision needs to be made he or she is unable to understand or to retain the information relevant to the decision, including information about the reasonably foreseeable consequences of failing to make that decision'. They recommended that the patient should have a basic comprehension of information where this was given 'in broad terms and simple language'.

Judicial approval of the approach of the Law Commission and of *Re C* was given in *Re MB (medical treatment)* (1997). Here a woman with a needle phobia, while agreeing to a Caesarean section that was clinically required, repeatedly refused the anaesthetic prior to the Caesarean section. Lady Butler-Sloss held that a person is not capable of making a decision where:

(a) the person is unable to comprehend and retain the information which is material to the decision, especially as to the likely consequences of having or not having the treatment in question: and (b) the patient is unable to use the information and weigh it in the balance as of the process of arriving at a decision.

The Court of Appeal in this case went on to consider the scope of capacity and the extent to which an individual may be regarded as incapable where the decision that is made can be regarded by some as irrational. This is discussed further below in the context of consent and refusal in relation to enforced Caesarean sections.

In a situation in which a patient has a fluctuating mental state it may be acutely difficult to decide whether she is capable of giving consent. In such a situation it is tempting to say that she lacks capacity to make treatment decisions. This is because English law allows the incapacitated patient to be given such treatment as those treating her believe to be in her best interests.[11] In *Re R (a minor: wardship: consent to medical treatment)* the Court of Appeal held that a child with fluctuating mental capacity was to be regarded as totally incapable of making a decision to consent or refuse consent.[12] However, in the later case of *Re T* the Court of Appeal held that the capacity of an adult patient is to be judged by reference to the particular decision to be made.[13] This is surely right. If a patient is capable today of understanding what treatment is proposed, the fact that yesterday she was not capable of understanding should not affect her right to make a decision. This approach was confirmed subsequently in *Re MB*.[14]

7.1.4 Reform of the law concerning mental capacity

The Law Commission's proposals were far more extensive than simply setting out one test and constituted a comprehensive review of capacity over the whole area of care and treatment of the mentally incompetent adult including such issues as advance directives (see Chapter 10A) and powers of attorney. After a period in which the Law Commission's report was left in abeyance the government finally undertook consultations on the report in their document *Who Decides?* in 1997[15] and in October 1999 issued a Green Paper, the document *Making Decisions*.[16] The ultimate proposals are considered in greater detail in other chapters in this book. While the Law Commission proposed a radical revision of the law, the government took a more limited approach, although *Making Decisions* did accept the need for a statutory definition of capacity. It was several years before the government finally introduced legislation leading to the passage of the Mental Capacity Act in 2005.

The Mental Capacity Act 2005 provides a statutory framework for decision-making concerning adults lacking mental capacity. The Act is due to come into force in April to October 2007 in stages. Like the common law, it roots decision-making in a 'best interests' test. It does not automatically provide for a third-party decision maker to act on behalf of an adult lacking capacity although in contrast to the common law it does allow for the appointment of a person to make treatment decisions on behalf of the person lacking capacity through a 'lasting power of attorney'.[17] Here we consider the main provisions concerning assessment of capacity. Further consideration is given in other chapters in this book to specific provisions concerning adults who lack mental capacity in relation to clinical research and end of life decision-making.

Section one of the Mental Capacity Act 2005 sets out a series of 'principles' that are to underpin decision-making. There is a statutory presumption in favour of decision-making capacity. In addition there is a requirement that all reasonably practicable steps are to be taken to ensure that the individual makes the decision. Furthermore, as at common law decisions must be reached on the basis of the 'best interests' of the individual. Section 2(1) states that a person will lack capacity where they are unable to make the decision themselves owing to 'an impairment of or a disturbance in the functioning of the mind or brain'. As at common law, the capacity test is decision-specific. A person may have the capacity to make one decision while at the same time being incapable of making another. Section 3(1) in effect codifies the *Re C* test and sets out the circumstances in which a person is unable to make a decision. It states that a person is unable to understand the information that is necessary in relation to this decision; unable to retain it; unable to use or weigh up the information as part of the decision-making process or unable to communicate the decision by any means (this includes talking and sign language). Information here includes information regarding the foreseeable consequences of the necessary decision.[18] Statutory safeguards are given to those caring for the person who lacks mental capacity, thus removing any legal uncertainty as to their actions. Section 5 of the Mental Capacity Act provides that where a person acts in the best interests of an adult lacking capacity they will not be subject to legal liability as long as first they have undertaken reasonable steps to ascertain that the adult lacks capacity; secondly, that they reasonably believe that the person lacks decision-making capacity; and thirdly, the decision that has been made is in the person's best interests.

The best interests test that exists at common law is codified and structured under the Mental Capacity Act 2005. Section 4 of the Act sets out some guidance as to what constitutes a person's best interests. The person must not simply take into account age or appearance or condition/aspect of behaviour which could lead to unjustified assumptions about his best interests. In addition relevant circumstances should be taken into account such as whether it is likely that the person will at some time have capacity in relation to this issue. Factors that should be taken into account 'as far as is reasonably practicable' include an individual's past and present wishes and feelings, any beliefs and values that would have been taken into account if they had capacity and any 'other factors that he would be likely to consider if he were able to do so' (section 4(6)). The legislation makes provision for the appointment of an Independent Mental Capacity Advocate under sections 35–7 to provide representation and support for a person who lacks capacity. Such a person should be appointed in a situation in which there is no close friend or family member who can be consulted and it is necessary to give 'serious medical treatment' to the adult.

Further guidance as to the operation of the legislation will be found in the Code of Practice issued by the Department for Constitutional Affairs (Now the Ministry of Justice) to accompany the legislation.[19]

7.1.5 Criminal law and consent to treatment

As a general rule, if a patient gives consent to a medical procedure being undertaken then no criminal liability will result. But the fact that consent has been given does not automatically mean that the treatment itself is lawful. The individual does not have absolute freedom in English law to do what he or she wishes with his or her body.[20] Some medical procedures such as female circumcision are expressly prohibited by statute.[21] Uncertainties surround the legality of certain other medical procedures. For example, while it appears that as long as organ transplant operations do not constitute an unjustified risk to the life of the donor they will not be held to be unlawful,[22] the lawfulness of animal to human transplantations is still to be resolved.[23] Where a major operation is undertaken without consent there is the possibility of a prosecution under section 18 of the Offences Against the Person Act 1861. This section makes it an offence to 'unlawfully and maliciously' cause grievous bodily harm to a person with the intention of causing grievous bodily harm. However, it is more likely that a nurse who has given treatment without the patient's consent will be prosecuted for the less serious crime of battery. This makes unlawful any non-consensual touching.[24]

7.2 Civil law liability

7.2.1 Battery

While treating without obtaining the patient's consent may lead to a criminal prosecution, it is far more likely that absence of consent will lead to an action in the civil courts. First, an action may be brought in the tort of battery. An action in battery arises if a patient is touched without her consent. Not every touching will lead to liability: for example, an action is unlikely to result from the nurse accidentally brushing a patient's shoulder as she passes in a corridor. There is no need to prove that the touching caused damage – the fact that it took place is sufficient for an action to be brought. In *Chatterton* v. *Gerson* Mr Justice Bristow held that no liability would arise as long as the patient was informed and understood in broad terms the nature of the procedure that it was proposed to undertake, and she had given consent.[25] If a broad general consent is given then any further claim that a patient has been given inadequate information should be brought not in battery but in negligence.[26]

7.2.2 Treating in an emergency where no consent can be obtained

There may be some situations in which it is lawful for the nurse to go ahead and treat a patient without obtaining her consent, most notably in an emergency situation as in the patient brought bleeding and unconscious into casualty. In such situations treatment can be given on the basis of necessity. In addition, if a patient has given initial consent to an operation but then, later, during the operation it is discovered that she is suffering, for example, from a life-threatening condition such as a cancerous tumour then this may be removed. But while necessity may justify the performance of a medical procedure in an emergency, exactly what is necessary is a matter of degree.[27] The nurse should ask herself if this particular procedure is immediately necessary or could it be postponed until the patient recovers consciousness and can make her own decision.

Consent and refusal

The patient has the right both to consent to and to refuse medical treatment. An action in battery may be brought if treatment is given in the face of an explicit refusal of consent. A well-known case often quoted as a warning to those who may be tempted to treat in the face of refusal is the Canadian case of *Malette* v. *Schumann*.[28] The claimant was brought into hospital following a road accident. A nurse found a card in her pocket that identified her as being a Jehovah's Witness and that requested that she was never to be given a blood transfusion. Despite the card the doctor performed the transfusion. On recovering her health the patient brought an action in battery. She succeeded and was awarded $20,000 damages. In a later English case, that of Ms B, continuation of treatment against the patient's wishes was held to be a battery. Ms B was quadriplegic. She was supported on a ventilator but wanted this support withdrawn.[29] The hospital refused to accede to her wishes. She went to court and ultimately her claim was successful. She was held to have decision-making capacity and she thus had a right to refuse treatment – which included the right to refuse ventilation. Nominal damages were awarded against the hospital for continuing to treat her. Subsequently the ventilator support was removed and she died. (See also Chapter 10.)

A further reason why patients may argue that their decision to refuse treatment should be upheld is because this is a fundamental human right, one that is now safeguarded under the Human Rights Act 1998. A number of the rights contained in the European Convention of Human Rights may be relevant in this context: for example, Article 3, because imposition of treatment upon a competent patient against their wishes may be held to constitute inhuman or degrading treatment or punishment. In addition, Article 8, which concerns the right to respect for privacy of home and family life, may be applicable – but as this right is not absolute it can be argued that there will not be an infringement of Article 8 where the patient is not in a position to give informed consent.[30] Article 9 of the Convention – freedom of religion – may also be used to support the refusal of treatment in a situation in which the reason why the individual is refusing treatment is because of a tenet of their particular religious belief. In the past in a number of cases refusal of treatment on religious grounds has been overruled by the courts, particularly in the context of refusal by child patients.[31] It will be interesting to see how these issues are considered in the future.

Overruling a refusal of treatment

While a clear refusal should be respected, there are situations in which a patient's refusal may be overridden. In *St George's NHS Trust* v. *S* the Court of Appeal set out guidance concerning cases in which patients refused treatment (case discussed further on pages 126–127 below).[32] Where a patient possesses capacity, they may refuse therapy; where a patient lacks capacity treatment may be given where it is in the patient's best interests. If there is a question mark over the patient's capacity then a proper assessment should be undertaken by an independent psychiatrist. If there is a serious doubt as to the patient's capacity and a declaration is sought, the patient's solicitor should be informed. Where the patient is incapable of instructing a solicitor, the official solicitor should be involved. The guidance notes that in a situation of acute urgency an application to the court may be inappropriate owing to time constraints. Nonetheless, it remains the case that judicial guidance may have advantages in such difficult cases.

7.2.3 Particular problems in overriding refusal of consent

Free not forced consent

A patient must reach her decision whether to consent or refuse treatment freely and without pressure being applied by relatives or by carers. In *Re T* in 1992 (discussed above) an important factor in the decision to authorise a transfusion was that T's refusal came after she had spent time alone with her mother, a confirmed

Jehovah's Witness. Ensuring that a patient gives free and full consent may be practically very difficult for a nurse working on a busy ward. Inevitably the amount of time that can be spent with a patient discussing the implications of a decision is subject to the time constraints of practice, but the patient must not be browbeaten by relatives or by medical staff into making the decision. In determining whether consent has been given in a particular situation the court will look to the circumstances. The fact that a patient is, for example, a prisoner does not mean that she is unable to give free consent. In *Freeman* v. *Home Office* the court held that whether the prisoner/patient had, in fact, consented was a question of fact for each individual case.[33] But in this type of situation it is of particular importance that when information is given to the patient it is made clear to her that she has a free choice.

7.2.4 Pregnant women refusing care

A midwife is faced with a pregnant woman in difficulties in labour who is refusing even to contemplate a Caesarean section. By rejecting treatment she is placing her life and that of the fetus in jeopardy. Should her refusal of treatment be respected? This issue came before the English courts in a series of cases during the 1990s. In *Re S* the case concerned a woman six days overdue giving birth where the medical team sought to undertake a Caesarean section.[34] To attempt a normal birth would have caused a very grave risk of rupture to the uterus because the fetus was in transverse lie, placing the lives of mother and child in grave danger. S, a born-again Christian, refused the operation because it was against her religious beliefs. The hospital went to court to obtain a declaration, which was controversially granted by Sir Stephen Brown. The judge made reference to the rights of the fetus, but English courts have in the past consistently rejected claims that the fetus has such rights.[35]

Sir Stephen Brown placed some emphasis on a US case, *Re AC*.[36] In a number of cases courts in the USA were prepared to order pregnant women to be given a Caesarean section despite their refusal of treatment.[37] In *Re AC* the court initially ordered a Caesarean section on a woman dying of cancer. This order was overturned on appeal after AC had died. The court said that in 'virtually all cases' a refusal could not be overridden; they did admit there may be exceptional circumstances in which a Caesarean may be ordered. An example given in discussion in the case was very similar to the facts in *Re S*. Nevertheless, *Re AC* is widely seen as the case that curtailed judicially ordered Caesarean sections in the USA.[38] In many ways *Re S* can be regarded as an exceptional case – an aberration.[39] After the decision the Royal College of Obstetricians and Gynaecologists (RCOG) published a consultation paper stating: 'It is inappropriate and unlikely to be helpful or necessary to invoke judicial intervention to overrule an informed and competent woman's refusal of a proposed medical treatment even though her refusal may place her life and that of her foetus at risk.'[40]

Despite this, in a number of subsequent cases judicial intervention was sought and the courts authorised the performance of Caesarean sections upon women who had refused such procedures.[41] The Court of Appeal was given an opportunity to rule on this issue in *Re MB*.[42] MB had a fear of needles. This had led her to refuse to have blood samples taken during pregnancy. In the late stages of pregnancy it was discovered that the fetus was in the breach position. A Caesarean section was proposed. MB initially agreed; however, she was opposed to administration of anaesthetic by needles. MB then went into labour. She agreed to a Caesarean section and the administration of anaesthetic by mask, but at the last moment refused the anaesthetic.[43] The hospital then sought a court order, which was given by Mr Justice Hollis. He found that MB was incompetent because of the effects of the needle phobia on her decision-making powers. She asked her lawyer to appeal. She then herself agreed to the Caesarean section and the operation was carried out the following day. MB challenged the legality of the procedure. On appeal to the Court of Appeal the right of the competent patient to refuse treatment was confirmed.[44] However, it was also recognised that, in an emergency, treatment could be given where a patient lacks capacity, as long as this was on the basis of necessity, the procedure not extending beyond what was reasonably required by the patient. Lady Butler-Sloss noted the judgment of Lord Donaldson in *Re T* where he stated that the doctor must assess carefully whether in that case the patient had the capacity 'commensurate with the gravity of the decision' she purported to make. The Court of Appeal referred to the three-stage test for capacity set out by Mr Justice Thorpe in *Re C* discussed above. Lady Butler-Sloss commented:

> A competent woman who has the capacity to decide may, for religious reasons, other reasons, for rational or irrational reasons or for no reason at all, choose not to have medical intervention, even though the consequence may be the death or serious handicap of the child she bears, or her own death. In that event the courts do not have the jurisdiction to declare medical intervention lawful and the question of her own best interests objectively considered, does not arise.

She went on to state:

> Irrationality is here used to connote a decision which is so outrageous in its defiance of logic or of accepted moral standards that no sensible person who has applied his mind to the question to be decided could have arrived at it . . . Although it might be thought that irrationality sits uneasily with competence to decide, panic, indecisiveness and irrationality in themselves do not as such amount to incompetence, but they may be symptoms or evidence of incompetence. The graver the consequences of the decision the commensurately greater the level of competence is required to take the decision.

Capacity may be eroded owing to temporary incompetence as indicated by Lord Donaldson in the earlier case of *Re T* as 'confusion, shock, pain and drugs'. The Court of Appeal on the facts of this particular case upheld the decision of the judge at the first instance that MB had lacked capacity. She was competent to consent to the Caesarean section. However, she did not have competence to refuse as she was 'at that moment suffering an impairment of her mental functioning which disabled her. She was temporarily incompetent'. Her phobia of needles impaired her ability to decide.

Two points arise here. First is the extent to which the circumstances of pregnancy itself served to erode the woman's capacity. In view of the fact that temporary factors may erode capacity, Kennedy is surely right to argue that '... there is an urgent need to establish the boundaries of the permissible' in this area.[45] Secondly, Butler-Sloss makes an important statement confirming that the law sanctions 'irrational' refusals. Nonetheless the judgment leaves unclear where the boundary can be drawn between 'acceptable' irrationality, which will not impact on respect for the patient's right to decide, and an 'irrational' decision, which may impact on capacity in such a way that an individual's competence to make that decision is affected. Having found MB to be temporarily incompetent the Court of Appeal then considered whether the procedure itself could be authorised. The House of Lords in *Re F* (1988) confirmed that medical procedures may be undertaken on an incompetent adult where it is in his or her best interests. The House of Lords indicated that best interests were to be determined with reference to the *Bolam* test:[46] what a responsible body of professional practice would authorise in such a situation – a medically based test. The difficulties with the application of such a test have been noted by academic commentators.[47]

It is questionable how far such a test formulated to determine issues of clinical judgement is appropriate in a broader context of determining the authorisation of treatment decisions.[48] A further point is that of the interrelationship of the 'best interests' test that applies in the case of the mentally incompetent adult, to the operation of the welfare principle in cases concerning the treatment of children. In *Re MB* Lady Butler-Sloss stated: 'In considering the scope of best interests, it seems to us that they have to be treated on similar principles to the welfare of a child since the court and the doctors are concerned with a person unable to make the necessary decision for himself.'[49]

These observations of Lady Butler-Sloss are interesting. However, is it the case that one overarching principle should be applied or do different considerations apply in the context of the (adult without capacity) and in relation to a child patient? There has been much cross reference between cases concerning children and adults (lacking capacity) at the end of life.[50] However, treatment decisions regarding vulnerable adults were notably the subject of considerable separate (and indeed extensive) consideration by the Law Commission in their report on mental incapacity. The complexities of such issues are excellently highlighted in that report. It is suggested that before the application of the best interest tests are further conflated the whole question of the interrelationship between treatment decisions of incompetent minors and adults requires reconsideration.

The Court of Appeal held that the treatment was in MB's best interests in this emergency situation. But in whose best interests was this procedure? The Court of Appeal took into consideration the fact that agreement had initially been given by MB for the Caesarean section. Furthermore, evidence from the consultant psychiatrist was to the effect that if the child had been born handicapped or had died, MB herself would have suffered long-term harm. In contrast, little harm would be caused by the administration of the anaesthetic against her wishes. What of the interrelationship between the best interests of both the fetus and the woman? The Court of Appeal upheld earlier cases such as *Re F (in utero)*[51] and *Paton* v. *British Pregnancy Advisory Service*[52] in confirming that the fetus has no independent status in English law. They were of the view that Sir Stephen Brown in *Re S* had reached an incorrect conclusion. The Court of Appeal stated:

Although it may seem illogical that a child capable of being born alive is protected by the criminal law from intentional destruction, and by the Abortion Act from termination otherwise than as permitted by the Act, but is not protected from the (irrational) decision of a competent mother not to allow medical intervention to avert the risk of death, this appears to be the present state of the law.[53]

Thus even at the point of birth itself the court could not intervene in the face of refusal of medical intervention by a competent woman with the aim of safeguarding the position of the fetus. The English courts may consider such future decisions in the light of Article 2 of the European Convention of Human Rights. However, the weight of authority makes it questionable whether a different approach will be taken.

Re MB also recognises that there may be circumstances (beyond the Mental Health Act 1983) when the use of forcible treatment may be justifiable. Lady Butler-Sloss stated:

> The extent of force or compulsion which may be necessary can only be judged in each individual case and by the health professionals. It may become for them a balance between continuing treatment which is forcibly opposed and deciding not to continue with it. This is a difficult issue which may need to be considered in depth on another occasion.[54]

One of the most important aspects of the decision in Re MB is that it provides guidance for future cases in this area by setting out procedures that should be undertaken. This includes the requirement that the woman should be represented in all cases save where, in exceptional circumstances, she does not wish to be so. This recommendation goes some way to meet concerns as to the manner in which such proceedings have been brought. This guidance has been subsequently incorporated into an NHS circular,[55] and is considered further in St George's NHS Trust v. S, discussed below.

7.2.5 Caesarean sections and the Mental Health Act

There have also been a number of cases in which the Mental Health Act 1983 was used to sanction the performance of Caesarean sections upon mentally incompetent women. Section 63 of the Act provides that:

> [t]he consent of a patient shall not be required for any medical treatment given to him for the mental disorder from which he is suffering.

The boundaries of section 63 – what amounted to medical treatment for mental disorder – came before the courts in Tameside and Glossop Acute Hospital Trust v. CH (1996).[56] CH was detained under section 3 of the Mental Health Act 1983. She was suffering from paranoid schizophrenia. She was then discovered to be pregnant. It was held that as she lacked capacity to consent to or refuse treatment a Caesarean section could be authorised, as the performance of a Caesarean section was treatment for 'mental disorder' and thus fell within the scope of section 63 of the Mental Health Act 1983. This was because if a stillbirth had occurred her health would have deteriorated, and she needed strong anti-psychotic medication which could not be given to her when she was pregnant. The court followed the approach in *B* v. *Croydon HA* that section 63 of the 1983 Act encompassed matters that related to the 'core treatment' (in that case including force-feeding).[57] Such a broad interpretation of this provision has been criticised.[58] For example, as Grubb has argued, section 63 does not cover any physical condition that impedes treatment of mental disorder. As he notes: 'The Government saw section 63 in far more limited terms covering perfectly routine, sensible treatment.'

A contrasting approach was taken by the Court of Appeal in the case of *St George's NHS Trust* v. *S.*[59] S was diagnosed as suffering from severe pre-eclampsia. She was advised that she should have an early delivery. S, who had intended a home delivery, refused treatment. She asserted that nature should take its course although she was informed as to the risk of death and disability to herself and the fetus. Her GP initiated steps that led to her detention in hospital under section 2 of the Mental Health Act 1983. She was subsequently transferred to another hospital. While she persistently refused treatment and sought legal advice, the hospital authority, without her knowledge, made an ex parte application to the High Court for a declaration to the effect that it would be lawful to undertake treatment, including a Caesarean section. Meanwhile, S had been in touch with solicitors with the intention of making an application to a Mental Health Review Tribunal. The declaration was granted. It appears that the judge was under an incorrect impression that S had been in labour for 24 hours. S gave birth to a daughter. The detention under the Mental Health Act was terminated. S discharged herself. While detained in hospital S was not offered treatment for her mental disorder. An action was subsequently brought for judicial review to challenge the legality of the action taken. The Court of Appeal again emphasised the fact that the competent adult is entitled to refuse treatment.[60] Lord Justice Judge stated:

> In our judgment while pregnancy increases the personal responsibilities of a woman it does not diminish her entitlement to decide whether or not to undergo medical treatment. Although human and protected by the law in a number of different ways as set out in the judgment in Re MB . . . an unborn child is not a separate person from its mother. Its need for medical assistance does not prevail over her rights.

These words are indicative of the tensions in drawing the boundaries between moral acceptability and legal enforcement in this area. While some may regard a pregnant woman as possessing moral responsibilities to the fetus in the latter stages of pregnancy, this still does not limit her legal rights. The orthodoxy of *Paton* and subsequent cases was again confirmed by the court. The court held that a battery had been committed on S. Lord Justice Judge stated:

> how can an enforced invasion of a competent adult's body against her will even for the most laudable of motives (the preservation of life) be ordered without irredeemably damaging the principle of self-determination?

The court examined the provisions of section 2(2) which provide that:

An application for admission for assessment may be made in respect of a patient on the grounds that (a) he is suffering from a mental disorder of a nature or degree which warrants the detention of the patient in a hospital for assessment (or for assessment followed by medical treatment) for at least a limited period; and (b) he ought to be so detained in the interests of his own health and safety or with a view to the protection of other persons.

The Court of Appeal emphasised that the criteria for detention under the section were cumulative. In this case the doctors had been justified in their assessment that the woman was suffering from depression that constituted 'mental disorder'. However, S was not being detained in order that treatment be given for her mental disorder. It was stated that:

> For the purposes of section 2(2)A such detention must be related to or linked with the mental disorder. Treatment for the effects of pregnancy does not provide the necessary warrant.

Thus the courts have affirmed that for treatment to be lawful under section 63 it must be crucial to the mental disorder. While here the treatment was not treatment for mental disorder within the provisions of the statute, as Bailey Harris notes, questions regarding the connection between the disorder and the treatment proposed are likely to arise in the future.[61] Finally, there had been irregularities in the documentation used by the hospital. Forms had not been completed when the woman was transferred between hospitals, as was required by regulations made under section 19 of the Mental Health Act. This would, in any event, have entitled S to discharge herself from hospital. While some might regard her decision as unjustifiable or even irrational, this did not mean that it was of no legal validity. The Mental Health Act cannot be used as a means of circumventing the competent woman's right to refuse a Caesarean section. Finally, the Court of Appeal criticised the procedure adopted in the case of the ex parte application; the application was made without the knowledge of S and her legal advisers, and as in *Re MB* they set out guidelines regarding the conduct of proceedings for a declaration.

The decisions of the Court of Appeal in *Re MB* and *St George's NHS Trust* v. *S* are in many respects welcome. The autonomy of the patient is confirmed. Judicial guidance is also given as to the correct procedures that should be adopted when making an application for a declaration and the need for pregnant women and their advisers to be provided with adequate information. Referring what appear to be insurmountable differences between the parties to the courts constitutes recognition that there are certain decisions that, because of their inherently difficult nature, may not be suitable for resolution by the parties alone because of their multifaceted nature and because there are broader issues of public policy that may arise. A conflict between the patient and her midwife or doctor over the conduct of childbirth may in fact be well suited to the involvement of an independent arbiter. It also provides safeguards for the patient. There are dangers in low-visibility of 'hard case' treatment decisions as evidenced by the concern of the courts to be involved, for example, in sanctioning certain invasive procedures on adults (lacking mental capacity) such as sterilisation or decisions at the end of life.[62]

Nonetheless, these controversial Court of Appeal decisions leave many issues to be resolved, in particular around the interpretation of 'capacity' to decide. The test for capacity is decision-relative. The graver the consequences of the ultimate decision, the more careful the scrutiny given to the capacity of the patient to make that decision. This is inevitable. The more serious the consequences of the refusal, the more important it is to ensure that the patient possesses the necessary competence to make the treatment decision. It is also the case that as temporary incompetence may invalidate capacity, it is important to ensure that the notion of capacity is not manipulated to deny individual autonomy. Nurses and midwives as patient advocates are likely to play important roles in this process.

7.2.6   Consent and civil law liability: negligence

For a general discussion of the law of negligence, see Chapter 6. Obtaining a broad general consent to medical procedures being performed is sufficient to avoid liability in battery. But in addition, for a patient to give full and effective consent she must have some appreciation of the risks that the medical procedure in question may go wrong. If a patient is not informed of the risk of complications and if one or more of these complications arises, then she may bring an action in negligence. The basis of her claim is first that those who are treating her are under a duty to provide her with information about the risks of the treatment; secondly, that this duty has been broken; and thirdly, that she has suffered harm because had she known of the risk (which did in fact materialise) she would not have consented to the treatment.

The leading case is *Sidaway* v. *Bethlem Royal Hospital Governors*.[63] Mrs Sidaway underwent an operation after having suffered for some time from a recurring pain in her neck, right shoulder and arm. The operation was performed by a senior neurosurgeon at the Bethlem Royal Hospital. Even if the operation had been carried out with all due care and skill there was a 1% to 2% risk of damage to the nerve root and the spinal column. Although the risk of damage to the spinal column was less than that to the nerve root, the consequences were more severe. The plaintiff was left severely disabled after the operation. She brought an action in negligence claiming that she had not been given adequate warning of the risks of the operation. During the hearing it was revealed that while the surgeon had told her of the risks of damage to the nerve root he had not told her of the risks of damage to the spinal column. In acting in this way he was conforming to what in 1974 would have been accepted as standard medical practice by a responsible and skilled body of neurosurgeons. The House of Lords rejected the claim that the surgeon had acted negligently. An 'informed consent' approach was rejected by all the Law Lords – except Lord Scarman. Some support was given to the suggestion that the test that a court should use in deciding whether the advice given was negligent was the same as that used in deciding whether medical treatment was negligent – the *Bolam* test.[64] This test provides that a health care practitioner:

> is not guilty of negligence if he has acted in accordance with a practice accepted as proper by a responsible body of medical men.

This approach was followed by Lord Diplock in the House of Lords. This obligation of disclosure applies to all types of medical procedure. A broader approach was taken by Lord Bridge, who said that a judge could disagree with the evidence given to him:

I am of the opinion that the judge might in certain circumstances come to the conclusion that disclosure of a particular risk was so obviously necessary to an informed choice on the part of the patient that no reasonably prudent medical man would fail to make it.

He commented:

The kind of case I have in mind would be an operation involving a substantial risk of grave adverse consequences, as for example, [a] 10 per cent risk of stroke from the operation . . . In such a case, in the absence of some cogent clinical reason why the patient should not be informed, a doctor . . . could hardly fail to appreciate the necessity for an appropriate warning.

Where the risk of an adverse effect was slight or insignificant, the information could be withheld where this was an accepted practice within the community of medicine. The risks disclosed must be reasonably foreseeable. Lord Templeman distinguished between general risks that would normally be known to the patient and special risks that might be required to be disclosed. Lord Templeman stressed that it was for the court to decide whether the practitioner had acted negligently or not. No distinction is drawn between therapeutic and non-therapeutic forms of care.[65] While the courts have traditionally been hesitant to scrutinise the responsible body of professional practice in the years following *Sidaway*, one example of a case in which they did do so was *Smith* v. *Tunbridge Wells*.[66] Mr Smith, a 28-year-old married man with two children, suffered a rectal prolapse. Surgery was proposed and was undertaken. While the operation was successful, the plaintiff suffered nerve damage during surgery and was left impotent. He brought an action claiming that he should have been informed of the risk of impotence. His claim was upheld by Mr Justice Morland who stated:

In my judgment by 1988, although some surgeons may still not have been warning patients similar in situation to the plaintiff of the risk of impotence, that omission was neither reasonable nor responsible.

Until relatively recently this case could be regarded as very much the aberration. However, over the last few years there have been indications that the courts are prepared to scrutinise the body of professional practice, and we return to this a little later.

'Informed' consent

An alternative approach to the professional practice standard which has been adopted in a number of other countries such as Australia, Canada and the USA is that of 'informed consent'.[67] Several states in the USA now require a standard of disclosure based upon the information that a 'prudent patient' would expect to receive. In *Sidaway* Lord Scarman, who delivered a dissenting judgment,

supported this approach, saying that the patient should be given such information as a prudent patient would wish to know. While at that time the majority in
the House of Lords rejected such an approach, today, while the judiciary itself
has still not explicitly imposed such a standard, in practice there has definitely
been a move towards its adoption. Health care professionals are now being
directed to give patients more information about certain types of treatment. There
is a perceived need for enhanced frankness and openness by health care professionals. One of the issues emphasised in the debate around the unauthorised
retention of human material including organs at Alder Hey and at a number of
hospitals up and down the country has been the failure to obtain adequate consent from relatives for the retention of such material.[68] In clinical research, following the controversy of the Griffiths inquiry, the new governance approach now
emphasises the need for informed consent.[69] In the inquiry into the events at
Bristol Royal Infirmary, Professor Ian Kennedy and his team have suggested
a number of ways in which the provision of information could be improved.[70]
The report emphasises in Chapter 23 the need for 'respect and honesty' in health
care. An important message is the need for the health care professional–patient
relationship to be seen as one of partnership. Consent is also to be seen as a
process:

> Trust can be only sustained by openness. Secondly, openness means that
> information be given freely, honestly and regularly. Thirdly, it is of funda-
> mental importance to be honest about the twin concerns of risk and uncertainty.
> Lastly informing patients and in the case of young children their parents must
> be regarded as a process and not as a one-off event.[71]

The report recommends: 'Patients must be given such information as enables
them to participate in their care.' It suggests processes for improving the con-
veyance of information such as ensuring that information is evidence-based, and
that, importantly, 'information should be tailored to the needs, circumstances
and wishes of the individual'. Such an approach if it becomes current in medical
practice will surely represent a critical shift to a 'prudent patient' test. It is also
reflected in the GMC guidance *Seeking Patient Consent: The Ethical Considerations.*[72]

While professional practice seemed to become increasingly responsive to an
'informed consent' as opposed to 'professional practice standard', this issue was
not subject to scrutiny by the courts for several years. Gradually in the 1990s there
were judicial indications that they were prepared to question the 'professional
practice' standard of the *Bolam* test. The decision of the House of Lords in *Bolitho*
v. *City and Hackney HA* signalled a different approach.[73] In this case Lord Browne
Wilkinson stated that:

> if in a rare case, it can be demonstrated that professional opinion is not capable
> of withstanding logical analysis, the judge is entitled to hold that the body of
> opinion is not reasonable or responsible.[74]

Admittedly this judgment is limited in scope and, despite some suggestions
made at the time, it does not at all mean that the *Bolam* standard in negligence –
the standard of the responsible body of professional practice – is dead. In addi-

tion, these comments relate to diagnosis and treatment. *Bolitho* itself did not address the question of disclosure of risk. However, it may be indicative of an increasing judicial willingness to take a 'hard look' at the view expressed by a body of professional opinion in the future. The application of *Bolitho* to diagnosis and risk disclosure was considered in the decision of *Pearce* v. *United Bristol NHS Trust*.[75] Here the Court of Appeal looked at the decisions in *Bolitho* and in *Sidaway*. Lord Woolf held that:

> if there is a significant risk which would affect the judgement of a reasonable patient then in the normal course it is the responsibility of a doctor to inform the patient of that significant risk, if the information is needed so that the patient can determine for him or herself as to what course she should adopt.

On the facts of the case the woman was advised against a Caesarean section and the child was delivered stillborn. There was a small risk of 1 to 2 in 1000 that the child would be stillborn. The claimant was unable to establish that this was 'significant'. Nonetheless, although the claimant was unsuccessful in this particular case the judgment itself can be seen as another step towards a patient-based approach to consent to treatment.[76]

The movement towards judicial recognition of enhanced disclosure was recently confirmed by the House of Lords in *Chester* v. *Afshar*.[77] Miss Chester, who suffered back pain, consulted a rheumatologist. She was found to have a significant deterioration of the spinal discs. She was referred to Mr Afshar, a consultant neurosurgeon, who advised her that surgery was needed to remove three discs. Miss Chester asked Mr Afshar about the 'horror stories' of such operations. At trial there was a dispute as to the information that actually had been given. Mr Afshar stated that he had informed her that there was a small risk of lower spinal cord nerve root disturbance, haemorrhage and infection. However, Miss Chester stated that she had not been given this information but rather had been told by the consultant that he 'hadn't crippled anybody yet'. Miss Chester stated that if she had been given the information as to the risk of treatment she would not have gone ahead with the information at the time, and she would have sought further opinions as to the best course of treatment.

At trial Miss Chester's evidence was preferred. The trial judge held that 'the defendant's failure to advise the claimant adequately was negligent'. In the House of Lords the discussion fundamentally concerned the causation point, which is discussed below at page 134. However, there was consideration 'obiter' of the risk disclosure issue by Lord Steyn. Importantly, he cast the issue of disclosure in terms of 'autonomy'.

> A surgeon owes a legal duty to a patient to warn him or her in general terms of possible serious risks involved in the procedure. The only qualification is that there may be wholly exceptional cases where objectively in the best interests of the patient the surgeon may be excused from giving a warning. This is, however, irrelevant in the present case. In modern law medical paternalism no longer rules and a patient has a prima facie right to be informed by a surgeon of a small, but well established, risk of serious injury as a result of surgery.

Secondly, not all rights are equally important. But a patient's right to an appropriate warning from a surgeon when faced with surgery ought normatively to be regarded as an important right which must be given effective protection whenever possible.

Thirdly, in the context of attributing legal responsibility, it is necessary to identify precisely the protected legal interests at stake. A rule requiring a doctor to abstain from performing an operation without the informed consent of a patient serves two purposes. It tends to avoid the occurrence of the particular physical injury the risk of which a patient is not prepared to accept. It also ensures that due respect is given to the autonomy and dignity of each patient.[78]

The judgments in the Court of Appeal in *Pearce* and the House of Lords in *Chester* v. *Afshar* can be seen as a broad 'patient-centred approach'. It thus appears that it is likely to become increasingly difficult to justify withholding information regarding the risks of treatment from patients. This may also be reflective of the fact that there is a tendency towards enhanced disclosure today on a routine basis in health care and that in many cases the responsible body of professional practice is likely to favour broader disclosure. Nonetheless, it does not mean that all risks will require disclosure. In a subsequent case of *Al Hamwi* v. *Johnston and Another* the action failed.[79] The trial judge, Mr Justice Simon, drew a distinction between giving information and ensuring that the patient understood that information. He stated that it was 'too onerous' to impose on the doctor a duty to ensure that the patient understood the information that had been given.[80]

Therapeutic privilege

While in the majority of cases providing a patient with information about her treatment can be seen as a positive step enhancing her autonomy, there may be some situations in which those caring for her believe that information may be withheld under what is known as the 'therapeutic privilege' where this is in the best interests of the patient. In *Sidaway* Lord Templeman said:

> [S]ome information may confuse, other information may alarm a particular patient . . . the doctor must decide in the light of his training and experience and the light of knowledge of the patient what should be said and how it should be said.

The application of this principle may be questioned in the light of recent medical practice with the movement towards providing a patient with full information and also in respect of what appears to be enhanced judicial willingness to scrutinise the provision of information to patients. Certainly if a therapeutic privilege exception does exist it needs to be exercised with extreme caution.

The courts, as indicated above, appear to be increasingly prepared to scrutinise the standard of disclosure proffered by health care professionals. It may also be the case that in the future, should information be withheld from patients, claims will be brought under the Human Rights Act 1998. The trend is towards disclosure and this should be welcomed as part of the nurse's partnership in clinical practice with her patient. Cooperation rather than conflict will surely facilitate better patient care.

The questioning patient

The nurse may give the patient some explanation of the procedures and potential risks of their treatment but the patient may later approach the nurse and ask for further information. How should the nurse respond? In the House of Lords in *Sidaway* some of the members of the court indicated that there might be an obligation to provide a full reply if questions are asked. Lord Bridge said:

> [W]hen questioned specifically by a patient of apparently sound mind about the risks involved in a particular procedure proposed, the doctor's duty must, in my opinion be to answer both truthfully and as fully as the questioner requires.[81]

But these statements were obiter and not binding. Subsequently in *Blyth* v. *Bloomsbury AHA* (1987), Lord Justice Kerr said that there was no obligation to disclose all information when a question was asked; it was sufficient if the information given was that which would be given by a responsible body of medical practitioners – the *Bolam* test. He stressed that the response of health care professionals to the patient's questions should depend on factors such as the circumstances, the nature of the information, its reliability and relevance and the condition of the patient. That case was, however, decided in 1987 and needs now surely to be placed in its historical context: recent judicial statements indicate a move towards willingness to recognise an obligation to answer questions.[82] The DH have suggested:

> If information is offered and declined, it is good practice to record this fact in the notes. However it is possible that patients' wishes may change over time and it is important to provide opportunities for them to express this.[83]

The recommendation of Professor Ian Kennedy in the Bristol Infirmary Inquiry Final Report, emphasising that patients should be given the opportunity to ask questions and to seek clarification and more information, should be noted in this context.[84] Following the Bristol Inquiry Report the Department of Health issued a *Reference Guide to Consent for Examination and Treatment* (2001) and new model consent forms. The government in their response to the Bristol Inquiry Report have stated that they endorse this guidance and confirm the principle that consent is a process and that the principle of consent is applicable to all clinical procedures, not simply to surgery; and moreover that 'patients should be given sufficient information about what is to take place, the risks, the uncertainties and possible negative consequences of the proposed treatment, about any alternatives and about the likely outcome, to enable them to make a choice as to how to proceed'.[85] Such an approach suggests that failure to answer patients' questions today is unlikely to be supported by a responsible body of professional practice. Today, it is submitted, a nurse should consider very carefully indeed before she decides to withhold information from a questioning patient, and any refusal will require very clear justification.

Causation

Even if a patient can establish that she should have been given more information, that by itself is not sufficient for an action in negligence to succeed (Chapter 6). The patient must go on to show that the failure to provide information caused the harm suffered. The present test used by the courts is subjective: would the patient have chosen differently had she been given more information?[86] In practice a patient may find it very difficult to prove causation since in many cases they would have taken the decision to choose the treatment even if provided with more information. However, a recent case has led to a reconsideration of the approach to causation in the context of informed consent: whether if, had the risk been disclosed, the person would still have gone ahead with the operation. There was some consideration of this issue in the House of Lords in *Chester* v. *Afshar* discussed above at pages 131–132. Miss Chester was not informed of the risk. However, she did indicate that there was a possibility that had she been informed of the risk she would ultimately have decided to go ahead. The House of Lords still held that the failure to inform was negligent. The decision of the House of Lords followed the approach taken in the Australian case of *Chappel* v. *Hart*[87] in finding that disclosure here was necessary in order to safeguard the patient's autonomy. Lord Hope held that unless such an approach was taken it 'would render the duty useless in the cases where it is needed the most'. If Miss Chester's claim had been rejected the consequence would have been that those persons who admitted that they would still have gone ahead with the surgery were placed in a worse position than those who were less straightforward.[88]

7.3 Conflicts in disclosure

There has been considerable debate in nursing surrounding the concept of the nurse as patient advocate.[89] One part of the role of the nurse as advocate is in helping her patients to exercise their rights. The ability to make a free choice regarding one's treatment is perhaps one of the patient's most important rights. If the nurse is acting as a member of a health care team and she believes that the information given by a doctor in the team to a patient is insufficient, what should she do? Does the law require her to advocate for her patient? There is no express recognition in English law at present of the role of the nurse as patient advocate, but there may be situations in which she would be held liable for failure to disclose.

The nurse may decide not to participate in a clinical procedure on the grounds that the patient has been inadequately informed, or she may decide to provide the patient with more information herself. But in taking either step she risks disciplinary proceedings and ultimate dismissal for disobeying orders.[90] In addition, in deciding to go ahead and disclose, the nurse runs the risk that her assessment of the amount of information the patient requires may be wrong. What if the patient is unable to cope with the information given and suffers a nervous breakdown? An action may be brought against the nurse claiming that she was negligent in disclosure. Whether such an action would succeed would depend on the test employed by the court. It is submitted that a court would assess whether she had acted negligently in disclosing, by reference to a professional body of nursing opinion.

A nurse may protest to a doctor that a patient has not been given sufficient information, but on being told by the doctor to obey orders she may decide not to give the patient more information about treatment risks. But what if the treatment risk materialised and the patient suffered harm? Any negligence action for failure to provide adequate information would probably be brought against the doctor rather than the nurse. If an action was brought against the nurse it might not succeed. In the past the courts have held that as long as a nurse is following a doctor's orders she will not be held liable.[91] But with the development of the role of the nurse as an autonomous practitioner and as advocate for her patient, this situation may change. If such an action were brought, a court would have to consider whether in remaining silent she had acted in accordance with a responsible body of professional nursing opinion. It has been suggested that a nurse may be found liable if she undertakes a task under instructions that she believes to be 'manifestly wrong', following comments made by the House of Lords in *Junor* v. *McNichol*.[92] It is possible that participation in treatment of a patient who has not been told of a very high risk of death or serious injury would come within this category. However, this would presumably only arise in the most exceptional case.

7.4 Conclusions

The law in relation to consent to treatment is evolving. Notable recent developments are the inclusion of decision-making concerning adults lacking mental capacity within a statutory framework (the Mental Capacity Act 2005) which will come into force in April and October 2007, and the evolution of the law in the area of informed consent to a more overtly 'autonomy-based' approach. The law in this area poses considerable challenges for the nurse. The nurse must confront the same difficult questions of disclosure as her medical counterpart when treating the patient as a sole practitioner. Determining whether the patient possesses capacity and determining what risks should be disclosed will be assessments for the nurse as for her medical counterpart. The role of the nurse is complicated, however, by the fact that she may feel that she has a role to play as advocate for her patient. The role of nurse as patient advocate has not yet been recognised in law and it remains to be seen to what extent this position will change in the future. At present, fear of placing her job in jeopardy and the risk of legal liability may constrain the nurse to do little more than simply protest. But the mere fact of disagreement may prompt reconsideration of what information should be given to the patient, a continued debate which must in the long term be to the patient's advantage. It is also important to note that both professional and legal developments are progressing in favour of fuller, franker disclosure and enhanced respect for patient autonomy. But the legal process is simply the tip of the iceberg of clinical practice in the area of consent to treatment. Many of these decisions involve considerable degrees of assessment and discretion, as for example in the operation of the capacity test. Nurses have a vital role to play in the actualisation of the reality of respect for consent to treatment on the ward and in the community.

7.5 Notes and references

1. Nursing and Midwifery Council, *NMC Code of Professional Conduct: Standards for Conduct, Performance and Ethics* (London, NMC, 2004).
2. See generally on consent to treatment: M. Brazier, *Medicine, Patients and the Law*, 3rd edn (London, Penguin, 2003), chapters 4 and 5; J.K. Mason & G. Laurie, *Mason and McCall Smith's Law and Medical Ethics*, 7th edn (Oxford, Oxford University Press, 2005); E. Jackson, *Medical Law Text and Materials* (Oxford, Oxford University Press, 2006), chapters 4 and 5; and also *Reference Guide to Consent for Examination and Treatment* (London, Department of Health, 2001).
3. See, for example, E. Wicks, The right to refuse medical treatment under the European Convention on Human Rights, 8 Med LR 17 (2001).
4. See, for example, Chapters 9a, 10a and 12a in this book.
5. See further A. Grubb, Consent to treatment: the competent patient. In A. Grubb (ed), *Principles of Medical Law*, 2nd edn (Oxford, Oxford University Press, 2004). See also note 2 above.
6. J. Keown, The ashes of AIDS and the phoenix of informed consent, 52 Med LR 790 (1989).
7. General Medical Council, *Serious Communicable Diseases* (London, General Medical Council, 1997).
8. *Re T (adult: refusal of treatment)* [1992] 4 All ER 649.
9. See generally M. Gunn, The meaning of incapacity, 2 Med LR 8 (1994).
10. Grubb (1994), 2 Med LR1.
11. *Re F (mental patient sterilisation)* [1990] 2 AC 1.
12. [1991] 3 WLR 592.
13. [1992] 4 All ER 649.
14. [1997] 2 FLR 426.
15. (1997) Cm 3803.
16. (1999) Cm 4465. J.V. McHale, Mental Incapacity: some proposals for legislative reform, *Journal of Medical Ethics*, **24** (1998), p. 322.
17. Sections 9–11.
18. Section 3(4).
19. Department for Constitutional Affairs, *Mental Capacity Act Code of Practice* (London, TSO, 2007).
20. See *R* v. *Brown* [1993] 2 All ER 75.
21. Prohibition of Female Circumcision Act 1985, section 1.
22. This was suggested by Lord Edmund Davies in a statement made extra judicially – see *Proceedings of the Royal Society of Medicine*, **62** (1969), pp. 633–4.
23. See M. Fox & J. McHale, Xenotransplantation, 6 Med LR 42 (1998).
24. P.D.G. Skegg, *Law, Ethics and Medicine* (London, Clarendon Press, 1984), p. 32.
25. [1981] QB 432.
26. See the comments of Mr Justice Bristow in *Chatterton* v. *Gerson*, and M. Brazier, Patient autonomy and consent to treatment: the role of the law, *Legal Studies*, **7** (1987), p. 169.
27. *Devi* v. *West Midlands HA* (1981) (CA Transcript 491).
28. (1990) 67 DIR (4th) 321 (Ont CA).
29. *Re B (adult: refusal of medical treatment)* [2002] 2 All ER 449.

30. See discussion in E. Wicks, The right to refuse medical treatment under the European Convention on Human Rights. 8 Med LR 17 (2001), and J. McHale & A. Gallagher, *Nursing and Human Rights* (Oxford, Butterworth Heinemann, 2004).
31. See, for example, *Re L (medical treatment; Gillick competency)* [1998] 2 FLR 810.
32. [1998] 3 All ER 673.
33. [1984] QB 524.
34. [1992] 4 All ER 671.
35. See further C v. S [1988] QB 135, and *Paton v. British Pregnancy Advisory Service* [1978] 2 All ER 987.
36. [1990] 573 A 2d 1235.
37. See further I. Kennedy, A woman and her unborn child; rights and responsibilities. In P. Byrne (ed), *Ethics and Law in Health Care and Research* (Chichester, John Wiley, 1990).
38. See discussion in I. Kennedy & A. Grubb, *Medical Law* (Oxford, Oxford University Press, 2000).
39. In *AC* itself an enforced Caesarean was rejected. The court did indicate that they may be used in suitable cases and mentioned a court decision very similar to *Re S*. However, they did not express an opinion on that case.
40. Royal College of Obstetricians and Gynaecologists, *A Consideration of the Law and Ethics in Relation to Court-Authorised Obstetric Interventions* (1994), and see also the revisions in *Supplement to a Consideration of the Law and Ethics in Relation to Court-Authorised Obstetric Interventions* (RCOG, 1996).
41. *Rochdale NHS Trust v. C* [1997]; *Norfolk & Norwich NHS Trust v. W* [1996] 2 FLR 613.
42. [1997] 2 FLR
43. It was suggested that anaesthetic should be given through a mask, but when the risks of this procedure – namely that there was a possibility that a patient on whom this procedure is used might regurgitate and inhale the contents of her stomach – were explained to her, consent was refused; [1997] FLR 426 at pp. 436–7.
44. Reference was made to the statement of Lord Justice Goff in *Collins v. Wilcock* [1984] 1 WLR 1172 as approved in *Re F* [1990] 1 AC 1, the judgment of Lord Templeman in *Sidaway v. Bethlem Hospital Governors* [1985] AC 871 at pp. 904–5 and Lord Donaldson in *Re T (an adult refusal to consent to medical treatment)* [1992] 4 All ER 649 CA.
45. I. Kennedy, A woman and her unborn child: rights and responsibilities. In P. Byrne (ed.), *Ethics and Law in Health Care and Research* (Chichester, John Wiley, 1990).
46. See *Bolam v. Friern Hospital Management Company* [1957] 2 All ER 118.
47. See, for example, P. Fennel, Inscribing paternalism in law: consent to treatment and mental disorder, *Journal of Law and Society*, **29** (1990).
48. See, for example, A. Grubb & D. Pearl, Sterilisation – courts and doctors as decision makers. CLJ 380, and Law Commission (1995), *Mental Incapacity* (London, The Stationery Office, 1989). See also now *Re SL (Adult Patient Medical Treatment)* [2001] 2 FCR 452.
49. [1997] 2 FLR 439.
50. See, for example, *Airedale NHS Trust v. Bland* [1993] AC 879, *Re R* [1996] 2 FLR 99.
51. [1988] Fam 122.
52. [1979] QB 276.
53. [1997] 2 FLR 441.
54. [1997] 2 FLR 439.
55. *Consent to Treatment*, NHS EL (97), 32. See also *Good Practice in Consent*, NHS HSC, 2001/023.
56. See also A. Grubb, Treatment without consent: pregnancy (adult). *Medical Law Review* **191** (1996).
57. [1995] 1 All ER 683.

58. See further discussion in Chapter 9A in this book.
59. [1998] 3 All ER 673.
60. Reference was made to the judgment of Lord Mustill in *Airedale NHS Trust* v. *Bland* and to Lord Reid in *S* v. *Mc* [1972] AC 24.
61. R. Bailey Harris, Pregnancy, autonomy and refusal of medical treatment. *Law Quarterly Review*, **550** (1998), p. 554.
62. For example, *Re B* [1987] 2 All ER 206 and the discussion in the Law Commission Report *Mental Incapacity* as to the involvement of judicial scrutiny of such treatment decisions, e.g. Part VI of the Report.
63. *Sidaway* v. *Bethlem Royal Hospital Governors* [1985] 2 WLR 503.
64. See *Bolam* v. *Friern Hospital Management Committee* [1957] 2 All ER 118.
65. *Gold* v. *Haringey Health Authority* [1987] 2 All ER 888.
66. [1994] 5 Med LR 334.
67. See, for example, in the context of Australia *Rogers* v. *Whittaker* ([1993] 4 Med LR 79 and Canada *Reibl* v. *Hughes* (1980) 114 DLR (3d) 1; also see A. Maclean, The doctrine of informed consent: does it exist and has it crossed the Atlantic?, *Legal Studies*, **24** (2004), 386.
68. *Report of the Inquiry into the Royal Liverpool Children's Hospital (Alder Hey)* (2001) http://www.rclinquiry.org.uk and *Bristol Inquiry Interim Report Removal and Retention of Human Material* (2000) http://www.bristol-inquiry.org.uk
69. *Report of the Review into the Research Framework at North Staffordshire* http://www.doh.gov.uk/wmro/northstaffs.htm and see Chapter 12A in this book.
70. See discussion in A. Gallagher & J. McHale, After Bristol: the importance of Informed Consent, *Nursing Times* **97** (2001), p. 32.
71. Bristol Royal Infirmary Final Report, p. 286.
72. General Medical Council, London, 1999.
73. [1997] 3 WLR 1151.
74. [1997] 3 WLR 1151.
75. [1999] PIQR P53. (CA) and see further M. Jones, Informed consent and fairy stories, *Medical Law Review*, **7** (1999), p. 103.
76. See further the discussion of this issue by A. Grubb, 7 Med LR 61 (1997).
77. [2005] 1 AC 234.
78. *Ibid*. Paras 16–18.
79. [2005] E.W.H.C. 206.
80. See further J. Miola, Autonomy rued OK? *Al Hamwi* v. *Johnston and Another*, *Medical Law Review*, **14** (2006), p. 108.
81.
82. For example, *Pearce* v. *United Bristol Healthcare NHS Trust* (1998) 48 BMCR 118 CA.
83. Department of Health, *Reference Guide to Consent for Examination and Treatment* (2001), para. 5.6.
84. Bristol Royal Infirmary Final Report (2001), chapter 23.
85. *Learning from Bristol: The Department of Health's Response to the Report of the Public Inquiry into Children's Heart Surgery at Bristol Royal Infirmary 1984–1995*. Cm 5363 (2002), pp. 139–40.
86. See *Chatterton* v. *Gerson* [1981] QB 432.
87. [1998] HCA 55.
88. For criticism of this case see M. Stauch, Causation and confusion in respect of medical non-disclosure, *Nottingham Law Journal*, **14** (2005), p. 66.
89. See generally G.R. Winslow, From loyalty to advocacy: a new metaphor for nursing, *Hastings Centre Report*, **32** (1984); E.W. Bernal, The nurse as patient advocate, *Hastings Centre Report*, **33** (1992).

90. See further as to the extent of the obligation of a nurse to obey a doctor's instructions, J. Montgomery, Doctors' handmaidens: the legal contribution. In S. McVeigh & S. Wheelar (eds), *Law and Medical Regulation* (Dartmouth, Aldershot, 1993).
91. *Pickering* v. *Governors of United Leeds Hospitals* (1954).
92. [1959], *The Times*, 26 March, House of Lords.

B   An Ethical Perspective – Consent and Patient Autonomy

Bobbie Farsides

Consent is a moral and legal cornerstone of contemporary health care. Interventions that proceed without the consent of the patient immediately require moral scrutiny, and even where it is claimed that consent has been given we want to ensure that this means much more than the mere fact that a form has been signed. It is important to show that far from being a protective mechanism for health care professionals, the primary role of consent is to protect patients, and particularly to protect their status as autonomous individuals who have an interest in remaining in control of their own lives.

In part A of this chapter, Jean McHale has given a very full account of consent in a legal context. However, she and other medical lawyers are quick to point out that the standards set by law are not necessarily those we would wish to reach through ethical argument. Nor indeed might the legally focused reasons for acquiring consent fully reveal why we consider it to be ethically important. In ethical terms consent is important because it demonstrates respect for autonomy, it protects the autonomous individual from certain harms, and through participating in a consent process the person's autonomy may be further enhanced.[1]

Autonomy is both a prerequisite for consent and a product of it. It is also representative of a relationship between a patient and a health care professional that is contractual rather than hierarchical, egalitarian rather than paternalistic, and patient-centred rather than medically determined. Consent, when properly conceived, will look something like the concept defined by Raanon Gillon in his book *Philosophical Medical Ethics*:[2]

> a voluntary un-coerced decision made by a sufficiently autonomous person on the basis of adequate information to accept or reject some proposed course of action that will affect him or her.

This definition offers what we might call a paradigm case or ideal type model, but Gillon is confident that it can be embraced by health care professionals and translated into practice. For this to happen, the health care professional must adopt a particular attitude to patients, and take seriously the duties implied by the definition.

7.6 Voluntariness, coercion and consent

Consent, Gillon tells us, is a 'voluntary and un-coerced decision'. By making this explicit he is not implying that health care professionals are in the business of directly coercing patients or forcing them into involuntary choices, but rather that the context within which decisions are made might not always enhance the voluntariness of the decision, and might sometimes be coercive. Furthermore the broader context within which the patient operates might have limiting effects of which the health care professional should be aware.

By definition patients have concerns about their health, and despite greater access to medical information the health care professional is still the expert upon whom they depend. Hospitals can be intimidating and alien environments within which people are stripped of many of their usual props, and where those aspects of their identity that give them confidence can be undermined. The sense of health care as a scarce resource might also have an impact, with individuals worrying about the consequences of their actions upon how and when they will be treated.

In broader terms patients do not shed their other social identities when they enter the hospital setting. For some individuals their ability to consent may be compromised by their position within their cultural group. For example, women within certain cultures might have the capacity to consent, but would not expect to have the right to determine what happens to them owing to cultural norms and expectations. Individual women might therefore be unpractised in exercising choices of the type involved in consenting within a health care setting.[3] This could pose difficulties when they are faced with difficult choices such as whether to accept an offer of pre-natal screening for genetically inherited diseases common among their ethnic group.[4]

It is of course important to avoid stereotypical assumptions and to determine in the particular case whether an individual is subject to such pressure. However, particularly in situations where consent is being discussed through an interpreter, it is important to explore whether a patient is being allowed to make a voluntary decision, or whether he or she is subject to coercive influences, be they overt or subtle.

7.7 Consent and autonomy

According to Gillon's definition, consent is the domain of 'sufficiently autonomous people'. This immediately affords us a class of patients unable to consent, but it also allows for less clear-cut cases where a person's autonomy might be compromised or undeveloped, but the question remains as to whether they are sufficiently autonomous to operate in the current situation. It also raises the profoundly important question of what to do in the absence of sufficient autonomy.

Autonomy is a fundamentally significant concept in Anglo-American bioethics, and the importance of respecting patient autonomy is clearly highlighted in the codes of ethics governing the main health care professions. There are many reasons why autonomy has become such a dominant concept – some historical, some cultural, and some to do with the success of particular models of analysis within bioethics.

In the latter part of the twentieth century an emphasis on individual autonomy sat happily with the prevailing political ethos that saw the breakdown of traditional socialism and communism, and a wide-scale shift towards market-driven libertarianism. In a political climate that favoured individualism over collectivism and personal effort over state welfare, it is hardly surprising that autonomy was what the advertising executives call a positive buzz word. The dominance of northern European and American culture with its emphasis on such notions as privacy, individual initiative and consumerism led to the individual being appealed to and represented in most areas of life as a potential exerciser of choice. To be autonomous was to fit into the picture of what it meant to be an effective and successful member of society.[5]

In terms of professional culture, within the health service the pendulum had swung against medical paternalism, and a general attack on the medical model of care led to a recharacterisation of the classic relationship between doctor and patient, and doctor and nurse. Instead of the all-powerful doctor and his hand-maid [sic] the nurse ministering to the sick patient, the relationship between carers and patient was now presented as a contractual model with each party having rights and duties. The patient became the client, and in some senses at least became indistinguishable from any other type of consumer. The nurse was encouraged to develop her own professional autonomy and where necessary act to promote that of the patient if it was under threat from the doctor.[6]

Given its high profile within both academic and professional literature, it is important to be clear about what one means by the term autonomy and what one assumes is involved in paying it due respect. To quote Beauchamp and Childress, 'respect for the autonomous choices of other persons runs as deep in common morality as any principle, but little agreement exists about its nature and strength or about specific rights of autonomy'.[7]

Here are just a few frequently quoted accounts of what it means to be autonomous, demonstrating the range of ideas theorists have seen in the concept:

'I am autonomous if I rule me and no one else rules I.'[8]

'A person is autonomous to the degree that what he thinks and does cannot be explained without reference to his own activity of mind.'[9]

'[A]cting autonomously is acting from principles that we would consent to as free and equal rational beings.'[10]

'I and I alone am ultimately responsible for the decisions I make and am in that sense autonomous.'[11]

The word 'autonomy' is derived from the Greek *autos* and *nomia*, and means self-rule. Most definitions remain true to this root, and include ideas of self-governance, sovereignty, control and quite often independence. To be autonomous is to be in control of your life in a very particular way, referring as it does to rationality as opposed to mere freedom. Responsibility is quite appropriately seen as a closely related concept and the autonomous person may be free or unfree to act upon their autonomous choices, but in doing so must accept some responsibility for the consequences.[12] More extreme definitions sometimes appear to suggest that one can only enjoy full autonomy if the choices one makes are completely unaffected by others. However, this is not the only way to think about autonomy, and more recently theorists have attempted to offer definitions that do not commit them to the substantive independence seen as necessary by many of the philosophers quoted above.

Gerald Dworkin, who quotes all the preceding definitions in his own work, characterises autonomy as 'the capacity of a person critically to reflect upon, and then attempt to accept or change his or her preferences, desires, values and ideals'.[13] To explain himself more fully he states:

> Putting the various pieces together, autonomy is conceived of as a second-order capacity of persons to reflect critically upon their first-order preferences, desires, wishes, and so forth and the capacity to accept or attempt to change these in the light of higher-order preferences and values. By exercising such a capacity, persons define their nature, give meaning to their lives and take responsibility for the kind of person they are. (p. 20)

Despite the variety in these definitions it is possible to glean the essence of the concept, and it is obvious that valuing and respecting autonomy entail respecting the person's right to give or withhold their consent to interventions that will affect them. By participating in the consenting process the autonomous person has the opportunity to judge the choice within the larger context of their life, goals and projects and make a decision consistent with the values they hold and the path they wish to pursue.

7.7.1 Sufficient autonomy to consent

By making the criterion 'sufficiently autonomous' Gillon demands that we judge the capacity of an individual to act autonomously in a given situation, rather than label groups and individuals capable of giving consent or otherwise. This is consistent with the approach advocated in law. Instead of making stereotypical assumptions that might lead us to classify some types of people as non-autonomous, we have to judge the capacity of individuals to make particular decisions and choices. And it is important to remember that the Mental Capacity Act requires us to start from an assumption of capacity and puts the onus upon professionals to demonstrate that capacity is lacking if they wish to deem the patient incompetent to make a particular decision. This is not to deny that some human beings fall outside the category of competent autonomous being, examples being the fetus, the neonate and the person in a persistent vegetative state.[14]

However, we now know that groups such as children[15] and the cognitively impaired benefit from closer attention and careful discrimination between individuals, and it is incumbent upon those dealing with these groups to judge each individual in relation to the capacity required in a particular situation.[16] People with quite severe learning disabilities or mental health problems could be seen as autonomous in certain respects and circumstances, and therefore able to give or withhold their consent.

In some types of case there will be heated debate over the extent to which people can be autonomous and thereby capable of consenting. Examples differ in kind but might include people with eating disorders or people with non-mainstream religious views such as the Jehovah's Witness cited in part A of this chapter. In the first case there may be a real difficulty in ascertaining the extent to which the underlying illness affects a person's autonomy, but the fact that it is an illness rather than a chosen way of life will be seen to make a difference. Just as the substance abuser's or alcoholic's first-order desire for their drug impairs their autonomy, the person with an eating disorder is disproportionately determined by the relationship they have with food. Having said this, it is important to remember that even those who find aspects of their life dominated by illness or addiction might remain capable of making autonomous choices in other areas of their life. One of the reasons that respect for autonomy and the prioritising of consent are seen as important in the context of health care delivery is that both are seen as a corrective for paternalistic attitudes. Whereas I have referred to autonomy as a positive buzz word, paternalism is often treated as a bioethical example of a dirty word. However, paternalism can be understood in a number of ways and it is at least possible to argue that some forms of paternalism are morally acceptable in certain circumstances. Hard paternalism is defined as acting or choosing on another's behalf because you feel qualified to do so, and because you believe it to be in their best interest that you do so irrespective of their past or future consent, and irrespective of their belief that they are perfectly able to act on their own behalf. Such paternalism is difficult to justify, and by underlining the importance of acquiring consent even in difficult circumstances we protect against paternalistic practices of this type being widespread.

Soft paternalism on the other hand involves acting on another's behalf and in their best interest because you believe them to be temporarily unable to exercise their autonomy, which could translate into a temporary inability to participate in the consenting process. In such cases one might protect against the unacceptable excesses of paternalism by introducing another notion of consent often referred to as hypothetical consent. In such a case one might choose in the patient's best interest and with reference to ideas about what they might or might not consent to were they able to participate. Thus we intervene only because we consider them to be unable to consent for themselves, and in deciding for them we attempt to make a choice that they will ultimately accept.

The nursing profession has played a significant role in challenging anachronistic models of medical intervention that were particularly prone to hard paternalism. However, in recent years it has become clear that some patients find the burdens associated with non-paternalistic models of health care quite difficult to bear. It is also true that in certain areas of medicine practices that were seen as paternalistic have been replaced with very different practices that may nonetheless be open to the same description. One could think of provision of information: where in the past the paternalist was understood to withhold painful truths in the interest of not upsetting the patient, now some would claim that we impose painful truths on some patients who would 'rather not know' because we feel it is better for them to do so.

7.7.2 Insufficient autonomy to consent

The question of how to proceed morally in the absence of consent is a difficult one. Now at least the legal position is clear and we have the power to appoint a medical proxy to make decisions on our behalf when we are no longer able to do so.[17] However, proxy consent is not unproblematic: for example, one has to decide how to decide for another. One option is to attempt to choose as you believe the person would have done had they been able to do so, often referred to as substituted judgement. This route was not advocated in the legislation; instead the proxy is advised to choose in the person's best interest. Naturally the hope is that the proxy will adopt a broad concept of best interest that will go beyond the physical needs of the patient to also address and incorporate some sense of what would be in keeping with the person's values and preferences.

As discussed earlier in the chapter, the Mental Capacity Act also clarifies the law regarding advance statements. However, even when their legal status remained ambiguous, the ethical principles behind such documents were clear, in that they attempt to allow an individual to give or withhold consent at a point at which their lack of capacity would usually exclude them. In practical terms they are a form of treatment refusal, and in order to ensure their legal validity they need to be carefully drawn up to adequately capture the context within which they could be used. One of the criticisms levelled at very medically oriented advance statements is that their enforcement is dependent on the patient finding themselves in the clinical situations they have anticipated. In response to this some end-of-life care projects have begun to work with rather different types of document that concentrate more on the issue of values, goals and priorities that the patient would wish to see reflected in the decisions made on their behalf.

Another important advance decision relates to the donation of organs after death, and a patient may have clearly stated their wish to donate and taken the trouble to register those wishes with the appropriate bodies and individuals. Recent changes in the law will ensure that these decisions cannot be overridden by relatives as has been the case in the past, and will thereby strengthen further the individual's ability to consent in advance to actions that will take place when they are no longer competent to make or enact their decisions.

7.7.3 Sufficient information

As clearly stated in Gillon's definition, the moral and legal requirement to acquire consent commits the health care professional to provide sufficient information to allow that consent to be given; therefore the room for negotiation is sometimes limited. However, as I began to suggest above when discussing paternalism, there are contexts within which the autonomous patient must be allowed to determine the amount of information they are given. On the issue of prognosis, for example, a health care professional might have good reason to assume that it is in the interests of the patient to know their predicted future, but it would be difficult to justify imposing the information upon an autonomous individual who has clearly stated that they do not wish to know.[19] Thus the autonomy of the patient and the need to respect this might have to trump the health care professional's commitment to fuller disclosure and their own beliefs about what is in the patient's best interest. Just as Jean McHale requires the nurse to justify withholding information, the nurse must also have valid reasons for imparting information that the competent patient does not wish to receive.[20]

The term 'adequate information' calls for judgement to be applied, and since at least the early 1990s there has been a great deal of debate around the issue of what counts as sufficient, with some commentators suggesting that the standards required in some contexts force doctors to be 'needlessly cruel' in imposing information upon people.[21] One area of concern relates to clinical experimentation, where we have come to believe that the information sufficient for consent must be particularly detailed. As a research nurse will often be the person involved in the process of providing information and acquiring consent, she must contribute to the complex decisions about how much information is sufficient, and when more information is unnecessary and may even be harmful.[22]

7.8 Deliberation

The requirement that a patient should have the time and opportunity to deliberate before making a choice seems common sense. Health care choices often have far-reaching effects, some of which will only become apparent upon reflection. Even in the most straightforward of decisions a patient would probably benefit from believing that they had been given time to decide rather than being rushed into a decision. Admittedly there will be emergency situations in which this will not be possible. For example, if an event occurs within childbirth that threatens the safety of the woman and the unborn child, a decision might have to be made with great haste. Furthermore, the practicalities of outpatient clinics might determine that certain choices need to be discussed and decided on in the course of one visit. However, generally speaking, time should be allowed for the patient to absorb the information given and think about the choice they might want to make. This could be particularly true, for example, when someone is faced with choices soon after receiving bad news. Many oncologists claim that once a patient has been given a cancer diagnosis little of what is said in the remainder of the consultation is heard, let alone taken in. Therefore to ensure that consent can be given to any treatment proposed, it seems particularly important to handle carefully the transition between the initial information about disease status and later discussion about treatment choices. Specialist nurses have an important role to play in such situations, and their experience will enable them to judge how to pace the information given and how to judge what the patient has heard and understood.

7.9 The right to refuse or accept

It could be argued that many health care professionals perceive consent as relatively unproblematic as long as people make the choices they expect them to make. However, it should be allowed that an autonomous patient might choose not to follow medical or nursing advice, hence Gillon's requirement that we acknowledge a right to accept and a right to refuse. Some refusals will be the product of misinformation, ignorance or cognitive impairment, but many will be the result of a difference of opinion or belief between the patient or patient's guardian, and the health care professional.

The reasons for the difference could differ. Some people might attach themselves willingly and strongly to cultural or spiritual/religious beliefs that place them under particular moral obligations, which in turn means that they accept a certain loss of control over their choices without necessarily losing their autonomy. So, for example, a devout Catholic might refuse an offer of antenatal screening for Down's syndrome because she knows that her beliefs exclude the possibility of terminating the pregnancy. Others might have very particular views about how they want their life to be shaped, and particularly how they want it to end, and they would make their choices consistent with these goals and standards, possibly even refusing life-saving treatments.

In the case of the person with religious views, the situation is complicated by the fact that we sometimes have a very narrow conception of the types of choices autonomous people make, and the types of belief that they can acceptably attach themselves to. We seem to have little difficulty in allowing some religions to determine the choices people make for themselves, yet in other cases we find the beliefs and consequent choices more difficult to accept. For example, a professional might allow that a devout Catholic would choose to risk a life-threatening tenth pregnancy rather than use contraceptives, whereas the same person might find it more difficult to accept a Jehovah's Witness's rejection of a life-saving blood transfusion. It could be argued that the difference here is not between the choices being made, both of which could have devastating effects, but in our attitude to the two bodies of faith, one of which is considered mainstream and acceptable, the other less so.[23]

In fact it could be argued that the perceived difference between these cases is the result of mere prejudice, given the equivalence of the consequences. Given this danger, it is worth remembering that one obstacle to respecting the autonomy of others and their right to refuse might be the fact that we operate in an ideological context that is quick to define ideas outside the mainstream as inappropriate subjects of rational choice.

Hence the need to combine a commitment to respect for autonomy and the valuing of consent with a commitment to tolerance, that is a willingness to accept that people will make choices we find unacceptable. For as long as these choices do not entail an unacceptable degree of harm to others we are obliged to accept what they choose and the reasons they give for doing so. The dilemmas we might face as a result of this are real, particularly when we see the demand that we should respect a patient's autonomy conflicting with the beneficently motivated duty of care we believe we have towards them.

7.10 The consent process: translating theory into practice

To translate a theoretical commitment to respect for autonomy into a practical reality requires that a nurse acquire certain skills and accept a responsibility to practise them. Given the contact the nurse has with patients and the situations within which they meet and interact, the nurse will be required at different times to assess competence and voluntariness and autonomy, enhance it where it is lacking, respect it where it is present, and find ways of promoting the patient's best interests and well-being where it is not present. The nurse will be a significant provider of information, and will often be best placed to judge the extent to which the patient has understood, digested and deliberated upon it. The nurse is often a key figure in the consenting process. Her involvement will require her to engage in a number of different types of activity and utilise a variety of skills. This is even more true since the advent of Nurse Consultants and Specialist Nurse Practitioners.

7.10.1 Communication

One of the prerequisites to acquiring a morally and legally valid consent is to communicate effectively with the patient and their family. Only by doing so will you understand them as an individual, and learn enough about the context from which they have come to the health care setting. Communication is a two-sided exercise. On the one hand, one needs to establish how the individual is coping with being in the health care setting, and what they hope to gain from their contact with health care professionals – this involves asking and listening. On the other hand, information needs to be effectively and appropriately communicated to the patient – this involves listening and then telling. It is also important to recognise the importance of good communication within the multi-professional team caring for the patient.

7.10.2 Cultural literacy

Given the earlier claims about the extent to which a person's autonomy might be compromised or simply overlooked as a result of their cultural context, there are important reasons for nurses to understand the cultural context within which they operate and the beliefs and practices of the different groups they live alongside. Cultural differences must be respected; however, tolerance and understanding do not necessarily commit one to permitting all choices because they are defended as culturally significant.[24] So, for example, the apparent willingness of a female minor to undergo circumcision and the clear wish of her parents that she should do so would not be sufficient reason for a UK-based health care professional to offer this procedure.

7.10.3 Clinical knowledge-base

Given the contemporary commitment to evidence-based practice, the nurse should be aware of what has been shown to be good practice in her field. The information that informs her own work should then be shared with patients in a manner that will assist in their decision-making. However, there might be situations in which the nurse's understanding of the situation will differ from the view offered to the patient by others involved in his or her care. In such cases it is important that these differences are resolved between the professionals, so that the patient is not given conflicting or contradictory messages.

7.10.4 Support

The nurse has an important supportive role in helping those who are unable or unwilling to engage in the consenting process. This might entail acting as the patient's advocate or supporting the person who has been appointed to this role, or it might often entail facilitating the patient in getting their own views heard, sometimes in situations where the patient is in conflict with both their family members and other professionals. To perform this role effectively the nurse will need to develop and enhance her own professional autonomy, and thereby increase her power to represent the patient's view to her medical colleagues. Thus her individual responsibility to a patient may feed in to a bigger professional and political issue.

When supporting a patient in this way the nurse needs to be non-judgemental and willing to convey views that may be very counter to her own and decisions that she may consider unwise and maybe even harmful.

One of the difficult balances to strike in such situations is that between being non-directive, which is seen as a good thing, and unsupportive, which is not. One of the most difficult questions a health care professional can face in such a situation is when the patient asks, 'What would you do nurse?' There is no easy way to say how one should respond. On the one hand to say what you the nurse would do is not strictly relevant and may even be counterproductive, but on the other hand it is an appeal to your expertise and knowledge to which you would feel some need to respond.[25]

7.11 Conclusion

The nursing profession has a valuable contribution to make in ensuring that patients understand the significance of the consent they are asked for, and the obstacles that might lie in the way of their giving it. Individual nurses can help patients to exercise their autonomy, and provide them with the information they need to make choices consistent with their interests and goals. They can support their patients in what is often an alien and intimidating environment, and where necessary can act as their advocates. The nursing profession should continue to challenge those aspects of the health care delivery system that work against the patient body being able to participate meaningfully in the decision-making processes that affect their care.

7.12 Notes and references

1. T. Beauchamp & J. Childress, *Principles of Biomedical Ethics*, 5th edn (Oxford, Oxford University Press, 2001).

2. R. Gillon, *Philosophical Medical Ethics* (Chichester, John Wiley and Sons, 1985; reprinted 1996), p. 113.
3. See T. Cullinan, 'Other societies have different concepts of autonomy', letter to the *BMJ*, republished in Len Doyal and Jeffrey S. Tobias (eds), *Informed Consent in Medical Research* (London, BMJ Books, 2001).
4. Rena Rapp, Testing women, testing fetuses, and Susan Wolf, Erasing difference: race, ethnicity and gender in bioethics. In Anne Donchin & Laura Purdy, *Embodying Bioethics: Recent Feminist Advances* (Lanham, MD, Rowman and Littlefield, 1999).
5. See C. Farsides, Autonomy and its implications for palliative care: a northern European perspective, *Palliative Medicine*, **12** (1998), pp. 147–51.
6. C. Farsides, Autonomy and responsibility in midwifery. In S. Budd & U. Sharma (eds), *The Healing Bond* (London, Routledge, 1994).
7. T. Beauchamp & J. Childress, *Principles of Biomedical Ethics*, 5th edn (Oxford, Oxford University Press, 2001).
8. Joel Feinberg, The idea of a free man. In R.F. Dearden (ed.), *Education and the Development of Reason* (London, Routledge and Kegan Paul, 1972), p. 30.
9. R.F. Dearden, Autonomy and education. In R.F. Dearden (ed.), *Education and the Development of Reason* (London, Routledge and Kegan Paul, 1972), p. 453.
10. John Rawls, *A Theory of Justice* (Cambridge, MA, Harvard University Press, 1971), p. 516.
11. J.L. Lucas, *Principles of Politics* (Oxford, Oxford University Press, 1966), p. 101.
12. B. Farsides, in S. Budd & U. Sharma (eds), *The Healing Bond* (London, Routledge, 1994).
13. G. Dworkin, *The Theory and Practice of Autonomy* (Cambridge, Cambridge University Press, 1989).
14. J. Harris, *The Value of Life* (London, Routledge, 1985).
15. P. Alderson, In the genes or in the stars? Children's competence to consent, *Journal of Medical Ethics*, **18** (1992), pp. 119–24.
16. A.E. Buchanan & D.W. Brock, *Deciding for Others: The Ethics of Surrogate Decision Making* (Cambridge, Cambridge University Press, 1989).
17. See British Medical Association Ethics Committee, *Consent, Rights and Choices in Health Care for Children and Young People* (London, BMA, December 2000). See also Department of Health, *Consent: What You Have a Right to Expect – A Guide for Children and Young People*, available at http://www.dh.gov.uk/assetRoot/04/11/69/03/04116903.pdf
18. See Chapter 7A in this book and also B. Dimond, Legal aspects of consent 4: the duty to inform patients of risks, *British Journal of Nursing*, **10** (8) (April/May 2001), pp. 544–5.
19. J. Jackson, *Truth Trust and Medicine* (London, Routledge, 2001), esp. chapter 9, pp. 130–46.
20. See Chapter 7A in this book on omitting information.
21. J. Tobias & R. Souhami, Fully informed consent can be needlessly cruel, *British Medical Journal*, **307** (1993), pp. 1199–201, reproduced in L. Doyal and J.S. Tobias, *Informed Consent in Medical Research* (London, BMJ Books, 2001).
22. See R. Buckman, *How to Break Bad News* (London, Pan Books, 1994), esp. chapter 4.
23. For an interesting discussion of this issue see Des Autels *et al.*, *Praying for a Cure: When Medical and Religious Practice Conflict* (Lanham, MD, Rowman and Littlefield Publishers Inc., 1999).
24. See R. Macklin, Against Relativism: Cultural Diversity and the Search for Ethical Universals in Medicine (Oxford, Oxford University Press, 1999), chapters 1–5; also David Heyd (ed.), *Toleration An Elusive Virtue* (Bognor Regis, Princeton, 1996).
25. C. Williams, P. Alderson & B. Farsides, Is non-directiveness possible within the context of antenatal screening and testing?, *Social Science & Medicine*, **54** (2002), pp. 339–47.

8 Responsibility, Liability and Scarce Resources

A   The Legal Perspective

Robert Lee

Arguments rage about the availability of resources for health care. In spite of government claims regarding additional resources and falling waiting times within the NHS, it is apparent that delivery of medical services takes place in a climate of resource constraint. Since its establishment in 1948, the NHS has been described as resembling a 'monument to institutionalised scarcity'.[1] In the light of the government's continued commitment to the provision of health services, the issue of NHS rationing finds itself high on the political agenda. As with a number of publicly funded services, NHS rationing centres on the restriction of supply by cost factors, coupled with increasing demand that is not curtailed by price.[2] A range of policy instruments, such as those generated by the National Institute for Health and Clinical Excellence (NICE), impose explicit restrictions on the delivery of services and treatments offered by the NHS. The limited allocation of resources raises interesting questions about the role of the judiciary in reviewing decisions taken by health practitioners.

There are a number of cases in which the courts have had to consider the level of resources made available by a National Health Trust. On the whole these cases, which often concern the denial or delay of life-saving treatment,[3] are beyond the scope of this chapter if only because such resource decisions are made at a senior management level rather than involving questions of the day-to-day issues of the responsibility of nurses. It can be lawful for a trust to refuse to fund certain forms of treatment,[4] but even then the trust might allow for exceptional circumstances that could justify making such treatment available. These issues arose in the litigation concerning the availability of herceptin for early-stage breast cancer – *R*

(*Rogers*) v. *Swindon Primary Care Trust*.[5] In that case, the Court of Appeal held that it was open to the Trust to decide not to support treatment with the unlicensed herceptin for early stage breast cancer, but having said that funding was irrelevant, any policy to treat with the drug could not be arbitrary or irrational. The policy adopted was found to be irrational, being based on treatment with the drug in 'exceptional circumstances', which, having ruled out financial considerations, included personal and social criteria. The better approach would have been to allow consultants to focus on the clinical needs and then fund the patients falling within the eligible group.

Rather than focusing on these strategic policies, the purpose of this chapter is to examine the legal problems that may arise for the nurse in attempting to provide patient care and maintain professional standards each day in the hospital under such economic pressures. The issues here include the possible allowances made by the courts if nurses are asked to perform duties that outstrip their competence or qualifications and the options for the nurse faced with such a request. In order to consider this, it is first necessary to explain the standard of care demanded of nurses by the law.

8.1 Standards of care

All nurses owe their patients a duty of care.[6] Liability is likely to follow if that duty is breached.[7] A breach will consist of a failure to meet the requisite standard of care. This may consist in failing to seek advice from someone better placed to assess the condition of the patient.[8] Famously, that standard is determined by the *Bolam* test[9] – 'the standard of the ordinary skilled man exercising and professing to have that special skill'.[10] This standard is objective. This is a well-established principle and was reiterated in the House of Lords in *Whitehouse* v. *Jordan* (1981),[11] on appeal from a judgment of Lord Denning in the Court of Appeal, which seemed to propound 'the near infallibility of clinical judgment'.[12] Lord Edmund-Davies stressed that if a surgeon (as it was in that case) fails to meet the *Bolam* standard in any respect – even while within the exercise of clinical judgement – then the surgeon must be adjudged negligent. He cited with approval the *Bolam* test as applied in the decision of the Privy Council in Chin *Keow* v. *Government of Malaysia* (1967):

> [W]here you get a situation which involves the use of some special skill or competence, then the test as to whether there has been negligence or not is not the test of the man on the top of the Clapham omnibus, because he has not got this special skill. The test is the standard of the ordinary skilled man, exercising and professing to have that special skill.[13]

One possible criticism of the *Bolam* test is that it might allow a body of specialists within medicine to attest that a particular practice is followed within the profession even though it may be less than desirable. The real fear is that the experts called as witnesses may dictate to the court what amounts to beneficial practice rather than the court upholding objective standards. In the judgments of the House of Lords in *Bolitho* v. *City and Hackney Health Authority*[14] it was emphasised that the body of opinion must be reasonable and must have a logical basis. Where this is in doubt it is open to the court to question the reasonable nature of the practice by taking into account whether the experts have addressed properly and adequately the risks and benefits to the patients of the practice before reaching a conclusion that is defensible. It should be said that it will be very rare indeed for the court to reach a conclusion that the views genuinely propounded by a medical expert were unreasonable.

The objectivity of the standard is crucial. The law will take no account of human failings in determining whether or not there has been a breach of the duty of care. Within any walk of life, people differ in their capacity to discharge a job: some are more innovative or energetic, others more thorough or painstaking. However, in imposing an external and objective standard, nurses are given some protection. Thus, there may be a reason why the nurse failed to meet the required standard – tiredness or inexperience, for example. Nonetheless, negligence can and will be found. No one need suggest that the nurse acted in bad faith. Decisions taken in good faith may lead to liability if the objective standard of skill and care is not met.[15] Equally, it will matter not that any failure is a single lapse in a long and trouble-free career. Liability may follow.

The point is well made in the judgment of Lord Justice Mustill in the case of *Wilsher* v. *Essex Area Health Authority* (1986), in which he speaks of the possible liability for injuries to a premature baby:

> If the unit had not been there, the plaintiff would probably have died. The doctors and nurses worked all kinds of hours to look after the baby . . . For all we know, they far surpassed on numerous occasions the standard of reasonable care. Yet it is said that for one lapse they . . . are to be found to have committed a breach of duty.[16]

It follows that medical personnel may be expected to perform at a standard that, in the circumstances, they would find difficult or impossible to meet. In the words of Brazier:

> [A] doctor who carries on beyond the point when fatigue and overwork impair his judgment remains liable to an injured patient. The fact that the doctor was required by his employer to work such hours will not affect the patient.[17]

This raises a host of issues. In *Johnstone* v. *Bloomsbury Health Authority* (1991),[18] the Court of Appeal held that the defendant health authority could require junior doctors, by an express term in their contract, to work an average of up to 48 hours per week overtime. However, in exercising its discretion to require that overtime be done under the contract, the health authority could not load work onto the plaintiff to such a level that it was reasonably foreseeable that his health might be damaged. This, however, does not answer a second problem, which is whether medical practitioners who feel that the work structure is such that adequate care cannot be delivered to the patient may then refuse to work further without incurring the risk that they would be held to be in breach of their contract of employment.

8.2 The problem of inexperience

One problem facing nurses is that much of their training is 'on the job'. In the case of *Wilsher*, a junior and inexperienced doctor wishing to monitor the oxygen in the bloodstream of a premature baby mistakenly inserted a catheter into a vein rather than an artery. Sir Nicolas Browne-Wilkinson VC accepted in that case that, under ordinary principles of *Bolam*, it would be generally futile to plead inexperience as a reason for failure adequately to provide specialist or technical medical services, since fault would lie in embarking upon the course of treatment in the first place. However, where, as in the instant case a first-year houseman is required to acquire the necessary skill and experience in order to qualify further, 'such doctors cannot be said to be at fault if, at the start of their time, they lack the very skills which they are seeking to acquire'.

This led Sir Nicolas Browne-Wilkinson to suggest that the standard should be fixed by reference to the post occupied by the person in question. Otherwise, 'the young houseman, or the doctor seeking to obtain specialist skill in a special unit would be held liable for shortcomings in treatment without any personal fault on his part at all'. He went on to argue that liability in English law rests upon personal fault so that liability should only follow if the acts or omissions of medical personnel fell short of their qualifications or experience.

This might give some consolation to nurses for it would mean that placed in situations in which their lack of experience exposed them to the threat of legal action, they could plead such inexperience and argue that they met the duty placed upon them personally. However, this judgment omits a vital part of the *Bolam* test and the majority of the Court of Appeal rejected it as a correct formulation of the law. The Court stated that the standard of care must be set in accordance with the special skill that the person professes to have. The patient is generally in no position to enquire whether (for example) a nurse actually possesses such a skill, hence the objectivity of the standard. If nurses hold themselves out to the patient as competent to undertake a particular procedure, a duty of care will arise and will be breached if the procedure is negligently performed.

Sir Nicolas Browne-Wilkinson's suggestion of a requirement of personal fault has appeared in earlier cases on medical malpractice.[19] It is worth noting where it leads. It would introduce a subjective standard, and in so doing might lead to the problem for nurses that a finding of liability would constitute a mark of personal failure. Whatever the perception of a medical negligence claim, fault is judged by an objective standard and persons found liable may not actually be at fault. In moving the standard towards gross negligence, Browne-Wilkinson's formulation would make it harder also for the patient to recover compensation for injury.

This, in part, may explain why the two other judges in the Court of Appeal preferred a more traditional pronouncement of the *Bolam* test. In the view of Lord Justice Mustill the duty ought not to be assessed in accordance with the actor performing the duty, but rather with the act performed. The standard should be set according to the post occupied. In the words of the judge:

> the standard is not just that of the averagely competent and well informed junior houseman . . . but of such a person who fills a post in a unit offering a highly specialised service.

Lord Justice Glidewell substantially agrees with this, saying:

In my view, the law requires the trainee or learner to be judged by the same standard as his more experienced colleagues. If it did not, inexperience would frequently be urged as a defence to an action for professional negligence.

The wording of both of these formulations is a little loose, but both are clearly intended to indicate that where a person holds out as possessing the requisite skill to provide a particular service, then the standard will be set in accordance with the reasonable skill of the average competent professional ordinarily providing that service. The case of *Djemal* v. *Bexley HA* (1995)[20] followed the judgment in *Wilsher* in discounting the actual experience of a senior houseman in an A & E unit in setting the required standard of care.

8.3 Risk and precautions

Although the standard itself is 'objective and impersonal',[21] the circumstances in which it is exercised will be highly relevant in determining breach. This is well illustrated by a Canadian authority, *Moore* v. *Large* (1932). The case concerned the alleged negligence of a doctor who had failed to X-ray the shoulder of a patient following that patient's fall so that a dislocation of the shoulder was overlooked. The court could find no negligence:

> It has not surely come to this that if the cause of the trouble is not apparent to the eye of the surgeon or physician he must advise an X-ray or take the consequences to his reputation and to his pocket for not having done so. Is the X-ray to be the only arbitrator in such a case and are years of study and experience to be cast aside as negligible?[22]

This would probably not be so today,[23] but what has changed is not the availability of X-ray (it was available in 1932) but societal expectation of the use of this device in checking against the risk of a particular disorder. To take an X-ray in such circumstances would now be almost standard practice although interestingly, with the link with cancer, attitudes are changing again. Further, the acknowledgment of the risk and any negligence disregarding it are judged by the standards of the time of the incident and not when any case comes ultimately to court. As Lord Denning said in *Roe* v. *Ministry of Health* (1954),[24] a case concerning contaminated anaesthetic:

> He did not know that there could be undetectable cracks, but it was not negligent for him not to know it at that time. We must not look at the 1947 accident with 1954 spectacles.

This raises the question of how a breach of the standard of care may be determined. Generally, it will require some balance between the good, which the practitioner seeks to achieve by intervention, and the risks run by a particular course of conduct in the light of the availability of precautions or safeguards. This may be illustrated by the case of *Mahon* v. *Osborne* (1939),[25] in which there was seemingly obvious negligence in terminating an operation without removing a swab, which was left under part of the liver and which caused a complication that eventually resulted in the death of the patient. Lord Justice Scott was prepared, however, to recognise circumstances 'where the patient has been taking the anaesthetic badly, and is suffering from shock' such that the doctor is anxious to terminate the operation and exercises discretion so that 'as soon as he has completed the removal of all swabs of which he is at that moment aware, he asks the sister for the count, and forthwith starts to close the wound'. In the judge's view, a finding of negligence would not be inevitable in such a situation. Here, the importance attached to preserving the life of a patient might outweigh the risk inherent in hastening the swab count.

It is possible to envisage a wide variety of situations within which risks, ordinarily intolerable in good medical practice, are run in situations of dire emergency. In the words of Lord Justice Mustill in *Wilsher*:

> [F]ull allowance must be made for the fact that certain aspects of treatment may have to be carried out in . . . 'battle conditions'. An emergency may overburden the available resources, and, if an individual is forced by circumstances to do too many things at once, the fact that he does one of them incorrectly, should not likely be taken as negligence.

Note that the absence of resources is not of itself a defence, but the fact of the emergency may change the circumstances in which nursing is conducted to the point that if an ordinarily competent nurse might reasonably have made a particular error under such pressure then the court will not find negligence. This is well illustrated by a case from Manitoba, *Roydch v. Krasey* (1971),[26] in which a doctor examined an intoxicated patient in a lorry at 1 a.m. in the morning with the aid of a torch. There was no negligence in his failure to diagnose injuries to the chest, ribs and lungs. One way of explaining this is to say that, under an objective standard, the difficulties in discharging the duty of care would have faced any practitioner working under such circumstances. Finally note that even where there may be a shortfall in the duty owed to the patient, it is necessary to show that the treatment administered led to the damage suffered by the patient – see *Aisha Qureshi v. Royal Brompton and Harefield NHS*[27] and *Anderson v. Heatherwood & Wexham Park Hospitals NHS Trust*.[28]

8.4 Staff shortages

This then raises the question of what will happen if, in the course of medical practice, a nurse is required to work under substandard conditions, or with an obvious shortfall in resources. Can such circumstances be taken into account in assessing breach of duty? In the following section, which considers shortages of nursing staff, the problem of inexperience will not be revisited; rather, attention is directed here to problems created by overall shortages in the nursing resources required to discharge the needs of the patients.

There are a series of cases concerning the provision of nursing staff, many of which involved relatively straightforward issues of patient supervision. *Dryden v. Surrey County Council* (1936) is a case involving two elements of medical negligence. One involved the failure to remove a swab, leading to a finding of negligence against the surgeon. However, an action was also brought against the Council on the basis that the nurses, whom they employed, had failed adequately to supervise the plaintiff, so that the error went unnoticed. This element of the claim seems to have been rejected by the court on the basis that, as a matter of evidence, the plaintiff failed to exhibit symptoms indicating a complication of this type. Nonetheless, the court did consider that element of the claim that argued that the responsibility of the Council lay in their failure to provide competent nursing staff as the ward was clearly understaffed. In fact, there were 54 beds in the ward and a nursing staff of one sister, one staff nurse and five probationers. This, as the judge admitted in a masterful piece of understatement, was not as good as 'the attention which a person will receive . . . if . . . he is fortunate enough to pay for the undivided attention of one nurse or . . . two nurses'. However, in the view of the judge, neither the presence of such a large number of probationers, nor the fact that the Matron had been seeking to gain an increase in staff established 'negligence by under staffing'.

This, at first glance, may seem rather surprising. In fact, however, it may be saying little more than, whatever the level of staff, there will be no finding of negligence unless some injury can be attributed to the lack of nursing care. Where this is so, the court will be required to consider the level of nursing provision. This must be done for the particular ward in question, for once again the courts are dealing with risk of injury, and the nursing provision required in an intensive care facility may not be that of the antenatal unit.[29]

This point is brought clearly home by the case of *Robertson* v. *Nottingham HA* (1997),[30] in which a series of errors of communication in the delivery of obstetric care resulted in the claimant (suing by her mother) bringing an action in negligence on the basis that her delivery at an earlier stage would have prevented the brain damage from which she now suffered. In fact the claimant both at trial and on appeal failed to prove that her brain damage resulted from the breakdown in communication. Nonetheless, the Court of Appeal emphasised that a health authority was under a duty to establish a proper system of care. That duty could not be delegated to others[31] and the standard of care would be judged in accordance with what might reasonably be expected of a hospital of the size and type in question. In that case the standard expected was that ordinarily exercised in a large teaching hospital and centre of excellence.

This point may be demonstrated also by cases in which known suicide risks have injured or killed themselves following admission to hospital. In *Thorne* v. *Northern Group Hospital Management Committee* (1964)[32] the patient's husband had informed the nursing staff of his wife's threats of suicide, and the patient, who had been undergoing treatment on a medical ward of a general hospital, was due to be transferred from the ward to an outside neurosis unit for further assessment. She was left unsupervised when both the nurse and the sister left the ward together. The patient left the ward, returned home and committed suicide. The husband failed in his action against the Hospital Management Committee. In the view of Mr Justice Edmund Davies:

> The duty owed by hospital authorities and staff to a patient is that of reasonable care and skill in the given circumstances. Whether a breach of that duty has

been established depends on the proven facts including what was known or should have been known about a particular patient and the fact that the defendants impliedly undertook to exhibit professional skill and administrative care of reasonable competence and adequacy towards their patient. They must take reasonable care to avoid acts or omissions which they can reasonably foresee would be likely to harm the patient entrusted to their charge; but they need not guard against merely possible (as distinct from reasonably probable) harm. On the other hand the degree of care which will be regarded as reasonable is proportionate both to the degree of risk involved and the magnitude of the mischief which may be occasioned to the particular patient in the absence of due care.

This case may be contrasted with that of *Selfe* v. *Ilford and District Hospital Management Committee* (1970),[33] in which the plaintiff, whose attempt at suicide by a drug overdose had failed, was admitted to a ward of 27 patients. The ground floor ward contained four known suicide risks – grouped at one end of the room. Selfe, a quiet and withdrawn man of 17, was left unattended on the ward when two of the three nurses on duty left the ward without informing the third. While that nurse was attending a patient elsewhere in the ward, Selfe climbed out of a window and made his way up to a roof from which he jumped. His attempt at suicide again failed, but he sued for his resultant injuries on the basis of negligent nursing supervision. Evidence indicated that, even with all of the nurses on the ward, an additional nurse was probably required. Mr Justice Hinchcliff found for the plaintiff, stressing that the high degree of risk on the ward required a commensurate increase in the care provided.

There are a number of cases that show, however, that where the staffing is adequate to meet the standard of care imposed upon the hospital or unit, a nurse will not be liable for every untoward incident on a ward. Examples of this principle include *Gravestock* v. *Lewisham HMC* (1955) (injury following fall of nine-year-old running in ward while nurse bringing food through to the ward);[34] *Cox* v. *Carshalton HMC* (1955) (inhaler slipped and scalded disabled minor as nurse away for matter of seconds);[35] and *Size* v. *Shenley HMC* (1970)[36] (nurse failed to reach mentally unstable patient before he attacked the plaintiff).

8.5 Lack of resources

Once a finding of fact is made that provision is in some way inadequate, a related issue arises of whether it can ever be a defence to plead lack of resources. The answer is simply no. If nursing staff meet approved nursing practice to a *Bolam* standard then this may refute a claim of negligence, but if they fall short of that standard then, once again, it does not matter why, and lack of resources is no better an argument than tiredness or inexperience.[37]

However, in spite of the objective nature of the standard, and the lack of any necessary element of personal fault in a finding of negligence, there is without question a move away from finding medical staff liable in situations in which lack of adequate resources makes it impossible to meet a required standard.[38] This is clear from the judgment of Sir Nicolas Browne-Wilkinson in *Wilsher*, in which he poses the following question:

> Should the authority be liable if it demonstrates that, due to the financial stringency under which it operates, it cannot afford to fill the posts with those possessing the necessary experience?

He goes on to say:

> [I]n my judgment, the law should not be distorted by making findings of personal fault against individual doctors who are, in truth, not at fault in order to avoid such questions.

Similarly, in *Robertson* v. *Nottingham HA*[39] Lord Justice Brooke in finding that the hospital system had been negligently run expressed the following view:

> It would be unjust and unfair to hold that Dr X, after being let down . . . by the negligence of others, was himself negligent . . .

One can quibble with this. It is not the law that is being distorted; rather it is the law that is distorting the concept of blame. Nonetheless, this move away from the concept of individual liability on the part of a medical professional, in favour of asking questions about the organisation as a whole, is significant, and it is important to understand what it represents.

8.6 From vicarious to direct liability

For many years, the view was taken that hospital authorities were not liable for actions of staff in discharging professional duties. This applied to nurses in the course of medical procedures under the guidance of the doctor, whose control was thought to be 'supreme'. However, the hospital authority remained legally responsible to patients for 'purely ministerial or administrative duties' and these included 'attendance of nurses in the ward'.[40] This artificial division, and the concept of control that underpinned it, was difficult to maintain, and in *Gold* v. *Essex County Council* (1942) Lord Greene expressed the view that:

> [n]ursing . . . is just what the patient is entitled to expect from the institution, and the relationship of the nurses to the institution supports the inference that they are engaged to nurse the patients . . . the idea that . . . the only obligation which the hospital undertakes to perform by its nursing staff is not the essential work of nursing but only so called administrative work appears to me . . . not merely unworkable in practice but contrary to the plain sense of the position.[41]

This case effectively established that a hospital authority would be vicariously liable for the negligence of an employee, such as a nurse. A mistake made by a nurse following the direct orders of a surgeon would probably not give rise to liability, but the surgeon no longer ruled 'supreme', even in the theatre. Following this case, a mistake by the nurse alone might mean that there would be no liability on the surgeon, but that vicarious liability might attach to the hospital authority.

It was established in cases such as *Cassidy* v. *Ministry of Health* (1951)[42] and *Roe* v. *Ministry of Health* (1954) that the test for vicarious liability was no longer one of control, but of whether the member of the medical staff was a permanent and integral part of the hospital staff. So fixed and well-settled was this body of law, that from 1954 to 1990, under a governmental circular, health authorities defended claims in negligence on behalf of all staff. At the date of judgment or settlement, damages would be apportioned, in accordance with the principles of vicarious liability, between the medical defence organisation and the health authority. Disputes as to the requisite shares of liability were rare.

In *Cassidy*, however, it had been suggested that certain liabilities might be direct, such that the duty of care could not be delegated 'no matter whether the delegation be to a servant under a contract of service or to an independent contractor under a contract for services'. For some years, this *dictum* of Lord Denning lay as an island of uncertainty in the stormy seas of medical malpractice litigation. In recent times, however, the concept of direct liability has received much greater attention. As Montgomery points out:

> In a modern system of healthcare . . . the responsibilities of doctors overlap with those of nurses, midwives, managers and others. Direct liability on the part of the health and hospital authorities may represent an important tool to unravel the complexities of modem health provision.[43]

Direct liability may have advantages in overcoming problems of where to place responsibility among health care teams. Equally, it may assist the law in keeping track of standards, as pressure on resources sees the devolution of tasks to nurses that were previously performed by doctors.

All of this is a way of saying that direct liability may arise out of the failure of structures of health care delivery that have been put in place in order to discharge duties towards the patient. Thus, in *Bull* v. *Devon Area Health Authority* (1989)[44] there was a gap of over an hour between the delivery of a first and a second twin. A significant passage of time prior to the case arriving before the court made it difficult for the defendant health authority to find evidence to dispute the claim of negligence, but Lord Justice Slade nonetheless stated:

> It is possible to imagine hypothetical contingencies which would have accounted for a failure without any avoidable fault in the hospital's system, or any negligence in its working, to secure Mrs Bull's attendance by any obstetrician qualified to deliver the second twin between 7.35pm and 8.25pm. In my judgment, however, all the most likely explanations of this failure point strongly either to inefficiency in the system for summoning the assistance of the registrar or consultant, in operation of the hospital, or to negligence by some individuals in the working of that system.

This point is supported also by Lord Justice Mustill, who speaks of a 'finding by the learned judge, amply supported by the evidence, that the system should have been such that the second twin would be delivered as soon as practicable after the first'. In considering the submission that the hospital 'could not be expected to do more than their best, allocating their limited resources as favourably as possible', Lord Justice Mustill makes the following response:

I have some reservations about this contention, which are not allayed by the submission that hospital medicine is a public service. So it is, but there are other public services in respect of which it is not necessarily an answer to allegations of unsafety that there were insufficient resources to enable the administrators to do everything they would like to do. I do not for a moment suggest that public medicine is precisely analogous to other public services, but there is perhaps a danger in assuming that it is completely *sui generis*, and that it is necessarily a complete answer to say that even if the system in a hospital was unsatisfactory, it was no more unsatisfactory than those in force elsewhere.

Cases like *Bull* and *Wilsher* demonstrate that there is an increasing number of instances in which there seems to be an organisational failure in the delivery of health care. If a health authority is at fault in the performance of its functions, this may be described as negligence, notwithstanding the difficulty in locating particular employees who might be said to be negligent. Arguably, this is the basis of the decision in the case of *Lindsey County Council* v. *Marshall* (1936),[45] and also other earlier cases such as *Collins* v. *Hertfordshire County Council* (1947),[46] which found negligence 'in the management and control of the hospital'. A number of Commonwealth authorities have also found negligence in the organisation of the hospital itself.[47]

This distinction between direct and vicarious liability was described by Lord Justice Brooke in *Robertson* when he stated:

> If effective systems had been in place . . . then the Health Authority would be vicariously liable for any negligence of those of its servants or agents who did not take proper care to ensure, so far as it is reasonably practicable, that the . . . systems worked efficiently. If on the other hand, no effective systems were in place at all . . . then the authority would be directly liable in negligence . . .

In either event, this should allow a patient suffering a medical accident to recover damages, but as we move towards more systems-based approaches (through clinical protocols and the like) this type of analysis may become more common.

Finally, it may be worth noting cases involving the administration of drugs and blood products. In the Court of Appeal decision in *Blyth* v. *Bloomsbury Health Authority* (1987),[48] the defendant health authority appealed against a judgment of Mr Justice Leonard, in which he found that the health authority was negligent in failing to follow a system put in place to monitor the use of the drug Depo Provera. The appeal succeeded, the Court of Appeal finding that the judge had reached the decision, not supported by the evidence, that there had been divergence from a system put in place within the hospital. Nonetheless, the Court of Appeal seemed to have accepted that the tests used by Mr Justice Leonard in looking at whether 'on a normal day an effective system existed by which patients could get advice on contraception from those who were equipped with the necessary information to enable them to give it fully' and whether 'exceptionally something went wrong' were acceptable tests within themselves. Implicit in the Court of Appeal's judgment is the necessity for a health authority to ensure that patients within the hospital are sufficiently well counselled in relation to drugs administered.

In *Re HIV Haemophiliac Litigation* (1990),[49] an application by the plaintiffs to the court for an order requiring the Department of Health and Social Security (DHSS) to produce departmental documents relating to its policies for the importation of blood products was resisted by the DHSS, on the basis that the plaintiffs did not have a good cause of action either by breach of statutory duty or in negligence. The Court of Appeal gave judgment on the preliminary issue of whether or not the DHSS might be in breach of statutory duty under section 3 of the National Health Service Act 1977, or otherwise negligent in the design of a system to secure the physical health of the people, and the prevention, diagnosis and treatment of illness within England and Wales. This was said to result from its failure to ensure a self-sufficiency in blood, as a result of which haemophiliacs were treated with factor VIII blood products contaminated with the HIV virus, imported from the United States. The Court of Appeal found that the relevant sections of the 1977 Act did not found an action for breach of statutory duty as it was not clear that Parliament had intended to allow individual enforcement and recovery.[50] However, in relation to negligence the Court of Appeal found an arguable case. In their words:

> It is obvious that it would be rare for a case in negligence to be proved having regard to the nature of the duties under the 1977 Act, and the fact that, in the law of negligence, it is difficult to prove a negligent breach of duty when the party charged with negligence is required to exercise discretion and to form judgments upon the allocation of public resources. That, however, is not sufficient . . . to make it clear for the purposes of these proceedings that there can in law be no claim in negligence.

It seems, therefore, that hospitals may increasingly have to face direct liability for their failure to organise adequate systems of health care delivery. Thus, in an era of resource constraint, if the delivery of health care is inadequate, it may become easier rather than more difficult for the patient to find a remedy. This is not least because the courts have traditionally been very protective of doctors (in particular), and when negligence alleged is that of the organisation, rather than of the medical professional, certain obstacles to medical negligence litigation may be removed.

8.7 Case study 1

The principles considered above can be illustrated by the use of a case study.

N is a sister on night duty and is in charge of a small rural hospital, which some time ago closed its accident and emergency facility. Shortly before midnight on a snowy winter's evening, two people arrive by car at the hospital. R says that he has found, on the roadside very near to the hospital, an injured person, V, who accompanies him. V has been the victim of a hit-and-run incident. V is fully conscious, but appears to have been hit in his upper body and may have broken a number of bones. He is also bleeding badly from the head. The nearest accident and emergency facility is ten miles away. There is no doctor currently on duty at the rural hospital, which has a sign at the gate advising that there is no accident and emergency unit within the hospital and that persons wishing for emergency treatment should report to their nearest accident and emergency hospital.

One interesting issue here is whether N must offer treatment to the patient. In *Barnett* v. *Chelsea and Kensington Hospital Management Committee* (1968),[51] three nightwatchmen had vomited continually since drinking tea in the early hours of the morning of New Year's Day. On finishing their shift they presented themselves to an accident and emergency department of a London hospital. They reported to a nurse who telephoned the casualty officer. Without examining the men, he told the nurse to send them home with instructions to call their own doctors in the morning. Five hours later, one of the men died from arsenic poisoning. Although the subsequent claim failed on the lack of proof of causation, it was said that where a person with obvious symptoms of illness presents himself to an accident and emergency department a duty of care arises so that skill and care should be employed in the diagnosis of any injury. This is so even though there will be no prior relationship with the patient. However, the general view taken by English law is that 'if a person undertakes to perform a voluntary act he is liable if he performs improperly, but not if he neglects to perform it'. It is for this reason that certain jurisdictions have enacted 'Good Samaritan' statutes, which either place a positive duty on doctors to stop at the scene of an accident, or offer immunity to medical staff who choose to render assistance.

Although there is a statutory duty to provide sufficient accident and emergency services to meet reasonable requirements within a locality, in practice this duty will prove very difficult to enforce before the courts. There is now a significant body of case law that demonstrates that the courts will rarely intervene to review a decision on resource allocation or enforce a claim to be admitted to treatment. Nonetheless, if a non-accident and emergency hospital chooses to admit a patient to treatment then a duty of care will arise. It follows that, in purely legal terms, N would be free to refuse treatment to V and urge R and V to present themselves to the nearest accident and emergency department. Nonetheless, once N opts to render care and assistance to V a duty of care arises, and the question then relates to the applicable standard of care. It is clear that liability may result from negligent treatment or advice rendered by N or any failure of communication in providing V with emergency treatment.

However, given that the unit is not an accident and emergency unit, in accordance with the case of *Roydch* v. *Krasey* (1971)[52] the circumstances in which treatment is rendered will be taken into account in determining the requisite standard of care. In *Knight* v. *Home Office* (1990) it was said that a prison hospital owes a duty of care to a mentally ill patient that is of a lower standard than that of a specialist psychiatric hospital. In that case, it was said:

> In making the decision as to the standard to be demanded the court must bear in mind as one factor that resources available for public services are limited and that the allocation of resources is a matter for Parliament . . . the facilities available to deal with an emergency in a general practitioner's surgery cannot be expected to be as ample as those available in the casualty department of a general hospital.

In *Phelps* v. *Hillingdon* L.B.C. (1998)[53] it was said that the only duty of a 'medical rescuer' was not to 'negligently create further danger or make the . . . situation worse'. What will prove of importance is that N adequately communicates, to anyone else rendering treatment to V, the steps she has taken and that she arranges for the necessary specialist care as expeditiously as possible.

8.8 Scarce resources and professional responsibility

Questions relating to the relevant standard of care are also significant for nurses in another context. As stated above, the law demands no more than a reasonable standard of care rather than standards of treatment that are at the cutting edge of medical science. But what should nurses do if they become convinced that patients are facing unacceptable levels of risk because the regime of treatment regularly falls short of reasonable standards? Two problems may arise for the nurse who decides to seek publicity in order to draw to the attention of the public the inadequacy of the care offered. The first is that the identification of a particular patient may breach principles of medical confidentiality. In addition, any public disclosure might amount to a breach of the contract of employment.

Neither the NMC's Code of Professional Conduct, *The NMC Code of Professional Conduct: Standards for Conduct, Performance and Ethics*, nor their Advisory Guidelines on Confidentiality suggests an absolute duty of professional confidence. Although clause 5 of the Code instructs the nurse 'to protect all confidential information concerning patients and clients . . . and make disclosures only with consent . . .', the Code does allow for exceptional cases of disclosure upon a court order or where this is necessary in the public interest.

This is in accordance with the general law although, following the Human Rights Act 1998, English Law has to conform with Article 8 of the European Convention on Human Rights and the right to respect for private and family life. In *Attorney General* v. *Guardian Newspaper* (No. 2) (1990)[54] Lord Goff stated that 'although the basis of the law's protection of confidence is that there is a public interest that confidence should be preserved and protected by law, nevertheless, that public interest may be outweighed by some of the countervailing public interest which favours disclosure'. However, in *X Health Authority* v. *Y* (1987)[55] any public interest in the disclosure of the fact that two practising doctors were being treated as AIDS patients was outweighed by the general public interest in retaining the confidentiality of AIDS-related information on a patient's file. The High Court in this case intervened to restrain the publication of the disclosure when leaked by employees.

However, in the case of *W* v. *Egdell* and Others (1990)[56] a consultant psychiatrist was employed by a patient's solicitor to prepare a report upon the patient for use in the consideration of the patient's release or transfer from a secure hospital. When no use was made of that report (which highlighted the long-standing nature, not previously drawn to the authorities' attention, of W's interest in home-made bombs), the psychiatrist himself disclosed the report to the medical director of the secure unit. In turn, the hospital forwarded the report to the Secretary of State. The Court of Appeal stated that while mental patients should be free to seek advice and assistance from independent doctors, nonetheless, given the wider public interest in public safety, this form of disclosure by the psychiatrist was thought not to be in breach of any duty of confidentiality.[57]

Thus, although it might be possible to argue that disclosure of patient-related information serves the wider public interest in highlighting the decline in the standard of care, this is by no means obvious. Where possible, particular patients should not be identified, or, if this is inevitable, the nurse should seek the permission of that patient to refer to the particular case. Note that the public interest in ensuring that patients are not inhibited from seeking treatment may mean that confidentiality can attach even to non-identifying information concerning medical treatment.[58]

Nurses may also be troubled that voicing opinions on the regime of care may lead to disciplinary action by their employer. Indeed, the fear of such disclosures leads to the introduction into contracts of employment of express requirements prohibiting disclosure to the media of matters relating to the working responsibilities of employer and employee. In certain instances it could be argued that, even in the absence of an express clause, implied duties of fidelity might dictate that any public disclosure would amount to a breach of the employment contract. Prior to 1999 there were well-documented incidents in which health service employees faced disciplinary proceedings or dismissal, apparently as a result of complaints concerning shortfalls in the standard of care. Where this led to the dismissal of an employee, that employee could consider redress by an industrial tribunal. However, this was unlikely to lead to reinstatement, even where the tribunal found in favour of the dismissed nurse.

This situation changed radically in 1999 following the passage of the Public Interest Disclosure Act 1998. This allows employees to make 'protected disclosures' without victimisation or dismissal.[59] All NHS employees are protected by these provisions, and there is not a ceiling upon the compensation that may be awarded if victimisation is proven. Among the categories of protected disclosure are failure to comply with legal obligations, and endangering the health and safety of any individual. This may cover past as well as ongoing malpractice. However, the Act also governs the manner of disclosure, encouraging initial internal disclosure if the 'whistleblower' is to receive the protection of the Act. Here a nurse may have a number of options if wishing in good faith to make a disclosure. It may be possible/appropriate for the nurse to speak directly to the persons retaining responsibility for the malpractice in question, or to his or her employer, to the Department of Health or some other relevant government department (if working in the NHS), or to an appropriate (prescribed) regulatory body – such as the Health and Safety Executive.

Where the elements of a protected disclosure, within the terms of section 103A of the Employment Act 1996, are present, in that a disclosure is made by a nurse in good faith and in the reasonable belief that an allegation of wrongdoing is made to the right person, at the right time, the employer is fixed with a duty both to act on the matter and to protect the nurse from suffering detriment because a disclosure has been made. It will be difficult indeed for the employer at that stage to raise issues of professional misconduct[60] though it is important that the nurse remains in employment in order to gain the protection of the Act – see *Fadipe* v. *Reed Nursing Personnel* (2001).[61]

Disclosure outside these categories will only gain the protection of the Act in limited circumstances. For example, disclosure for personal gain (such as a payment from the media) will not be protected. Moreover, the nurse would have to show that internal disclosure would have been ineffective as leading to the concealment or destruction of evidence, or victimisation, or because previous, similar disclosures have been ignored. Where there is public disclosure, a court or tribunal can take into account a number of factors relating to the seriousness of the incident, issues of patient confidentiality, the workings of internal proceedings and so on in deciding whether the disclosure is protected by the Act.

In the case of exceptionally serious disclosures, it is possible to make public disclosure immediately without the need to show fear of victimisation, likely cover-up or previous inaction. However, it would be rare indeed for a nurse to be justified in going immediately to the media, when other options, such as a Member of Parliament or a professional association, are available. Unfortunately there is nothing in the Act to require internal procedures to deal with complaints by nurses concerning the inadequacy of patient care. This may mean that disclosure is no easy matter for a nurse as she or he informs immediate supervisors, then the employer, only to witness prevarication or inaction. This may drag the nurse into the uncomfortable territory of increasingly public disclosure, where she or he is already unpopular and may fear more subtle forms of prejudice – such as failing to gain promotion.

Nonetheless, increasingly, there are professional demands made upon nurses. The NMC Code of Conduct suggests that the nurse must report circumstances that could jeopardise standards of practice and also report circumstances in which an appropriate standard of care cannot be provided. Such reporting should be to 'an appropriate person or authority'. Again, the NMC Code suggests that nurses should 'obtain help and supervision from a competent practitioner until they and their employer consider that they have acquired the requisite knowledge and skill'. Increasingly, it seems that nurses cannot merely stand by and ignore declining standards of patient care. It is the nurse who is seen as occupying the role as patient advocate, and arguably nurses find themselves under a more direct professional duty to take action in relation to resource shortfalls than do doctors.

8.9 Case study 2

W is a night duty charge nurse on a ward for acutely ill patients. She believes that the standard of care for these patients has dropped dramatically owing to two events: (1) the withdrawal of one night nurse, on a permanent basis, from ward duty, and (2) the replacement over time of a number of more experienced nurses by junior staff. Matters came to a head when a patient died in distressing circumstances, in a situation that W believes was largely a consequence of lack of adequate supervision on the ward.

Under the NMC's Code of Conduct, W here should 'report to an appropriate person or authority, having regard to the physical, psychological and social effects on patients and clients, any circumstances in the environment of care which would jeopardize standards of practice'. Similarly it is said that she should 'report to an appropriate person or authority any circumstances in which safe and appropriate care for patients and clients cannot be provided'. W clearly finds herself in this situation, and if the hospital in which she works operates a complaints procedure she would be advised to follow that procedure and voice her concerns accordingly. If no response is forthcoming, or if such complaints are swept aside, then W may wish to raise the matter with persons further up the management ladder, even through to the chair of the health authority or Trust where that appears to be appropriate. Alternatively, at some point W may wish to report to the Royal College of Nursing (RCN).

On a strict interpretation of confidentiality rules it could be argued that the passage of information even between those in the health care system should take place only to serve the treatment of the patient. However, if this principle were to be followed rigorously, investigations into medical accidents might be inhibited. The General Medical Council allows that doctors must judge whether it is appropriate to pass on patient information to others within the health care system so that they can perform their duties. Here the permission of the patient cannot be obtained, and public disclosure might cause distress to relatives. Arguably, however, disclosure within the health care system ought to be permissible. Further problems may arise where, instead of effecting any remedy, the disclosure by W leads to further problems at work. If W finds herself the subject of formal disciplinary proceedings, or indeed victimised in some way by line managers as a result of the complaint, how should W react? Prior to the 1998 Act there were few available remedies here. Section 27B of the Employment Rights Act 1996 (as amended by the Public Interest Disclosure Act 1998) allows that W should suffer no detriment as a result of her actions. If W can show any element of detriment as a result of her actions she will be able to bring a claim for compensation.

This course of action may also invite press comment, whether or not W actually instigates this. At this point, W will have to take care to avoid breaching professional confidentiality rules in any statements to the press. However, in so far as W and those giving evidence on behalf of W need to give evidence as to the particular events that led to the complaint, the disclosure will generally be permissible under professional conduct rules. Under the NMC Code disclosure is allowed 'where required by the order of a court'. This does not exactly cover the situation of a tribunal, which will not generally proceed by witness summons or the subpoena of witnesses. Nonetheless, it is difficult to see that a health authority or Trust would have much success in seeking to restrain by court action the disclosure of information where that information is being legitimately used to pursue a remedy in an industrial tribunal. Indeed one in-built advantage of the 1998 Act is that it is in the long-term interests of employers to ensure that internal complaints are dealt with in a speedy and responsible manner.

8.10 Conclusion

The continual pressures to meet targets and to cap spending have had a dramatic and radical impact not only on the methods of service delivery but also on the demands and expectations placed on various health care professionals and the allocation of resources. The development of responsibility at all levels, financial, administrative and professional, down the line from the hospital administrator to the individual nurse implies that issues surrounding professional accountability and autonomy require closer examination.

This change in the underlying philosophy of the delivery of health care in some ways is running in tandem with the growth of legal problems that may arise for the nurse. Problems arise in attempting to provide patient care and maintain the professional standards expected of the 'ordinarily skilled' practitioner. The changes have had, and continue to have, resource implications. The reduction in resources may increase the number of instances in which nurses are placed in situations that require them to perform duties that it could be argued are beyond their level of competence or qualification. The development of professional skills and qualifications is directly dependent on the training received 'on the job'.

If resources are stretched the qualified nursing staff will be fully utilised in the delivery of patient care, with time for training limited. Unrealistic demands may be placed on the student or newly qualified nurse yet, in the eyes of the law, the standards required will remain objective. The spectre of liability demands that attention be given to demonstrable training for, and the maintenance of standards of, the professional nurse. It will be up to individual nurses to show that their qualifications and training are sufficient to the role and task in each and every situation.

Of necessity, the changes in the NHS will have not only personal and professional implications for the nurse but also implications of a systemic nature. The role of the nurse in relation to the patient as well as to the nurse managers will be tested. The nurse has been seen to be the advocate on behalf of the patient and also accountable to a manager. However, the nurse could possibly be placed in a situation where there is a conflict of interest. The NMC Code deals with the obligatory reporting by nurses when witnessing poor standards of patient care. The 1998 Act offers some protection where the nurse chooses to act in the patient's interests. Yet at the heart of the matter is the relationship between cost, quality and quantity of treatment, which it is not open to the individual nurse to resolve.

8.11 Notes and references

1. R. Klein *et al.*, *Managing Scarcity* (Buckingham, Open University Press, 1996), p. 37.
2. K. Syrett, Impotence or importance? 'Judicial review in an era of explicit NHS rationing, *Modern Law Review*, **67**(2) (2004), pp. 289–304, at pages 292–3.
3. For a review, see R.G. Lee, Judicial review and access to health care'. In T. Buck (ed.), *Judicial Review and Social Welfare* (Toronto, Carswell, 1998).
4. *R* v. *North West Lancashire Health Authority, Ex p A* [2000] 1 WLR 977.
5. [2006] EWCA Civ 392; on 23 August 2006, NICE issued guidance recommending that herceptin be funded for use in early-stage breast cancer, and see note by K. Syrett, *Public Law*, **664** (2006).
6. See *Barnett* v. *Chelsea and Kensington HMC* [1968] 1 All ER 1068; *Gold* v. *Essex CC* [1942] 2 All ER 237; *Urbanski* v. *Patel* [1978] 84 DLR (3d) 650; R. Lee, Hospital admissions: duty of care, *New Law Journal*, **567** (1979).
7. Liability will not inevitably follow for a number of reasons. There may be no resulting damage, or the medical error may not be the causative factor of later injury, or the damage may be too remote.

8. *Satwat Rehman* v. *University College London Hospitals NHS Trust* (High Court, 28 May 2004, Judge Eccles QC).
9. [1957] 1 WLR 582.
10. Note the incorporation of this principle into statute: Congenital Disabilities (Civil Liability) Act 1976, section 1(5).
11. [1981] 1 All E.R. 267. See also R.L. Deutsch, Medical negligence reviewed, *American Law Journal*, **87** (1983), p. 674.
12. M. Brazier, Patient autonomy and consent to treatment: the role of the law, *Legal Studies*, **170** (1987), and for a wider review of Lord Denning's approach to standards of care, see S. McLean, Negligence: a dagger at the doctor's back? In P. Robson & P. Watchman, *Justice, Lord Denning and the Constitution* (Aldershot, Gower, 1981).
13. [1967] 1 WLR 813.
14. [1998] AC 232.
15. See *Whitehouse* v. *Jordan* [1981] 1 All ER 267, and in the USA, *Demmer* v. *Patt* 788 F2d 1387 (8 Cir 1986).
16. [1988] AC 1074.
17. M. Brazier, *Medicine, Patients and the Law*, 2nd edn (Harmondsworth, Penguin, 1992).
18. [1992] QB 333.
19. Most famously by Lord Denning in *Whitehouse* v. *Jordan* [1980] 1 All ER 650.
20. [1995] 6 Med LR 269.
21. Per Lord MacMillan in *Glasgow Corporation* v. *Muir* [1943] AC 448.
22. Lord MacMillan in *Glasgow Corporation* v. *Muir* [1943] AC 448, at p. 183, quoted by E. Picard, *Legal Liability of Doctors and Hospitals in Canada* (Toronto, Carswell, 1984).
23. See, for example, *Leake* v. *Targett* [2005] EWHC 956 (QB).
24. [1954] 2 QB 66.
25. [1939] 2 KB 14.
26. [1971] 4 W.W.R. 358 (Man. QB).
27. [2006] EWHC 298 (QB).
28. (High Court, 16/05/05 – Judge Eccles QC).
29. *Knight* v. *Home Office* [1990] 3 All ER 237.
30. [1997] 8 Med LR 1.
31. See also *M* v. *Calderdale & Kirklees HA* [1998] Lloyd's Rep. Med. 157.
32. *The Times*, 6 June 1964.
33. *The Times*, 26 November 1970.
34. *The Times*, 27 May 1955.
35. *The Times*, 29 March 1955.
36. Unreported.
37. For further discussion on the issue, see *Ball* v. *Wirral HA* [2003] WL 117143, and also *Clinical Risk*, **9**(3) (2003), pp. 123–4, and note that the application of the *Bolam* standard is important – in *Hardaker* v. *Newcastle HA* (2001) Lloyd's Rep Med 512, the police owed a duty of care in providing a decompression chamber in the event of diving accidents, but the requisite standard was not that of a hospital facility.
38. See, for example, the statement in *Smithers* v. *Taunton and Somerset NHS Trust* [2004] EWHC 1179 (QB) to the effect that it is impossible for maternity services always to guarantee a safe outcome for a baby.
39. (1996) 8 Med LR 1.
40. Per Lord Justice Kennedy in *Hillyer* v. *St. Bartholomew's Hospital* [1909] 2 KB 820.
41. [1942] 2 KB 293.
42. [1951] 2 KB 343.
43. J. Montgomery, Suing hospitals direct: what tort? *New Law Journal*, **137** (1987), p. 703, in response to J. Bettle, Suing hospitals direct: whose tort is it anyhow?, *New Law Journal*, **137** (1987), p. 573.

44. [1993] 4 Med LR 117.
45. [1937] AC 97.
46. [1947] KB 598.
47. See *Commonwealth* v. *Introvigne* (1982) AWR 749, *Kandis* v. *State Transport Authority* [1984] 154 CLR 672 (both Australian HC); and *Albrighton* v. *Royal Price Albert Hospital* [1980] 2 NSWLR 542 CC.A). *Yepremian* v. *Scarborough General Hospital* [1980] 110 DLR (3d) 513 seems to accept this possibility of negligence; also A. Dugdale & K. Stanton, *Professional Negligence*, 2nd edn (London, Butterworths, 1989), at paragraph 22.22, who speaking of duties to provide treatment under the National Health Services Act 1977 state that 'it is undoubtedly the case that the effect of basing this duty on statute is to ensure that it is non-delegable in its nature'.
48. *The Times* 11 February 1987 (Court of Appeal); quotes that follow are taken from the report at [1993] 4 Med LR 151, 156.
49. (1990) 41 BMLR 171.
50. See also *Danns* v. *Department of Health* [1996] PIQR P69.
51. [1969] 1 QB 428.
52. See above at section 8.3.
53. [1999] 1 WLR 500.
54. [1990] 1 AC 109.
55. [1987] 2 All ER 648.
56. (1990) Ch. 359.
57. See also the interesting case of *Woolgar* v. *Chief Constable of Sussex Police* [2000] 1 WLR 25, in which the court allowed that the police could pass information about a nurse on to (what is now) the NMC where public safety so required.
58. See *R* v. *Department of Health ex p Source Informatics Ltd* [2001] QB 424.
59. Indeed in certain cases this allowance of disclosure has been described as a 'duty' to whistleblow – see *RBG Resources plc (in liquidation)* v. *Rastogi and others* [2002] EWHC 2782 (Ch).
60. *Trustees of Mama East African Women's Group* v. *Dobson* (EAT 23 June 2005 – unreported).
61. [2001] EWCA Civ 1885, reported at (2005) ICR 1760; but note now the refusal of the Court of Appeal to follow this case – see *Woodward* v. *Abbey National PLC* [2006] EWCA Civ 822.

B   An Ethical Perspective – How to Do the Right Thing

David Seedhouse

8.12 Introduction

Health care resources are scarce. This is an unfortunate fact of life. In those cases where there are not enough to go round, difficult choices must be made. Sometimes nurses must make these choices. This may mean that they cannot help everyone they would like to. It may mean that they will not be able to offer as much to each patient as they would ideally wish to, but this is not a perfect world. In order not to waste resources, and in order to be as fair as possible across the health service, all nurses must be aware that rationing is sometimes necessary. Nurses must recognise these facts; nurses must do the right thing.

This, at least, is the official position: it is held (and fostered) by governments preoccupied by the need to keep health care costs in check,[1] by several health economists,[2] some of whom devote considerable energy to the production of technical 'rationing formulae', and it is increasingly (though often grudgingly) accepted by many nurses. Slowly but surely the 'official line' has also come to be believed by many of the general public, who listen to the various experts and – not unreasonably – conclude that if those in the know see the need to ration then there must indeed be such a need.

But is the official position true? Certainly not everyone accepts it. For instance, it has been argued that the basic duty of any government must be to defend its people against threats to life and safety, and that since in normal circumstances health care does this much better than any other sort of public provision (and is infinitely more useful than an idle army), governments must – as a matter of obligation to their subjects – switch military funding to health services.[3] It is also claimed that in the USA, where spending on health care consistently consumes around 14% of the gross domestic product, there are already more than enough health services to go round; the problem is that not everyone who needs them can get access (millions of Americans do not have health insurance and cannot afford to pay privately to get the help they need).[4]

It is further argued, against the official view, that the belief that the development of new medicines and technologies must fuel growing patient demand ad infinitum is based on a myth.[5] It is argued that just as a doubling of public toilets or public bus services would not automatically double the desire (or need) of the public to make use of them, so too there is a finite amount of kidney disease, a limit to the number of people who can benefit from coronary by-pass surgery, and so on. Perhaps if more buses were supplied very cheaply, or even at no cost to the user at all, their use would increase, but even so there will always be a natural limit on the number of people who would like to travel from A to B at any one time.

It is not easy to judge which one of these positions – the 'official line' or that of the 'rebel camp' – is correct. Clearly, both are at least partly true. For instance, where there are more potential recipients than donated organs, there is an undeniable scarcity of this particular resource. On the other hand, it is equally incontrovertible that if money were to be taken from some expensive 'high-tech' or over-provided medical services, and spent instead on the provision of better and more comprehensive 'preventive services', many 'health needs' now not met because of scarcity could be provided for.

What is clearest of all, however, is that there are considerable philosophical and practical uncertainties underlying the 'resources debate', most of which are unlikely to be resolved in the foreseeable future. The nature of 'health care cost' and 'health care benefit' is not agreed in theory.[6] Nor is it yet physically possible to collate even the simple financial costs of many modern health services.[7] And even if credible classifications and calculations were to be developed, even if someone were to invent a comprehensive 'health service slide rule', the accuracy and appropriateness of these taxonomies and methods of calculating would inevitably be challenged. It would, for instance, remain the case that different individuals would value even identical services (and identical results) in different ways. For one person a few more days of life, even in great pain, might be of immense value – while for another there would be no point at all.

8.13 Nursing in scarcity

What can nurses do when faced with such intangibles? These days almost all nurses work in environments where managers, and others, are openly concerned about efficiency, avoiding waste and reducing cost wherever possible.

What is the nurse, concerned about how best to use scarce resources, to do? How can she be fair? How can she deal with perceived injustice? How can she make any difference at all?

Whether or not any individual can make a difference within massive, complex systems depends on two factors. First, and obviously, what she can do depends on whether or not she is in a position of any power and influence. Secondly, and less obviously, what she can do depends upon the clarity with which she has formulated her goals. Philosophy (or clear thinking) can do nothing about the first factor, but it can help (albeit only a little) with the second. With practice a nurse can improve her understanding of both general situations and her own circumstances, she can learn to define the meaning of key terms (such as 'resource', 'rationing' and 'fairness'), and she can become better able to identify her role (and the limits of her role).

It is not possible in this chapter to provide a philosophical education. In order to learn philosophy there is no substitute for a carefully formulated programme of study undertaken over several years. However, it is possible to show how a philosophically informed nurse might at least begin to react to resource allocation problems, and in so doing to offer insight into one method of coping with seemingly impossible situations.

8.14 A number – or a free person?

Nursing is a hierarchical and often authoritarian profession. All groups of nurses have a 'pecking-order', and those nurses who do not toe the line can, in some circumstances, suffer severe reprimand. This is a deep-seated aspect of nursing culture. It is an equally long-established tradition that most nurses are of a lower rank than doctors. These circumstances are changing somewhat nowadays, with the advent of nurse managers and as nursing is increasingly thought of as a profession. However, for very many nurses it remains the case that they are able to exert only a very limited influence on health service policy.

So, when it comes to 'doing the right thing', most nurses apparently have very little choice; the 'right thing' is defined by 'the system' in which they are a 'cog' or a 'number' and their only option is to implement it. The 'right thing', in other words, is handed down to them (this might be called 'doing the right thing 1'). Of course, there is an alternative form of 'doing the right thing', which can be defined as a nurse taking the course of action that she has, after careful deliberation, deemed to be the best – whether or not this is the action recommended by the system. The 'right thing', in this form, is a matter of conscience and intelligent reflection (and might be called 'doing the right thing 2').

How might the nurse 'do the right thing' in the two case studies offered by Robert Lee in part A of this chapter?

8.14.1 Case study one

Consider again the first case study of the nurse, N, on night duty in charge of a small hospital where R brings V, the victim of a hit-and-run accident, despite the sign at the gate advising that there is no accident and emergency unit there (section 8.7).

As far as 'doing the right thing 1' is concerned, Robert Lee has already given part of a possible answer that 'in purely legal terms, N would be free to refuse treatment to V and urge R and V to present themselves at the nearest accident and emergency department'. Officially the hospital does not provide accident and emergency services, so there is no legal obligation on the nurse to do anything. Furthermore, if this hospital is cost-conscious, and if the management have made it clear that emergency cases are not to be treated, then to 'do the right thing 1' the nurse must turn the potential patient away – and must do so whatever her feelings about it, and whatever help she might have been able to give. Since she would have 'done the right thing', there would be no sanction 'the authorities' could take against the nurse.

However, in this case (as in all cases) the nurse might instead consider 'doing the right thing 2' – that is, she might not simply follow the regulation course, but might first take the trouble to analyse the situation for herself, and then act according to the result of her own reasoning. Of course, if she decides that she must advise V and R that she cannot help them, and that they must attend the nearest accident and emergency hospital, then the practical outcome will be the same. However, the nurse herself will have thought more thoroughly than if she had merely obeyed the rules, and may well feel more confident (and more in charge) as a result.

But how is she to carry out this analysis? How might she structure her thinking if she decides to 'do the right thing 2'? N does have the option to help the injured person, but if she does so she might well place herself at greater personal risk than if she were simply to turn V and R away. As stated in section 8.7, 'once N opts to render care and assistance to V, then a duty of care arises and the question then relates to the applicable standard of care. It is clear that liability may result from negligent treatment or advice rendered by N or any failure of communication in providing V with emergency treatment.' So what should N do?

Certainly, 'doing the right thing 2' is the more complicated – and potentially more fraught – option. What factors should the nurse take into account? How might she begin to think clearly about this case? If she does decide to deliberate on the situation she must do so quickly, and under considerable emotional pressure – neither of which are conducive to clear reasoning. Given this, the nurse might find it helpful to organise her thinking under three distinct headings: context, outcomes and obligations.

Context

First, N must assess the risk. 'Risk', of course, is a general term that might be interpreted in several ways. The nurse might, for instance, think about the risk to the injured party (if he is not instantly helped, how will he be affected?); the risk to her conscience (what if she begins to help and the patient dies – or what if she does not help and the patient dies?); the risk to her future career, and so on.

She must also, prior to any further deliberation, decide whether any intervention she could make would do any good. If it would not, and if it is clearly better that V attends a working clinic, then obviously that is where he should go. If, on the other hand, she decides she could give some help, she must also work out how effective she would be and how certain she is of her judgement about her effectiveness. Also, if there are other patients whom she might be helping instead of V, she must consider whether she should assist them before she turns her attention to V.

The context, in this case as in most cases that nurses have to deal with, is one of uncertainty. N simply does not know for sure what the outcome of any of her options will be. Because of this it is very important that she reflects, in the abstract, on her priorities.

Outcomes

Is she, for example, most concerned with the reputation of the hospital? Is she concerned for the safety of her other patients, who may be endangered if she devotes herself solely to the care of V? Or is her priority the injured person directly in front of her? She may not, in a short space of time, be able to think through all the ramifications, but it will help her considerably if she feels she understands which of these possible goals are, in principle, the most important.

Obligations

Does she have any obligations or duties that override the context? Must she, for instance, as a 'caring professional', do all she can to help V, who is clearly suffering? This is for her to decide. However, as she thinks about this she must be aware that not only must she justify her decision to herself but she may also have to justify it to others. So if she decides she is obliged to intervene wherever she sees suffering, she must also be able to say whether this is a general obligation and is always incumbent on her, or whether there are factors (such as context and outcome) that may sometimes cancel out such a duty.

8.14.2 Case study two

Consider now the second case study (set out in section 8.9) of W, the night duty charge nurse believing that the standard of care had dropped prior to a patient's dying in distressing circumstances. In this case, even more than the first, there are evidently two distinct 'right things' to do. 'Doing the right thing 1' in this case is either to do nothing because the context is so overwhelming (the nurse may know that similar staffing difficulties are being experienced across the country – how can her situation be made an exception?), or to pursue the matter through the 'official channels', as explained in section 8.9. However, since all the 'official channels' are themselves part of the system that allows (or is forced to allow) such a situation to arise, it is extremely unlikely that this course of action will bring about an improvement in the situation on the nurse's ward. 'Doing the right thing 1' would almost certainly mean that little would change.

  However, if the nurse were to 'do the right thing 2' it might be a different matter. Although she might in the end reach the same conclusions as generated by 'doing the right thing 1', the nurse must first try to think as an individual uninfluenced by the system. What, she might ask, ought to be done in these circumstances? The questions she must address are similar to those considered by N in Case one, and again might usefully be divided into the three categories.

  What are the risks in this context? Will 'whistle-blowing' be effective? How important is the nurse's career? (There are well-known examples of nurses destroying their careers in the pursuit of causes they believe to be just.) Are the nurse's obligations to her patients paramount, or does she have wider duties (to her colleagues or to those future patients she might not be able to care for if she is suspended from work or sacked)? In principle, what outcomes does she value most highly? Is her own happiness paramount? Or is it crucial that the patients on her ward get the best possible service? If the latter, does it matter that if she succeeds in getting what she wants for her ward, resources may be moved from other hard-pressed parts of the hospital – so decreasing the quality of service to other patients? If she finally decides that the context is simply unacceptable, and that something must be done to improve it, then 'doing the right thing 1' may very well cease to be an option.

8.15 Principled solutions?

Some nurses may find it helpful to try to apply 'ethical principles' to resource allocation dilemmas. This approach has been widely recommended in recent years, and most texts on 'nursing ethics' contain sizeable sections on 'basic', 'ethical' or 'philosophical' principles.[8] A quartet of principles are regularly advocated, and it is likely that most nurses will at least have heard of them. They are 'non-maleficence' (do no harm), 'beneficence' (do good), 'respect autonomy' (respect the patient's choice) and 'justice' (see Chapter 2).[9] The attraction of this group of principles is that they seem to offer an uncomplicated structure within which to organise one's thoughts. Moreover, it seems possible to seize on just one of these principles in order to 'solve' a dilemma. If, for instance, a nurse feels that a doctor is not taking the wishes of a patient seriously she might describe this as 'unethical' behaviour purely because the doctor is not 'respecting autonomy' (so ignoring or overriding any alternative justifications the medic might have). Most nurses will have personal experience of cases in which this has happened – and might well consider it fair criticism – but it is very important not to confuse the assertion of single principles (however justifiable) with 'ethical analysis'. The latter is a much more complicated procedure which – if it is to be done at all properly – must involve reflection upon a range of 'ethical principles' together with the other considerations (context, outcomes, obligations) already mentioned in this section.

This is not to say that the use of the principles is unhelpful. The point is that any thoughtful ethical analysis is bound to place considerable intellectual demands on the health care analyst. In Case two it might appear that the hub of the matter is a straightforward clash between the ideal of 'efficiency' and the principles of 'justice'. It might, in other words, seem to nurse W that her patients are being unjustly treated, and that their interests are regarded as secondary to those of the hospital as a whole (which must be run as 'efficiently' as possible). However, if W is seriously to argue this case then it is not enough for her merely to cry 'unjust!' since 'justice' can be understood in more than one way, and can even be interpreted in ways that contradict each other.

For example, there are those who think that the key to understanding 'justice' is to treat people first and foremost in accord with what they deserve; others disagree, arguing that the basic criterion of justice is need; and there is a further group who believe that justice can come about only when people's rights are upheld.[10] What is more, sophisticated analysts tend to blend and adapt these different understandings in subtle ways, depending on the matter under scrutiny. Any contemplative analysis of the merits (or justice) of the management of the acutely ill patient must consider and explain what justice means in this case (whether the patients have the same right to treatment as other patients in the hospital, and so no special priority; whether they have needs of such gravity that they are entitled to treatment before those with lesser needs; whether this set of patients merits privileged attention and so deserves priority treatment for some reason).

Philosophers are used to such discussions, and often spend much time trying to disentangle the various issues, only to see them knot together again the moment they move their attention elsewhere. Such detailed reflection requires a fair amount of expertise – and countless hours – neither of which are usually available to the nurse. And this can place the nurse who sees that these are complex matters, and who recognises that they can be properly dealt with only by careful analysis, at a considerable disadvantage. If she tries to protest in an intelligent way it is very easy to defeat her. Her opponent can say: 'We don't have the time for this sort of reflection'; or, 'What you are suggesting requires an analysis of everything we do, and this is not a practical proposition' (which of course means that everything can continue unchanged – inertia is not only a natural tendency but also a powerful weapon in the hands of those who are happy with the status quo). Her opponent might also ask: 'What do you mean by justice?', knowing full well that any credible answer must take more time and effort than almost any nurse can give (and knowing that even if the nurse does attempt an answer it will be very easy to say later: 'Please spell out your interpretation of need/rights/equity,' or whatever other terms she has not fully explained).

In such circumstances the nurse has three strategies open to her. She might spend many hours developing her case (she might even enlist the help of a trained philosopher); she might take a simpler course and analyse her work problems using the 'context, outcomes and obligations' framework (in the knowledge that this is by no means all there is to ethical analysis); or she might take her opponent on, on his own terms. Whenever he says, 'Could you expand on that?' or 'What do you mean?', the nurse might ask in turn, 'What do you mean by efficiency?', 'How do you justify removing resources from this ward and increasing them on that?' or 'What are your principles for resource allocation within this hospital, and on what grounds do you justify these?'

8.16 Conclusion

This part of the chapter has raised questions, but only sketched out answers to them. The rest is for the individual nurse to decide, and there are many books and papers available to which she might turn for more detailed guidance. What is most important is that each nurse realises the complexity of any resource problem she is facing and, if she so decides that she is able to tackle it in a systematic manner. If she genuinely tries to do this, and if she feels she has arrived at a defensible decision, then there is probably little more she can do. She cannot change the world, and whatever she does she is hardly likely to unsettle governments focused so intently on financial balance sheets.

Nevertheless, there will always – if only occasionally – be times when the nurse can do something to change things for the better. If, for example, she decides not only to treat V (in Case one) but to publicise the fact in local newspapers (so both promoting the hospital as a compassionate organisation and letting it be known that were funds available an accident and emergency service could be provided or reinstated) then she might have an impact. Moreover, if the nurse were to contact the relatives of the patient who died 'in distressing circumstances' (in Case two) and enlist their support she might campaign intelligently and effectively for more resources. On both strategies she would face very significant risks – indeed, she could expect censure from the system were her involvement to become known – but she would at least stand a chance of making a desirable difference.

She would, in other words, be working for justice as a combination of meeting needs and deserts and upholding rights – through positively discriminating in favour of those patients closest to her.

In general, a great deal rests on the following question, and how it is answered in the coming years: whether nurses in general continue mostly or only 'to do the right thing 1' or whether the profession increasingly aims 'to do the right thing 2' (and commits its own resources to ensuring this). If the former, then it is hard to see how nurses will be able to justify their claim to professional status, but if the latter, and the majority of nurses become able and willing to think through the question 'How best might I act in this situation?' (rather than asking 'What am I supposed to do here?'), then nurses, as a group, might perform an enormous service: they might open up the health service to internal debate, to genuine conversation (without fear of sanction and reprisal) about how best to deliver public health services – not least when there are not enough of them to go round. And it is certain that it is only by continually considering whether to 'do the right thing 1' or to 'do the right thing 2' that nurses will exercise their 'moral muscles' sufficiently to effect resource allocation injustices for the better, since never to consider 'doing the right thing 2' eventually and inevitably destroys the capacity for moral reasoning.[11,12]

8.17 Notes and references

1. See *Health Care Analysis*, **1**(1) (1993), passim.
2. A. Williams, Cost-effectiveness analysis: is it ethical? *Journal of Medical Ethics*, **18** (1992), pp. 7–11.
3. J. Harris, Unprincipled QALYs: a response to Cubbon, *Journal of Medical Ethics*, **17** (1991), pp. 185–8.
4. C. Hackler, Health care reform in the United States, *Health Care Analysis*, **1**(1), (1993), pp. 5–13.
5. A. Smith, Qualms about QALYs, *The Lancet*, **1**(X) (1987), pp. 34–6.
6. D.F. Seedhouse, *Fortress NHS: A Philosophical Review of the National Health Service* (Chichester, John Wiley and Sons, 1994).
7. A. Culyer, The morality of efficiency in health care: some uncomfortable implications, *Health Economics*, 1(1) (1992), pp. 7–18.
8. I. Thompson, K.M. Melia & K.M. Boyd, *Nursing Ethics* (Edinburgh, Churchill Livingstone, 1988).
9. R.P. Gillon, *Philosophical Medical Ethics* (Chichester, John Wiley and Sons, 1985).
10. D. Miller, *Social Justice* (Oxford, Oxford University Press, 1976).
11. D.F. Seedhouse, *Practical Nursing Philosophy: The Universal Ethical Code* (Chichester, John Wiley and Sons, 2000).
12. D.F. Seedhouse, *Health: The Foundations for Achievement*, 2nd edn (Chichester, John Wiley and Sons, 2001).

8.18 Further reading

Seedhouse, D.F. (2007) *Ethics: The Heart of Healthcare*, John Wiley and Sons, Chichester.
Seedhouse, D.F. (2005) *Values Based Health Care: The Fundamentals of Ethical Decision-Making*, John Wiley and Sons, Chichester.

9 Mental Health Nursing

A   The Legal Perspective

Michael Gunn and M.E. Rodgers

While there are many issues that face nurses working with people with mental illness or a learning difficulty, this chapter will consider some of the more commonly encountered problems. The chapter will deal with treatment under the Mental Health Act 1983 (MHA);[1] treatment falling outside that Act; the use of the nurse's holding powers under section 5(4) of the MHA; the care and management of violent or aggressive patients; treatment in the community; and the nurse's role in relation to Mental Health Review Tribunals. Readers should be aware that a comprehensive review of the MHA has been in progress for a period. At one time this was to take the form of a new piece of legislation but now it will take the form of significant amendments to the Mental Health Act 1983 by way of the Mental Health Bill 2007. That bill will come into force at about the same time as the Mental Capacity Act 2005 (MCA), to which it introduces some amendments. Both the amended Mental Health Act and the MCA will be in force during 2007. Some of the changes to the Mental Health Act are of sufficient significance and independence that they are dealt with separately.

Two such changes must be mentioned at the outset. First is the move away from local social services authorities only being able to appoint approved social workers (ASWs) to a position where they can appoint sufficient 'appropriate mental health professionals' (AMHPs). This group of professionals is likely to include nurses, occupational therapists and psychologists. The key to appointment will be that they have the right skills, experience and training. Should nurses be appointed, they will be centrally involved in, for example, admission to hospital in a way that they have not been before. The AMHP, like the current ASW, can be an applicant, as an alternative to the potential patient's nearest relative, and so must understand the compulsory admissions procedure in terms of both the substantive issues and procedure that have to be satisfied.

Second is the other change to professional roles proposed in the Mental Health Bill 2007. This is the move away from the 'responsible medical officer' (a role that can only be fulfilled by a doctor) to that of the 'responsible clinician'. The responsible clinician may be any practitioner who has been approved (that is, an 'approved clinician'), and not only doctors may be approved but also practitioners from other professions such as nursing, psychology, occupational therapy and social work. If an approved clinician is the patient's responsible clinician, he or she has the same functions as those currently reserved to the doctor who is the patient's responsible medical officer, which include the power to detain an inpatient under section 5, the grant of leave of absence under section 17, the renewal of the section 3 authority to detain under section 20, the power of discharge under section 23, and similar powers in relation to patients detained through the criminal justice system under Part 3 of the Mental Health Act 1983.

These two changes will significantly affect the status of those nurses so functioning and have the potential dramatically to affect the status of mental health nursing in general. For nurses with such roles, this chapter will provide some insight into some of the issues but not all.

9.1 Treatment under the Mental Health Act 1983

Treatment for mental disorder may lawfully be given under the MHA provided the patient is detained under the Act by means of a non-emergency section. It is important to stress that treatment for purely physical problems is not under consideration here. Further, this part of the discussion deals with patients detained in hospital. In the future, there are new provisions relating to community patients, which are dealt with below.

Before looking at the provisions of the legislation, it is important to stress that there are European Convention on Human Rights requirements that must be met.[2] The reality is that these will, usually, be met if the requirements of the legislation are satisfied by people exercising appropriate professional judgements. This is presumably why the Mental Health Bill 2007 contains no provisions to amend Part 4 of the Act to deal with a series of cases about the topic.

If nurses are to be involved in the treatment of a patient, they must first be able to satisfy themselves whether the patient is detained under a relevant section. The Fifth Biennial Report of the Mental Health Act Commission[3] stressed the importance of the nurse's role, and it is the nurse's legal and ethical input to this area of law that will be covered in this chapter.

9.1.1 First stage: is the patient a detained patient?

A nurse must be able to make sure that the appropriate detention documentation for a non-emergency section is present in the patient's ward file. The nurse is, therefore, looking for documentation that indicates that the patient is detained under any of the following: .

- section 2 (for assessment including medical treatment)
- section 3 (for treatment)
- section 36 (remand of accused person to hospital for treatment)
- section 37 (hospital order, with or without a restriction order under section 41)
- section 38 (an interim hospital order)
- section 46 (an order relating to a member of the armed forces)
- section 47 (a transfer of a prisoner, with or without restrictions under section 49)
- section 48 (transfer of a civil or remand prisoner, with or without restrictions under section 49).

It is not necessary for the nurse to be sure that the patient is lawfully detained. The function of ascertaining the legality and appropriateness of detention is for the hospital managers, a function that is normally delegated to the medical records department. In any case, section 6(3) of the MHA ensures that it is appropriate to rely on the forms since it provides:

> Any application for the admission of a patient under this Part of this Act which appears to be duly made and to be founded on the necessary medical recommendations may be acted upon without further proof of the signature or qualification of the person by whom the application or any such medical recommendation is made or given or of any matter of fact or opinion stated in it.[4]

What is usually required, therefore, is that the nurse files and then is able to find in the notes, the relevant forms indicating that the patient has been admitted under one of the sections to which reference has already been made. If the patient has been admitted under section 2, the nurse is looking for:

(1) the application form that must be either Form 2 (where the nearest relative was the applicant[5]) or Form 3 (where an approved social worker was the applicant[6])
(2) a form for the medical recommendation (either one copy of Form 4 where the recommendation was done jointly or two copies of Form 5 where the recommendations were done separately)
(3) Form 15, which indicates that the patient has been accepted by the hospital as a detained patient.

If the patient has been admitted under section 3, the nurse is similarly looking for:

(1) the relevant application form (Form 8 where the applicant is the nearest relative and Form 9 where the applicant is an approved social worker)
(2) the relevant form stating the medical recommendations (one copy of Form 10 where there is a joint medical recommendation and two copies of Form 11 where there are separate recommendations)
(3) a copy of Form 15.

If the patient is detained under section 36, section 37, section 38 or section 46, there must be documentation from a court indicating the imposition of the section. If the patient is detained under section 47 or section 48, there must be a warrant from the Home Secretary directing the transfer of the patient to the hospital.

Some significant changes will be introduced to detention procedures when, and if, the Mental Health Bill 2007 comes into force. First, it will remove all specified mental disorders (MHB 2007, clause 1) and only use the concept of mental disorder, defined as any disorder or disability of mind. All other conditions will still have to be met, but how significant a change this means remains to be seen. It will, though, mean that people with personality disorder not satisfying the current definition of psychopathic disorder could be compulsorily detained, as could people who suffer brain damage later in life. It will not, however, become easier to admit people with learning disability as such a person does not have a mental disorder unless their disability 'is associated with abnormally aggressive or seriously irrespons-ible conduct' on their part (MHB 2007, clause 2). Also the only exclusions from the concept of mental disorder will be dependence on alcohol or drugs (MHB 2007, clause 3). This means, for example, that people with a sexual deviancy would be able to be detained under the Act on the basis of that deviancy, provided all the other criteria are satisfied. Whether this happens remains to be seen.

Secondly, the old so-called 'treatability' test will be replaced by a requirement for appropriate medical treatment to be available on admission: treatment must be appropriate in a patient's case 'taking into account the nature and degree of the mental disorder and all other circumstances of his case' (MHB 2007, clause 4). If there is no treatment that is appropriate, there is a belief that admission may still be possible. There is no requirement in the Act (even as amended) or under the European Convention on Human Rights (as currently interpreted by the European Court) that a condition must be treated when in hospital provided there is a mental disorder and the place of detention is suitable. Thus people with a personality disorder (not limited to psychopathic disorder as defined in the 1983 Act when and if the changes of the Mental Health Bill 2007 are implemented) could be compulsorily detained even if there was no treatment available, but detention in hospital would have to be appropriate for that individual. Finally, there are significant changes to the definition of nearest relative both to equalise civil partners with married couples and to allow the county court to replace any-one found to be unsuitable to act as such (MHB 2007, clauses 21–24). All these changes will enable the Mental Health Act 1983 as amended to be more compliant with the European Convention on Human Rights.

9.1.2 Second stage: does the treatment fall within the MHA?

Nurses must be able to satisfy themselves that the treatment proposed is treat-ment that may lawfully be carried out under the MHA. Medical treatment is widely defined by the Act in section 145(1):

> [M]edical treatment includes nursing, and also includes care, habilation and rehabilitation under medical supervision . . .

When, and if, the changes introduced by the Mental Health Bill 2007 are implemented, the definition in section 145 will be clarified so that the definition reads that medical treatment 'includes nursing, psychological intervention and specialist mental health habilation, rehabilitation and care'.

For the purposes of assessing the legality of the particular activity in question, treatment is classified into three different groups covered by sections 57, 58 and 63, which are found in Part IV of the MHA. The following discussion will deal with these sections in reverse order since section 63 is, in most cases, the first that would be considered to permit treatment of a detained individual. Sections 58 and 57 deal with what can be suggested to be more invasive treatments or treatments that are recognised as giving rise to greater concern. For these treatments to be given, either the procedure stated in section 57 or 58 must be followed or the urgent treatment provisions in section 62 must be applied. It is worth noting that where a patient is detained under the MHA and treatment is provided under the treatment sections in Part IV of the MHA the MCA will have no effect,[7] and it is important also to take into account the impact of the introduction of supervised community treatment by the Mental Health Bill 2007, which is considered below.

Treatment without consent

Treatment provided under the remit of section 63 is treatment for mental disorder given by or under the supervision of the patient's responsible medical officer (RMO) (this role will be performed by the responsible clinician when, and if, the Mental Health Bill 2007 is implemented and underlines the point made earlier about the significant impact on professional roles, including those of nurses), and does not require the patient's consent. Patients, therefore, can be provided with any form of medical treatment that is for their mental disorder without their consent. This proposition does not apply to the special forms of treatment that fall under sections 57 and 58 (that is, psychosurgery, surgical implantation of hormones to reduce male sexual drive, electro-convulsive therapy and medication continued after the first three months of administration); for these the special procedures outlined below must be followed. Patients can be given medication for their mental disorder, under section 63, for three months before the special procedure under section 58 has to be followed. The three-month period runs from when medication was first given, which will not necessarily be the same time as when the patient was first detained.

For the nurse participating in the administration of medication, it will be necessary to establish, first, that the patient is detained; second, that the medication is being given for the patient's mental disorder; and third, that the treatment is being given less than three months since it started. It will not usually be possible to check the notes for a form, since none is required under section 63. Thus, clearly recording the first administration of medicine is vital, as is ensuring that the legally relevant information and documentation are readily available for inspection.

In recent years it has become apparent that one particular issue on the application of section 63 can cause difficulty. This is in determining whether a particular treatment is, indeed, for the patient's mental disorder as opposed to a physical disorder or condition. Two situations highlight the difficult and controversial boundary between treatment for a physical condition and for a mental disorder. The first concerns the treatment of anorexia nervosa, particularly where the patient is an adult (where the patient is a child the treatment might be given without recourse to the MHA in some circumstances). The Mental Health Act Commission, in its Fourth Biennial Report, stated that in its view 'severe anorexia nervosa falls within the definition of mental disorder'.[8] If this is the case an individual may be admitted to hospital, provided all other criteria are satisfied, under section 2 MHA for assessment (which may be followed by treatment), or alternatively section 3 MHA for treatment, where an assessment has already been carried out and reflects the current situation.[9] It is also the view of the Mental Health Act Commission that 'treatment of anorexia nervosa necessary for the health or safety of the patient, including involuntary feeding and maintenance of hydration, is permissible in patients whose anorexia is causing serious concern'.[10]

The only basis on which this opinion may be predicated is that these forms of activity fall within the definition of treatment within the Act and that section 63 is the relevant section authorising treatment. No one, it is submitted, can dispute that, given the wide definition of medical treatment in the Act, involuntary feeding does fall within 'treatment'. Anorexia nervosa is a mental disorder. But the essential question, as required by the wording of section 63, is whether the treatment is *for* the mental disorder from which the patient is suffering. The Court of Appeal has held, in B v. *Croydon Health Authority* (1994), that, if treatment is capable of being ancillary to core treatment – that is, it is nursing care 'concurrent with the core treatment or as a necessary prerequisite to such treatment or to prevent the patient from causing harm to himself or to alleviate the consequences of the disorder' – it will be upheld as lawful under section 63.[11]

The second area is in relation to compulsory Caesarean sections. A series of cases has been presented to the courts where the question of whether treatment is for a physical problem or for a mental disorder has been the issue.[12] While different outcomes have resulted from these cases, there appears to be an adherence to the principles put forward in B v. *Croydon Health Authority* (1994) in that the treatment for the physical condition must be ancillary to the treatment for the mental disorder for it to be regarded as treatment for the patient's mental disorder and thus the treatment can be given under section 63 (to a detained patient) without her consent. Hence in *Tameside and Glossop Acute Services Trust* v. CH (1996), the Caesarean was sanctioned on the basis that:

> an ancillary reason for the induction and, if necessary, the birth by caesarean section is to prevent a deterioration in [the patient's] mental state. Secondly, there is the clear evidence . . . that in order for the treatment of her schizophrenia to be effective, it is necessary for her to give birth to a live baby. Thirdly, the overall structure of her treatment requires her to receive strong anti-psychotic medication. The administration of that treatment has been necessarily interrupted by her pregnancy and cannot be resumed until her child is born. It is not, therefore, I think stretching language unduly to say that achievement of a successful outcome of her pregnancy is a necessary part of the overall treatment of her mental disorder.[13]

By contrast in R v. *Collins, Pathfinder Health Services Trust, St George's NHS Trust ex parte S* (1998),[14] despite the patient being detained under the provisions of section 2 of the MHA, the court refused to accept that the caesarean section was lawful:

Section 63 of the [MHA] may apply to the treatment of any condition which is integral to the mental disorder . . . provided the treatment is given by, or under the direction of, the responsible medical officer. The treatment administered to S was not so ordered; she was neither offered nor did she refuse treatment for mental disorder . . . In the final analysis, a woman detained under the Act for mental disorder cannot be forced into medical procedures unconnected with her mental condition.[15]

With respect, this appears to be much the more appropriate approach. It is difficult to imagine that, when Parliament passed section 63, it expected that its interpretation would be so wide as to include Caesarean sections. If there is an inability to treat under the MHA owing to lack of nexus between the disorder and the treatment required, that will necessitate an understanding of the common law or new statutory provisions affecting patients who lack capacity to consent. These will be considered later in this chapter and have also been dealt with in Chapter 7.

Treatment under section 58

The second group of treatments for mental disorder consists of electro-convulsive therapy (ECT) and the continuation of the administration of medication, by any means, for mental disorder three months after the person was first administered that medication when a detained patient. As can be seen, this latter situation follows on from the treatment that can lawfully be given under section 63. The treatments covered by section 58 are very common,[16] with continuation of medication being the most frequently used. For nurses, it is essential that they ensure their involvement is lawful, whether they are involved in the distribution of medicine for self-administration or are actually undertaking the administration of the medication.

Once the nurse has identified that the patient is detained, the nurse must then establish whether the administration of medication requires a form in the patient's notes. Having ascertained that the section 63 three-month time frame has expired, a formal record must exist before further medication can lawfully be provided. Alternatives exist for the legality of administration to be established. First, the patient must have consented to it. For that consent to be valid under section 58, it must be verified by either the patient's own doctor (the RMO or – when and if the Mental Health Bill 2007 is implemented – the patient's responsible clinician) or a Second Opinion Approved Doctor (a SOAD, who will be appointed as such by the Secretary of State for Health, but whose day-to-day involvement is monitored by the Mental Health Act Commission). To verify the consent, they will have 'certified in writing that the patient is capable of understanding [the] nature, purpose and likely effect [of the treatment] and has consented to it' (section 58(3)(a)). Alternatively, if the patient cannot, or will not, consent, the medication may continue, but only if a SOAD has 'certified in writing that the patient is not capable of understanding the nature, purpose and likely effects of that treatment or has not consented to it but that, having regard to the likelihood of its alleviating or preventing a deterioration of [the patient's] condition, the treatment should be given' (section 58(3)(b)). When, and if, the Mental Health Bill 2007 is implemented, what will have to be certified is that it is appropriate for the treatment to be given and a new section 64(3) will state that it is appropriate for treatment to be given if it 'is appropriate in his case, taking into account the nature and degree of the mental disorder from which he is suffering and all other circumstances of his case'. The simplest means of ensuring that one of these alternatives exists is for the nurse to check which form, if any, is in the patient's file. If the patient is consenting to treatment, it must be covered by a Form 38; if the patient is not consenting, a Form 39 must be present. The question for the nurse, initially, is not whether the patient is consenting but whether there is a form apparently proper on its face that entitles the nurse to be involved in the treatment of the detained patient.

In most hospitals, where thought has been given to the issue, a copy of the relevant form is kept with the medicine card, so that the legal authorisation for the treatment of the patient may be checked every time a drug is administered. This is a simple procedure that enables an easy check to be made. It is surprising, however, how frequently the relevant form is not kept with the treatment card and how frequently the nurse does not realise the significance of the form, and the importance of checking that it covers the treatment in question.

In addition to the issue of checking the lawfulness of treatment, the nurse may be involved in other matters relating to treatment of the detained patient. Treatment covered by Form 38, where the patient consents, does not give rise to a statutory review of the need for treatment.[17] The MHA Code of Practice, however, at paragraph 16.35 requires that, as a matter of good practice, 'all treatments . . . should be regularly reviewed and the patient's treatment plan should include details of when this will take place'. The Code of Practice, while not specifying intervals for review, suggests that a new Form 38 should be completed when:

(1) there is a change in the treatment plan from that recorded
(2) consent is re-established after being withdrawn
(3) there is a break in the patient's detention
(4) there is a permanent change of RMO
(5) the patient's detention is renewed (or annually, whichever is earlier)
(6) there is change in the hospital where the patient is detained.[18]

As well as being good practice, reviewing treatment regimes will enable regular consideration to be given to the question of the patient's continued consent. A patient retains the right to withdraw consent to treatment at any time (section 61), and nurses should be aware of the need to assess continuing consent whenever delivering medication. In the event that consent is withdrawn the nurse should request the attendance of the RMO, who may be able to encourage the patient to accept the treatment. By so doing, the nurse will ensure compliance with their own professional code of practice, and will also act in accordance with the MHA Code of Practice, which states:

Where a patient withdraws consent he or she should receive a clear explanation, which should be recorded in the patient's records:

[. . .]

(7) of the likely consequences of not receiving the treatment;

(8) that a second medical opinion . . . may or will be sought, if applicable, in order to authorise treatment in the continuing absence of the patient's consent;

(9) of the doctor's power to begin or continue urgent treatment under [the emergency provisions] until a second medical opinion has been obtained, if applicable.[19]

The need to check Form 38 is not only relevant to continued consent, but assists in highlighting those cases where the drug or its dosage listed has changed since the form was originally signed. In this situation the treatment may be unlawful. While the MHA itself does not require specific drugs to be named, or specific dosages, the Code of Practice does suggest that medication should be listed by name. However, the Code of Practice goes on to state that the RMO should '[ensure] that the number of drugs authorised in each class is indicated, by the classes described in the British National Formulary (BNF). The maximum dosage and route of administration should be clearly indicated for each drug or category of drug.'[20] Where specific drugs are named, no further drug may be administered unless a new Form 38 is completed. To avoid this problem most SOADs when signing Form 39 do not list specific drugs but categories according to the BNF, and do not specify the dosage unless it will exceed the recommended BNF upper limit.

Little mention has been made so far of ECT, and it is true that ECT is in a minority of section 58 treatments insofar as SOAD activity is concerned, since the most likely need for a SOAD is with regard to consideration of medication.[21] There has been a very significant increase in the work of SOADs. In 2004/2005, SOADs acted in 10,500 cases. Of those, the RMO's plan was unchanged in 80.0% of cases, the plan was slightly changed in 9.3%, the plan was significantly changed in 2.2% and the matter, surprisingly and worryingly, was not recorded in 8.5% of cases.[22] This does not necessarily suggest a weakness in the system since it cannot be measured simply by outcomes as the system builds in a desire to ensure that the treatment provided will be acceptable,[23] but whether it implies improper collusion or an acceptable recommendation for treatment at the outset is not clear. The Mental Health Act Commission's Eleventh Biennial Report also highlights a striking difference in the usage of ECT between the genders, with 69% of requests being for women.

For ECT, clear indicators for its use are documented. The National Institute for Health and Clinical Excellence (NICE) published guidelines in 2003.[24] The Royal College of Psychiatrists published its revised ECT Handbook in 2005, which indicates that individual responsibility cannot be overridden by the NICE guidelines, although these must be taken into account.[25] Further, the Royal College's approach expects the NICE guidelines to be followed with non-consenting or incapacitated patients.

The nurse may not play a major role in the administration of ECT but will clearly have a role in the assessment of whether the treatment should take place or, after the Mental Health Bill 2007, whether the treatment is appropriate. As with the administration of medicine, the patient may consent to ECT. If so, and the nurse were concerned about the patient's capacity to consent, the first step would seem to be to raise it with the RMO. If this has no effect, the suggestion of seeking the involvement of a SOAD would seem sensible. If, however, this is not done, recording dissent may be the only step left that the nurse feels able to take. This dissent should be identified by the Mental Health Act Commission and, potentially, investigated. An alternative may be to utilise the Public Interest Disclosure Act 1998,[26] although how willing a nurse may be to take this route is uncertain.

Treatment under section 57

The treatments covered by section 57 are psychosurgery and the surgical implantation of hormones to reduce male sexual drive. In order for them to be performed the patient must consent, and this must be verified by a SOAD and two people appointed by the Mental Health Act Commission. These three must 'have certified in writing that the patient is capable of understanding the nature, purpose and likely effects of the treatment in question and has consented to it' (section 57(2)(a)). Also, the SOAD must certify that, 'having regard to the likelihood of the treatment alleviating or preventing a deterioration of the patient's condition, the treatment should be given' (section 57(2)(b) – when, and if, the Mental Health Bill 2007 is implemented, this requirement will change to a determination of whether the treatment is appropriate, as defined above). These requirements are certified as being satisfied by the completion of a Form 37. If there is no Form 37, the treatment cannot go ahead. The presence of a Form 37 will also be required if the treatment is planned for an informal patient, being a patient who is not detained under the MHA by virtue of a section. When the MCA 2005 is in force, the provisions for proxy decision makers will not impact upon this section since this form of treatment is clearly permissible only under Part IV of the MHA and hence is excluded from the scope of the MCA 2005. These two forms of treatment, which raise considerable ethical and legal issues, are carried out relatively rarely on detained patients.[27] Owing to this limited use, more attention has been spent on the preceding treatments authorised by sections 58 and 63.

Emergency treatment under section 62

Before moving on to consider treatment outside the MHA, it is worth noting that the requirements in the Act relating to sections 57 and 58 may be sidestepped in an emergency by virtue of section 62. In these cases it is important for nurses to ensure that they are satisfied that the criteria for section 62 are met, since reliance upon another person's view (that is, the doctor's) may not be sufficient to protect the nurse from action if the treatment turns out to be unlawful. At the very least, it is necessary for the nurse to ensure that there is documentation that the section has been satisfied. This may be done via a local form (as suggested by the Code of Practice in paragraph 16.41) or some other recording system.

It may be necessary for the nurse to assess whether the treatment actually satisfies section 62, as part of the nurse's duty to account to the patient. The section provides:

(1) Sections 57 and 58 above shall not apply to any treatment –
   (a) which is immediately necessary to save the patient's life; or
   (b) which (not being irreversible) is immediately necessary to prevent a serious deterioration of his condition; or
   (c) which (not being irreversible or hazardous) is immediately necessary and represents the minimum interference necessary to prevent the patient from behaving violently or being a danger to himself or others.
[. . .]
(3) For the purposes of this section treatment is irreversible if it has unfavourable physical or psychological consequences and hazardous if it entails significant hazard.

Frequently, this section has caused debate. However, it should very rarely be used. It can only apply where the patient is detained and where one of the four forms of treatment is proposed: that is, psychosurgery, the surgical implantation of hormones to reduce male sexual drive, the administration of medicines after the first three months and ECT. The provisions of section 62 apply to no other form of treatment. It would appear difficult to see how neurosurgery is likely to be necessary in an emergency, especially in the light of the few cases that are considered for section 57 treatments. Additionally, it is difficult to see how the requirements of the section can ever be satisfied in relation to the administration of medicines, since the end of a three-month period ought to be predictable. Even if a patient has only once been administered a medicine for mental disorder the three-month rule operates, at which point an assessment of that patient's needs for medication, including PRN (as required) medication should be made and, depending on the outcome, a Form 38 or 39 brought into being. It is, therefore, the case that section 62 may only be of any real use with regard to the provision of ECT in an emergency, where, for example, a patient is in a catatonic stupor and might otherwise die. Despite the stringent conditions for using section 62, and the requirement in the Code of Practice to monitor why and for how long section 62 treatment is continued, the Mental Health Act Commission has often commented on the inappropriate use made of this section.[28]

9.2 Treatment outside the Mental Health Act 1983

For the nurse, the questions are often fairly straightforward when the person is a detained patient and the treatment falls within the MHA. However, the position is not so clear-cut where the treatment falls outside the remit of the Act. The nurse may be involved in the care of a person who is an informal patient, or who is detained under an emergency section of the MHA, or who is a patient for whom treatment is proposed for a physical disorder. In these situations, the MHA treatment provisions will be of no assistance. Until the introduction of the Mental Capacity Act 2005 in 2007, the answers lie in the common law. The common law and the MCA follow similar lines. On the meaning of competency, the MCA provides greater clarity and one source of reference, and on what to do if someone is incompetent the MCA provides a clearer set of prioritised options.

9.2.1 First stage: is the patient competent?

If treatment is to be provided in these circumstances, it must be ascertained whether the person is competent to consent to treatment. It must always be assumed that the patient is competent, regardless of their medical history or any 'label' that may be attached to them. It is only if it is shown that the patient is not competent that anything other than the consent of the patient may be relied upon. Despite the clear importance of this requirement, the matter did not receive judicial attention until the 1990s. The issue of competence was considered peripherally, and in relation to children, in *Gillick* v. *West Norfolk and Wisbech AHA and the DHSS* (1985). Subsequently, a series of cases considered the matter in relation to adults, primarily *Re T (adult: refusal of medical treatment)* (1992)[29] and *Re C (adult: refusal of treatment)* (1994). In the latter case the court adopted the following test, which was then approved by the Court of Appeal in *Re MB (Medical Treatment)*[30] and which requires that the patient must 'sufficiently understand the nature, purpose and likely effects of the proffered' treatment. In so doing, the judge adopted a proposal by an expert witness that the decision-making process should be divided into three stages:

> first, comprehending and retaining treatment information, second, believing it and third, weighing it in the balance to arrive at choice.

This test for capacity has been adopted by the Code of Practice, but with a little more by way of explanation:

> 15.10 An individual is presumed to have the capacity to make a treatment decision unless he or she:
>
> is unable to take in and retain the information material to the decision especially as to the likely consequences of having or not having the treatment; or
> is unable to believe the information; or
> is unable to weigh the information in the balance as part of a process of arriving at the decision.

The Code of Practice also makes it clear that capacity can be variable, and so should be assessed at the time the treatment is proposed.[31] It is also important to remember:

> Mental disorder does not necessarily make a patient incapable of giving or refusing consent. Capacity to consent is variable in people with mental disorder and should be assessed in relation to the particular patient, at the particular time, as regards the particular treatment proposed.[32]

When the Mental Capacity Act 2005 is fully in force, there will exist statutory provisions in relation to the presumptions of capacity and the assessment of lack of capacity. Section 1 sets out the relevant presumptions:

- the patient must be assumed to have capacity unless it is established that capacity does not exist
- a patient should not be treated as unable to make a decision unless all practicable steps have been taken to assist them make the decision

- a patient should not be treated as lacking capacity simply because the decision made is 'unwise'
- any acts done on behalf of a patient without capacity must be done in their best interests
- before any act is done it must be considered to be the least restrictive intervention.

The definition provided to establish where a patient does lack capacity is set out in section 2 thus:

[A] person lacks capacity in relation to a matter if at the material time he is unable to make a decision for himself in relation to the matter because of an impairment of, or a disturbance in the functioning of, the mind or brain.

Section 3 then goes on to provide criteria to establish whether the patient is unable to make a decision: that is, if they are unable:

- to understand the information relevant to the decision
- retain that information
- use or weigh that information as part of the process of making the decision
- to communicate that decision.

The nurse's involvement may well include assisting in the assessment of whether the patient has the necessary capacity to make the decision. While the common law has been reasonably clear since the decisions in *Re C* (1994) and *Re MB* (1997), the MCA 2005 sets out clearer guidelines for an assessment of capacity, although they do not differ greatly from the current legal position.

Regardless of whether the nurse is involved in making the assessment of capacity, she or he must be able to check the records to see whether the patient is regarded at the time of the treatment as being not competent to consent to the particular treatment in question. To be involved in these various activities, therefore, a nurse needs to be professionally qualified and skilled to assist in determining capacity and to be capable of identifying the warning signs that the patient may not be competent to consent. The nurse also needs to be sufficiently aware to consider the legal situation prior to being included in the treatment of the patient.

9.2.2 Second stage: where the patient is competent

It is quite clear that, where patients are competent, their decisions must be respected and followed. This is so even where the patient is dying and it is life-saving treatment that is refused, and this is a principle propounded in numerous cases: for example, *Re MB (medical treatment)* (1997) and *R v. Collins, Pathfinder Health Services Trust, St George's NHS Trust, ex parte S* (1998).[33] In the event of a dispute or uncertainty surrounding capacity, the courts have indicated that they should be involved in deciding the issues, and this should be done as soon as possible. The procedure for seeking the court's view will be much simpler once the MCA is in force in 2007. However, the fact that a decision by a patient is deemed 'irrational' or 'contrary to what is to be expected of the majority of adults'[34] should not automatically give cause to doubt as to the patient's competence, and this is confirmed in the MCA 2005. The nurse clearly has a role to play in identifying potential problems of this nature and in so doing will be complying with their professional code of ethics, which requires the nurse to act as advocate for their patient.

9.2.3 Third stage: where the patient is not competent

If a patient is not competent, treatment may be given provided it is in their best interests. At common law, 'best interests' means that the treatment is that which is the best that can be provided to someone, taking into account all relevant factors (including medical, welfare, emotional . . .).[35] In certain situations a reference to the court to confirm the validity of treatment may be required, for example where an incapable patient is to be sterilised, or a patient in a persistent vegetative state is to have any life-maintaining equipment disconnected or treatment stopped.[36]

Where reference to the court is not required, the treatment provider must ascertain whether the treatment is in the patient's best interests. The question that may arise is whether the nurse is required to comply with the doctor's request that treatment be provided. This places the nurse in a difficult position if he or she is not satisfied that the treatment being proposed is indeed in the best interests of the patient according to proper nursing standards. In a case such as this (and as is considered more fully elsewhere in this book) it is submitted that the nurse should be wary of simply following the doctor's instructions without at least raising and recording any doubts there may be about the proposed course of action.

A best interests approach is not a surprising one where the patient is not, and has not been, capable of expressing any treatment wishes. But defining a person's best interests may be problematical. It may fail adequately to achieve the proper balance, as Fennell points out, between the obligation to show respect for persons (that is, concern for the person's welfare and the sanctity of life) and the obligation to respect the wishes of the person – that is, the balance between paternalism and autonomy.[37] It should be noted that the current best interests test does not solve the 'ethical differences which may occur within care teams concerned with the treatment of incapable patients'.[38] However, when the MCA 2005 is fully in force, a statutory test to determine best interests will be in place. Section 4 sets out the issues that need to be taken into account in order to determine what is in the patient's best interests. Hence the following factors will have to be considered:

- the person's past and present wishes and feelings (and any relevant written statement executed when the patient had capacity)
- the patient's beliefs and values if these would be likely to have influenced his decision if he had capacity
- other factors that the patient would have been likely to take into consideration.

In addition there is a statutory role for others in determining best interests, and where practical and appropriate the following should be consulted:

- anyone named by the person as someone to be consulted on the matter in question or matters of that kind
- anyone engaged in caring for the patient or interested in their welfare
- a donee of a lasting power of attorney granted by the patient
- a deputy appointed by the court.

The scope of consultation is such that deciding what is in a patient's best interests may still remain problematical and result in conflict between the medical team and the patient's carers.

Under the MCA, there is a range of routes whereby decisions may be made on behalf of an incapable adult. First, that adult may have put in place a decision or procedure that will take priority. Where a person has made a decision in advance, that decision must be respected. It is widely accepted by the courts and, following the implementation of the MCA 2005, will be covered by statute, that a competent patient can make a valid statement as to treatment in advance of the treatment situation arising. Such 'Advance Directives' are subject to restrictive interpretation in current case law:[39]

- the patient must have had capacity at the time of making the statement
- only clear refusals of specified treatment will be upheld
- if there is any doubt as to validity, a declaration may be obtained or treatment given in line with the best interests test
- basic care cannot be refused (there is uncertainty as to what constitutes basic care)
- requests for specified types of treatment cannot be binding
- refusal of treatment that would fall within the remit of the MHA treatment provisions cannot be refused by way of an advance directive.

Some form of investigation should therefore be carried out to ascertain whether an advance directive exists, although the lengths to which medical professionals should go to comply with this have not been the subject of judicial consideration.

The restrictions in relation to advance decisions under the MCA 2005 are similar.

The other way in which the adult can have greater impact upon the decision made when they are incompetent is through the appointment of a donee with the power to make personal welfare decisions for an incapable patient.[40] The appointment of this 'proxy' decision maker may occur via the patient themselves in a lasting power of attorney, created when the patient was competent, or by the court. The donee is required under section 9 of the MCA 2005 to act in accordance with the principles of the Act, and in particular to make welfare decisions with regard to the best interests test laid down in section 4. It will be interesting to see whether a donee is able to take treatment decisions on behalf of a patient for a mental illness.

As a general rule, if neither of the above is present, action that is in the best interests of the patient can be taken under section 5 of the MCA, unless it gives rise to the need for extra protections (thus requiring an additional procedure or the view of an independent mental capacity advocate) or is challenged (and thus the issue of capacity or what is in the individual's best interests is to be determined by the new Court of Protection, which will have the power to decide those questions and may, for example, appoint someone to make decisions on behalf of the incompetent adult).

It should be noted that section 28 of the MCA 2005 seeks to exclude treatment under Part IV of the MHA 1983 from the working of the MCA. However, if the patient is informal, treatment for their mental health will not fall within Part IV, with the exception of psychosurgery under section 58 MHA 1983, meaning that the MCA powers will be available to make the decision on treatment.

It should be noted that an incompetent patient who may be compliant in the sense of remaining in hospital does not need to be detained formally in order that treatment is provided. The provisions of section 131 prevail, in that detention should only occur where it is needed in accordance with the relevant criteria of the detention section. Any treatment provided will need to comply with the concept of best interests under the common law or, when in force, the Mental Capacity Act 2005.[41]

9.3 The nurse's holding power

Section 5(4) of the MHA has provided nurses with a specific power to detain patients for a short time[42] although this power may only be exercised within the limits of the section. Section 5(4) provides:

> If, in the case of a patient who is receiving treatment for mental disorder as an in-patient in a hospital, it appears to a nurse of the prescribed class[43]
>
> (a) that the patient is suffering from mental disorder to such a degree that it is necessary for him to be immediately restrained from leaving the hospital; and
> (b) that it is not practicable to secure the immediate attendance of a [doctor] for the purpose of furnishing a report under [section 5(2)], the nurse may record that fact in writing; and in that event the patient may be detained in the hospital for a period of six hours from the time when that fact is so recorded or until the earlier arrival at the place where the patient is detained of a [doctor] having power to furnish a report under [section 5(2)].

This power presents a nurse who has the appropriate training and qualification with an important professional responsibility. The power is to be exercised by the nurse making a professional judgement as to whether the power should be utilised – as stated by the Code of Practice: '[i]t is the personal decision of the nurse who cannot be instructed to exercise this power by anyone else'.[44] If, following an assessment by the nurse, the power is not exercised and the patient either comes to harm, or harms someone else, it does not follow that the nurse is necessarily liable to any legal action.[45] What will be assessed is whether the decision not to exercise the power was taken reasonably. If it was a reasonable decision – that is, it was a decision that a group of responsible qualified nurses would have made in the same situation – no liability will follow. It is a power in which there is an element of risk-taking, and following guidance will reduce, although not eliminate, the risks. Hence it is wise for nurses to be familiar with the guidance in the Code of Practice, paragraph 9.2, which states:

Before using the power the nurse should assess:

(a) the likely arrival time of the doctor as against the likely intention of the patient to leave. Most patients who express a wish to leave hospital can be persuaded to wait until a doctor arrives to discuss it further. Where this is not possible the nurse must try to predict the impact of any delay upon the patient;

(b) the consequences of a patient leaving hospital immediately – the harm that might occur to the patient or others – taking into account:

the patient's expressed intentions including the likelihood of the patient committing self-harm or suicide;

any evidence of disordered thinking;

the patient's current behaviour and in particular any changes in usual behaviour;

the likelihood of the patient behaving in a violent manner;

any recently received messages from relatives or friends;

any recent disturbances on the ward;

any relevant involvement of other patients;

(c) the patient's known unpredictability and any other relevant information from other members of the multi-disciplinary team.

As section 5(4) is written, it appears that the holding power can only be invoked after the completion of the written record (on Form 13) and hence restraint would not be permitted until after the making of the record. However, this in some cases would be wholly impractical, for example where the patient unexpectedly leaps out of bed and runs out of the ward. In these situations, it can be argued that the common law will permit restraint for one of a number of reasons: for example, to prevent crime, to safeguard the well-being of others, or to fulfil the duty owed to the patient. The filling out of Form 13 would therefore take place as soon as possible after the restraint being used. The Code of Practice is somewhat ambiguous on this point. In paragraph 9.6 it seems to suggest that the power may be invoked without completion of Form 13, but paragraph 9.4 indicates that to use the power the Form must be completed. The case law on the subject is also unclear and unhelpful. In *Black* v. *Forsey* (1988) the House of Lords decided, in the context of Scottish Mental Health Act provisions, that a common law power to 'arrest the insane'[46] could not be used because of the specific statutory limitation. In addition, in *R* v. *Bournewood NHS Trust ex parte L*[47] the Court of Appeal suggested that de facto detention was unlawful where Mental Health Act powers to detain were available. The fact that the House of Lords overruled the Court of Appeal would suggest that it will still be permissible to detain a patient while invoking section 5(4) with completion of the documentation afterwards.

In addition, it is clear that section 5(4) is a power that assumes an appropriate level of staffing. Indeed, paragraph 9.9 of the Code of Practice states that a 'suitably qualified, experienced and competent nurse should be on all wards where there is a possibility of section 5(4) being invoked'. Hence appropriate staffing will be an essential prerequisite for the use of the power, but also, adequate staffing may lessen the likelihood of the power's being used. Failure to staff the ward adequately will mean the section cannot be exercised at all, or only with great difficulty. The MHA therefore implicitly requires wards to be staffed with at least one nurse who is appropriately qualified, and it may be the case that many hospitals/wards will fail to reach this standard. Whether the nurse has knowledge of the particular patient or is trained in the specific area of mental disorder before being able to use section 5(4) is a matter of good practice only. The legislation requires only qualification and adherence to the process.

The use of the holding powers available under the MHA has been a source of concern for many years. The Mental Health Act Commission commented in both its Seventh and Eighth Biennial Reports on the high, and then increasing, use made of the powers. That there is '[h]igh usage does not necessarily imply misuses',[48] but raises the question of whether more patients should be detained under sections 2 or 3 of the MHA. If the usage is lowered, it may be that more dubious methods are being used to prevent patients leaving hospital care. In its Eleventh Biennial Report the Commission noted that there had been a decline in the use of section 5, which 'should *probably* be welcomed, since the drop in its use could be reflective not in any lessening of coercion in mental health services, but by a greater use of de facto detention'.[49] The latter, of course, becomes less likely with the introduction of new procedures in the Mental Health Bill 2007 to deal with such detention since the *Bournewood* case and as mentioned in the following section. The Commission found that a section 5(4) was most likely to be followed by a section 5(2), which is as expected since it should be used to prevent a patient leaving hospital while a doctor is called.[50]

9.4 Detention by informal methods

Ever since the introduction of the Mental Health Act 1959, most patients have been present in hospital without formal powers. Section 5 of the 1959 Act, which is section 131 of the 1983 Act, permits this. However, some of the patients in hospital are not capable of deciding whether to be there; some of those patients are compliant. The consequence is that those patients in hospital through detention under the Act have their legal position clear and their rights and protections clearly laid out; the legal position of patients in hospital without such formal powers depends upon their capacity to decide whether to be there and what to accept when in hospital. The latter legal position can only be operated by a capable patient. Thus there is a group of patients whose legal position is not adequately protected as they are not detained under the Act and are not capable of making decisions. This is what is known as the Bournewood gap, after the case in which the issue was determined.[51]

The presence of this gap has been found to be in breach of the European Convention on Human Rights and amendments to the MCA in the Mental Health Bill 2007 are designed to meet the demands of the ECHR. In effect, the court decided that compliant, incapable patients who would be prevented from leaving if they tried to depart from the hospital are deprived of their liberty, which is a breach of

Article 5, unless there are sufficient substantive and procedural protections that the intervention is permitted under Article 5(1)(e). At the time of *Bournewood*, the problem was that the only law was the common law, which, in these circumstances, was felt to be too unclear for someone to know the grounds upon which it might be decided that they should live in hospital, and the procedural protections were minimal (since the only real way to resolve the matter was to seek a court declaration, which was expensive and a relatively limited remedy). The Mental Health Bill introduces a set of procedures that certainly clarify the position and will meet ECHR scrutiny. However, they may go too far, as it is entirely possible that applying the MCA to this issue would have provided sufficient substantive and procedural protections since the law is much clearer than it was and the power of the Court of Protection to decide on matters of controversy would be sufficient access to a court. It is likely that such challenges will be forthcoming as necessary, given that some people have an automatic right to take a case to the court and others may do so with the permission of the court. Whether the new procedure, under the Mental Health Bill 2007 is overly complex remains to be seen, but since it may well apply to all informal patients who are not capable of deciding whether to stay in hospital, it could become a very burdensome and, arguably, overly complex means of dealing with the Bournewood gap. The new legislative provisions will clarify the status of such patients in hospital, but questions about treatment will have to be answered through the MCA. The key for nurses will be to ensure that any concerns about the legal status of an informal, incompetent patient are raised with the appropriate authority.

9.5 The management of violent or aggressive patients

For some considerable time patients who present violently or aggressively have been a matter of concern for the staff most closely involved with their care and treatment. As long ago as 1977, the Confederation of Health Service Employees in its report *The Management of Violent and Potentially Violent Patients*[52] attempted to address this thorny issue. More recently it has come to the fore in relation to handling a group of patients perceived to be particularly problematic – that is, patients suffering from personality disorder. These issues are covered in the proposed reforms to the MHA and are discussed below.

9.5.1 The informal or detained patient

Common law justifications

It is submitted that reliance on the common law indicating that people may defend themselves or others is the proper basis upon which to authorise activity to deal with a violent or aggressive patient, whether that be by way of physical force, seclusion or medication. Where some sort of physical response is necessary, the least force necessary safely to contain the problem that the patient presents should be used. In many cases this may be holding the patient, or properly trained staff

using control and restraint techniques. Where such force is unlikely to be sufficient or where its use may be harmful to the patient, staff and/or other patients,
seclusion may be necessary. In some cases an appropriate alternative may be
medication (possibly by way of sedation). These activities have not been justified
on the basis that they are 'medical treatment' within the MHA (where the patient
is detained) or part of a treatment programme to which the patient has consented.
Where the person is detained, it is submitted that regarding these activities as
'treatment', even in the light of the very wide definition of treatment permitted
by the MHA, is not correct. Treatment, regardless of the definition, should always
be intended to have some curative or ameliorative purpose or expectation, which
will not be the case with the techniques mentioned. As regards an informal patient
the same is true, but as the patient may consent to treatment it may be tempting to
use the patient's consent as justification for restraint. While this is not impossible,
it is suggested that it is difficult and also poor practice.

Seclusion

It is assumed that seclusion, albeit controversial, is lawful and will continue to be
used even if only rarely. 'Seclusion is the supervised confinement of a patient in
a room, which may be locked to protect others from significant harm.'[53] There is
nothing inherent in seclusion that makes it unlawful, but it is subject to abuse by
being used for too long, or as a means of punishment, and then it becomes an
unlawful interference with a patient's freedom of movement or bodily integrity.
Hence the Code of Practice emphasises in paragraph 9.16 that seclusion should be
seen 'as a last resort' and be 'for the shortest possible time'. In addition, seclusion
should not be used:

- as a punishment or threat;
- as part of a treatment programme;
- because of shortage of staff;
- where there is any risk of suicide or self-harm.

If seclusion is imposed on informal patients, it should be a trigger to consider the
formal detention of the patient.

The Code of Practice also offers guidance as to the need for each hospital to
have a policy on seclusion and for the procedure to be applied. Paragraph 19.18
provides that the decision to use seclusion may be made by the nurse in charge
of the ward. If seclusion is initiated without the involvement of the patient's
RMO, he or she must be notified at once in order that they may attend. Having
placed a patient into seclusion, the duty of care owed to the patient demands that
account be taken of the change in circumstances, and thus the Code of Practice
further provides:

19.19   A nurse should be readily available within sight and sound of the seclusion room at all times throughout the period of the patient's seclusion,
and present at all times with a patient who has been sedated.

19.20   The aim of observation is to monitor the condition and behaviour of the
patient and to identify the time at which seclusion can be terminated . . .

the patient should be observed continuously. A documented report must be made at least every 15 minutes.

19.21 The need to continue seclusion should be reviewed every 2 hours by 2 nurses (1 of whom was not involved in the decision to seclude) and, every 4 hours by a doctor. A multidisciplinary review should be completed by a consultant or other senior doctor, nurses and other professionals, who were not involved in the incident that led to seclusion if the seclusion continues for more than 8 hours consecutively; or 12 hours intermittently over a period of 48 hours.

Regarding where the seclusion takes place, the Code of Practice provides:

19.22 The room used for seclusion should:

- provide privacy from other patients;
- enable staff to observe the patient at all times;
- be safe and secure;
- not contain anything which could cause harm to the patient or others;
- be adequately furnished, heated, lit and ventilated;
- be quiet but not soundproofed and with some means of calling for attention; the means of operation should be explained to the patient.

Staff may decide what a patient may take into the seclusion room, but the patient should always be clothed.

The Mental Health Act Commission collates information on the usage made of seclusion and this has been an area that merited 'particular attention'. Their Eighth Biennial Report indicated that nearly 5000 episodes of seclusion were used in 1997/1998 in relation to just under 2000 patients. In addition, and perhaps of more concern, is the statement that 'there is a considerable number of units where policies are either inadequate or out of date and the guidance in the Code is not followed'.[54]

The best advice is that the Code of Practice be followed, although it is possible for a positive decision to be taken, for good reason, to have an approach to seclusion (or indeed another issue within the Code) that is not consistent with the letter of the Code.[55]

9.6 Treatment in the community

The context of the above discussion has been the treatment and care of the person with a mental illness within a hospital or nursing home. However, many people with mental illnesses are perfectly able to live in the community and receive treatment with only outpatient visits or short inpatient stays. For these individuals treatment will be with their consent since the treatment provisions in the MHA only permit compulsory treatment when the patient is in hospital or when they are on leave of absence under section 17 MHA. The courts have accepted that provided a person is receiving treatment in a hospital (whether on a ward, or through outpatient provision) a detention section can be renewed, as can section 17 leave of absence.[56] While this has, in effect, provided a community treatment order, it has not been regarded as the solution to a long-running debate about treatment in the community. Indeed, one consequence of the Mental Health Bill 2007 may be to limit the length of time for which the continuing section 3 and its renewal and continuing grant of section 17 leave will be permissible. The government seems to expect that section 17 leave of absence will only underpin hospital admission, so where hospital admission is not appropriate longer term, other provision must be considered. When, and if, the Mental Health Bill 2007 is introduced, supervised community treatment (SCT) will be available (in addition to guardianship).

In the past, there were arguments for compulsory community treatment orders, as when the Department of Health examined the issue of community treatment and produced an internal review report[57] and the Royal College of Psychiatrists recommended a new supervision order that would enable compulsory treatment to be given in the community.[58] However, despite the calls for compulsory treatment orders, these provisions were not introduced. Instead, a form of supervision order, aftercare under supervision, was introduced through the Mental Health (Patients in the Community) Act 1995, which gave certain powers to the supervisor. Crucially, however, the supervisor's powers fall short of compulsory treatment and arguably the supervision order is less effective for this omission. Indeed, the powers differ only slightly from the powers of guardians appointed under section 7 MHA, the difference being that the supervisor can require the patient to attend at specified places for medical treatment. This may in all possibility be an outpatient clinic or the community psychiatric nurse's clinic. If the patient does not attend, the supervisor may take or convey the patient to the place for medical treatment – a form of community arrest perhaps? However, having got the patient to the medical practitioner, there is no method prescribed in the amended MHA to force the patient to comply with the treatment. Instead of a compulsory community treatment order, what has been produced is a watching power that, in reality, merely enables the supervisor to consider whether re-admission to hospital is warranted in the event of failure to comply with treatment.

For the community nurse, the aftercare under supervision presents very little change in the way patients must be treated, since ongoing consent must be checked and refusal complied with where the patient is capable. When a patient refuses treatment, and is subject to supervision, the only additional duty will be to inform the supervisor in order that they may consider the options. However, how this will fit with the duty of confidentiality is a further ethical dilemma, but one that would generally fall in favour of disclosure in the public interest.

Through the Mental Health Bill 2007, the government intends to introduce supervised community treatment. As the government's explanatory memorandum to the bill explains as an overview:

> The SCT provisions will allow some patients with a mental disorder to live in the community while still subject to powers under the 1983 Act. Patients subject to SCT remain under compulsion and liable to recall to hospital for treatment. Only those patients who have been detained in hospital for treatment will be eligible for SCT. In order for a patient to be placed on SCT, various criteria need to be met. An AMHP also needs to agree that SCT is appropriate. Patients who

are on SCT will be made subject to conditions while living in the community. Conditions will depend on their individual and family circumstances. Conditions will form part of the patient's community treatment order which is made by the responsible clinician. Patients on SCT may be recalled to hospital for treatment should this become necessary. Afterwards they may then resume living in the community or, if they need to be treated as an in-patient again, their responsible clinician may revoke the SCT and the patient remains in hospital for the time being. SCT differs from after-care under supervision, which it will replace, in that it will allow patients who do not need to continue receiving treatment in hospital to be discharged into the community, but with powers of recall to hospital if necessary. It is different from leave under section 17 of the 1983 Act, which remains suitable for a patient as a means to give shorter term leave from hospital, as part of the patient's overall management as a hospital patient.

How effective this will be remains to be seen, as it will not override the patient's right to refuse treatment while in the community. There has been a consistent theme during the law reform process not to introduce compulsory treatment in the community. What this new power provides is perhaps a more streamlined relationship between hospital and community. It also provides significant opportunities for the engagement of nurses if they are appointed as approved mental health professionals or as responsible clinicians.

9.7 The Mental Health Review Tribunal

It is increasingly the case that nurses involved in the care of detained patients are asked to participate in hearings in front of the Mental Health Review Tribunal (MHRT), whether by way of oral or of written evidence. It is therefore helpful to know the purpose of the MHRT and also to be aware of the procedures adopted.

The MHRT is created by virtue of the MHA 1983,[59] and derives all its powers from the MHA 1983 or secondary legislation (for example, the MHRT Rules). There will be a panel of three to hear any applications to the MHRT, and this panel will comprise a legal member, a medical member and a lay member.[60] The legal member acts as the chair of the panel. In some cases there will also be a Tribunal Assistant whose role is to ensure that the administration of the hearing goes smoothly: they do not play any part in decision-making or discussion of the law.

There are two main situations where an MHRT hearing will take place: either the patient themselves will have applied for a hearing,[61] or the patient will have been referred for a hearing by the Hospital Managers.[62] It is possible for the patient's nearest relative to apply for a hearing,[63] although this is not a very common occurrence. Only detained patients can apply for a hearing; an informal patient is not so entitled, and this inequality has been the subject of debate in the context of the *Bournewood* case.

A patient cannot make repeated applications for a hearing. They are restrained by section 66 of the MHA 1983 to applying once in each period of formal detention; hence if the patient has been detained under section 2, then under section 3 for six months, renewed for another six months, they will have three opportunities to seek a hearing. It should also be noted that with regard to section 2 detentions any application must be made within the first 14 days of the detention[64] owing to the short time limit of the detaining provision. Having made an application, an MHRT should sit within seven days where a section 2 detention is concerned, or within eight weeks where a section 3 detention is concerned, although it may well be the case that these time limits are not met. Where a patient has not exercised their right to seek an MHRT hearing and the patient is detained under section 3 or has been transferred to hospital under section 19 having been subject to section 7 guardianship, the hospital managers must refer the case after the expiry of the first period of detention and thereafter every three years.[65] It is worth noting that state funding is available to patients subject to an application or reference to enable them to have legal representation.

Once an application has been made, the responsible authority is required to file reports before the hearing[66] insofar as is reasonably practicable. These reports are:

● the Part A Statement – being basic information about the patient
● a medical report on the patient, normally prepared by the RMO
● a social circumstances report on the patient, prepared by a social worker, although not always an approved social worker.

In addition, many hospitals will also provide a nursing report in relation to the patient, and these are normally of great assistance to the MHRT.

The time frame for filing these reports is set out in the MHRT Rules[67] as being three weeks before the hearing, which in the case of an application against a section 2 detention is clearly impractical. Hence in this situation it is normal for the reports to be provided to the Tribunal panel before the hearing commences.

If a nurse is asked to provide a written report for an MHRT hearing there may well be local guidance available as to its format, since this is not covered by guidance from the MHRT itself. Normally a nursing report will focus on the patient's behaviour and management on the ward, including information about willingness to take medication and ability to engage with staff and other patients. If the patient has been treated before by the same staff and hence is known to the hospital, it can be helpful to highlight how the patient's presentation has changed. The Tribunal panel will not always expect an opinion as to whether the patient should be detained, but it can sometimes be helpful to include this if the author has sufficient knowledge and experience.

Nurses are also increasingly expected to participate in the Tribunal hearing itself, and it is always worth observing a hearing before being asked to attend to give evidence, in order to gain familiarity with the procedure. The process in an MHRT is primarily inquisitorial rather than adversarial – hence the Tribunal panel will be taking an active role in the questioning of the individual witnesses rather than being the legal representative for the patient. It is also worth noting that it is generally the case that the hospital, via the RMO and the nursing staff, do not have a legal representative and do not therefore have an automatic right to question the patient or other witnesses. The purpose of the hearing is to review the justification for the continued detention of the patient at the time of the hearing – they are not reviewing the situation when the patient was first detained. It is for the hospital to prove to the Tribunal panel that detention is justified, not for the patient to prove they should be removed from section,[68] and questioning will focus on the reason for detention.

If the evidence does not support the case for continued detention, the MHRT will discharge the patient immediately.[69] If the criteria for detention are not met and the Tribunal wishes to discharge, there also exists a power to defer discharge until a later date.[70] This is often used where community support/housing and so on need to be put in place. However, a deferred discharge does not mean the hospital must keep the patient in their care until the date specified; they can discharge earlier if this is appropriate. It is important that the time between the hearing and the date of deferred discharge is not excessive since this may fall foul of the European Convention on Human Rights Article 5, hence deferred discharges will often only amount to a few days.

Where the Tribunal has found that the patient is not suffering from a mental disorder, and hence does not need to be detained in hospital, they are required to discharge, but the Tribunal also has several discretionary powers. Even if the criteria for discharge under section 72(1) are not met, the Tribunal will have discretion to discharge in any event. Here they must consider the extent to which treatment will alleviate or prevent deterioration in the patient's mental condition, and the question of the patient's ability to care for themselves.[71] It is not common for the Tribunal to use this discretionary power. It is more likely that the Tribunal will exercise its powers, if not discharging the patient, to make recommendations under section 72(3) and (3A). Hence the Tribunal can, to facilitate discharge at a future date:

- recommend that the patient be granted leave of absence under section 17
- recommend that the patient be transferred to another hospital
- recommend that the patient be transferred into guardianship
- recommend that the RMO consider making a supervision application in respect of the patient.

Where such a recommendation is made, the Tribunal, under the MHRT Rules[72] shall specify a date whereby, if the recommendation has not been acted upon, the Tribunal may reconvene to hear the case anew. If the Tribunal does reconvene, new reports will need to be filed and the Tribunal will have all the powers it would have had if the case were being heard for the first time.

9.8 Notes and references

1. See generally, B.M. Hoggett, *Mental Health Law*, 4th edn (London, Sweet & Maxwell, 1996); L.O. Gostin, J.V. McHale & W. Bingley, *Gostin on Mental Health Law* (London, Shaw & Sons, 2005); R.M. Jones, *Mental Health Act Manual*, 9th edn (London, Sweet & Maxwell, 2004); and P. Bartlett & R. Sandland, *Mental Health Law Policy and Practice* (London, Blackstone Press, 2000).
2. Numerous English court decisions have built upon the jurisprudence of the European Court. The latest decision, which provides a summary and reference to the jurisprudence, is *R (on the application of B)* v. *Haddock* [2005] EWHC 921.
3. Mental Health Act Commission, *Fifth Biennial Report 1991–1993* (London, The Stationery Office, 1993), at para. 7.15.

4. See *R* v. *South Western Hospital Managers, ex parte M* [1994] 1 All ER 161.
5. The definition of a patient's nearest relative can be found in section 26 MHA, and will, as indicated, be amended, when and if the Mental Health Bill 2007 is introduced, to include civil partners at the same stage as married partners.
6. The MHA requires each local authority to appoint sufficient approved social workers, and also the Mental Health Act Code of Practice (London, Department of Health, March 1999) suggests at para. 2.35, that an approved social worker should be the preferred applicant. Note, as indicated in the text, that the role of approved social workers will be replaced by that of approved mental health professionals when and if the Mental Health Bill 2007 is implemented.
7. Section 28 of the Mental Capacity Act 2005.
8. Mental Health Act Commission, *Fourth Biennial Report 1989–1991* (London, The Stationery Office, 1991), at para. 6.18. A Guidance Note (No. 3) was subsequently issued by the Commission in August 1997.
9. See further the discussion by R.M. Jones, *Mental Health Act Manual*, 9th edn (London, Sweet & Maxwell, 2004), on the ability to use section 2 where a patient is already well known to the health care professionals and approved social workers.
10. Mental Health Act Commission, *Fifth Biennial Report 1991–1993*, at para. 7.0, and see the Mental Health Act Code of Practice 1999, at para. 16.5.
11. *B* v. *Croydon Health Authority* [1995] 2 WLR 294, per Lord Justice Hoffman, at p. 298.
12. For example, *Re S* [1994] 4 All ER 671, *Tameside & Glossop Acute Services Trust* v. *CH* [1996] 1 FLR 762, *Re MB (Medical Treatment)* [1997] 2 FLR 426 and *R* v. *Collins, Pathfinder Health Services Trust, St. George's Healthcare NHS Trust ex parte S* [1998] 3 WLR 936. It should be noted that not all of these were decisions under the MHA, but came under the common law provisions of 'best interests'.
13. Per Mr Justice Wall, at p. 773.
14. See note 12 above.
15. Per Lord Justice Judge, at p. 958.
16. This is indicated by the fact that 20,934 requests for second opinions were completed by the Mental Health Act Commission in the period 2003/2005, with 80.9% being in respect of medicine and 18.2% for ECT only: Mental Health Act Commission, *Eleventh Biennial Report 2003–2005* (London, The Stationery Office), at fig. 60.
17. This is in contrast to treatment provided under section 57 and section 58(3)(b) where section 61 places a duty on the responsible medical officer to review the necessity of treatment.
18. Mental Health Act Code of Practice 1999, at para. 16.35.
19. Mental Health Act Code of Practice 1999, at para. 16.19.
20. Mental Health Act Code of Practice 1999, at para. 16.14.
21. Mental Health Act Commission, *Eleventh Biennial Report 2003–2005*, para. 4.64.
22. Mental Health Act Commission, *Eleventh Biennial Report 2003–2005*, fig. 63.
23. Mental Health Act Commission, *Eleventh Biennial Report 2003–2005*, para. 4.67.
24. National Institute for Clinical Excellence, *Guidance on the Use of Electroconvulsive Therapy*, Technology Appraisal 59 (London, NICE, 2003).
25. Royal College of Psychiatrists, *ECT Handbook*, 2nd edn (London, Gaskell, 2005).
26. This Act seeks to protect individuals who disclose information in the public interest and to enable the individual to claim legal redress in the event of victimisation following disclosure. It is important to note that the Act only covers certain types of information disclosure and specifies how the disclosure should be carried out. For example, if a nurse were to make disclosures to the local media this would not be within the terms of the Act and no protection from victimisation would be granted.

27. Over the two-year period 2003/2005 covered by the latest Mental Health Commission Biennial Report, only seven referrals for neurosurgery were made – a figure that is lower than for any previous period: Mental Health Act Commission, *Eleventh Biennial Report 2003–2005*, at fig. 65.

28. For example see the Eighth Biennial Report 1997–1999 (London, The Stationery Office), at para. 6.22.

29. Per Lord Donaldson, at p. 798.

30. [1997] 2 FLR 426.

31. Mental Health Act Code of Practice 1999, at para. 15.11.

32. *Mental Health Act Manual*, 9th edn (London, Sweet & Maxwell), para. 15.12. See also Gunn *et al.*, Decision-making capacity, *Medical Law Review*, 7 (1999), p. 269.

33. See note 12 above.

34. Per Lord Donaldson in *Re T* [1992], at p. 796.

35. See, for example, *Re F (mental patient: sterilisation)* [1990] 2 AC 1 and *Airedale NHS Trust v. Bland* [1993] AC 789.

36. These issues are covered by a Practice Note: *Practice Note (Official Solicitor: Declaratory Proceedings: Medical and Welfare Decisions for Adults who Lack Capacity)* [2001] FLR, p. 158.

37. P.W.H. Fennell, Inscribing paternalisation in the law: consent to treatment and mental disorder, *Journal of the Law and Society*, **17**(29) (1990), p. 29.

38. *Journal of the Law and Society*, **17**(29) (1990), p. 43.

39. See further Mental Health Act Code of Practice, para. 15.11, and the BMA (1995) Code of Practice on Advance Statements about Medical Treatment (London, BMA).

40. Sections 9 & 16.

41. *R v. Bournewood Community and Mental health NHS Trust, ex parte L* [1998] 3 All E.R. 289.

42. See B. Dimond, The Right of the nurse to detain informal patients in psychiatric hospitals in England and Wales, *Medical Law* (1989), pp. 535–47.

43. The Mental Health (Nurses) Order 1998 (SI 1998 No 2625) defines who will be a nurse of prescribed class as a 'nurse registered in any part of the register maintained under section 7 of the Nurses, Midwives and Health Visitors Act 1997 which is mentioned in paragraph (2)'. Paragraph 2 refers to nurses in Part 3 (first-level nurses trained in the nursing of persons suffering from mental illness), Part 4 (second-level nurses trained in the nursing of persons suffering from mental illness (England and Wales)), Part 5 (first-level nurses trained in the nursing of persons suffering from learning disabilities), Part 6 (second-level nurses trained in the nursing of persons suffering from learning disabilities (England and Wales)), Part 13 (nurses qualified following a course of preparation in mental health nursing) and finally Part 14 (nurses qualified following a course of preparation in learning disabilities nursing).

44. Mental Health Act Code of Practice, 1999, at para. 9.1 (London, Department of Health).

45. *Palmer v. Tees Health Authority* (1999).

46. As it was described by David Lanham in an article of that title in *Criminal Law Review* (1974), p. 515.

47. See note 17 above.

48. Eighth Biennial Report 1997–1999, para. 4.26, and see also Table 4.

49. Mental Health Act Commission, *Eleventh Biennial Report 2003–2005* (London, The Stationery Office, 2005), at para. 4.26.

50. Mental Health Act Commission, *Eleventh Biennial Report 2003–2005* (London, The Stationery Office, 2005), at para. 4.27.

51. See note 41 above; the decision of the European Court of Human Rights is *H.L. v. U.K.* (2004), Application No. 45508/99.

52. Confederation of Health Service Employees, *The Management of Violent and Potentially Violent Patients* (1977).
53. Mental Health Act Code of Practice 1999, para. 19.16 (London, Department of Health).
54. Mental Health Act Commission, *Eighth Biennial Report 1997–1999*, para. 10.18 (London, The Stationery Office).
55. *R* v. *Mersey Care NHS Trust, ex parte Munjaz* [2005] UKHL 58.
56. See the latest case, in which the previous ones are also considered, *R (on the application of CS)* v. *MHRT* [2004] EWHC (Admin) 2958.
57. Department of Health, *Legal Powers on the Care of Mentally Ill People in the Community* (London, Department of Health, 1993).
58. *Royal College of Psychiatrists Community Supervision Orders* (London, Royal College of Psychiatrists, 1993).
59. MHA 1983, section 65.
60. MHA 1983, section 65, and see also Schedule 2.
61. MHA 1983, section 66.
62. MHA 1983, section 68.
63. MHA 1983, section 66.
64. MHA 1983, section 66(2)(a).
65. MHA 1983, section 68.
66. MHRT, Rule 6 and Schedule 1.
67. MHRT, Rule 6.
68. MHA 1983, section 72.
69. MHA 1983, section 72(1)(2).
70. MHA 1983, section 72(3).
71. MHA 1983, section 72(2).
72. MHRT, Rule 24(4).

B   An Ethical Perspective – Compulsion and Autonomy

Harry Lesser

In mental health nursing, one ethical issue predominates: that of when the use of compulsion, whether as compulsory hospitalisation, compulsory treatment or compulsory restraint, is justified. For compulsion in these cases can be justified, it is commonly thought, only if the client's mental judgement is so impaired or underdeveloped that they lack the competence to decide for themselves how they should be treated. This does occur in physical illness, as with children, people who are unconscious, people who are drunk or drugged. But in mental illness it is probably more common – by no means all mental illnesses affect a person's judgement in this way but many do – and it is certainly more problematic: the decisions are often, though not always, very difficult to make, because of uncertainty as to whether the client is or is not competent. Moreover, though the decisions have to be made on the facts, it is also vital that they be made in the proper ethical spirit and on ethically justifiable grounds.

Gunn and Rodgers, in their excellent survey of the law and the changes that are likely at the time of writing, show that, with regard to these decisions, two very important changes are imminent. The first is that nurses are going to be more involved, perhaps much more involved, in making decisions about admission, discharge and treatment; and the authority of the nurse is going to increase accordingly. The second is that the law is going to provide less guidance as to the criteria for making these decisions: the guidance will be in general terms, and the nurse will have to decide how they apply to the particular client. The power of the nurse will be increased, and so the need to exercise this power ethically will become that much stronger.

9.9   The ethical use of compulsion

It is widely agreed nowadays, in theory if not always in practice, that in dealing with adults, even if they are mentally disturbed, the presumption should be that compulsion should be avoided if possible, and it is the use of compulsion that requires to be justified. There are two reasons for this. One is that individual autonomy is valuable in itself, and is to be preserved unless it thwarts other important values: some people would go so far as to say that it should be preserved except when its restriction is needed to maintain future autonomy, so that people should be left alone unless they propose to do, or not do, something that will destroy or seriously harm either their own autonomy or that of others. The second reason is that people are normally the best judges of their own interests, even though they are not perfect judges. This is particularly the case when there is no objective answer to what is in their best interests, but only a subjective preference: for example, while sometimes it seems obvious that the benefits of treatment outweigh the disadvantages, at other times only the client can decide whether, for them, the pain of the side effects (for example) is worth enduring for the sake of the improvement in their condition. Hence the conclusion, for both ethics and the law, that competent adults must not be subjected to compulsory treatment or compulsory hospitalisation.

However, it seems clear that not all adults are, in the required sense, competent, and that lack of competence can be caused not only by being unconscious (the paradigm case), or by being temporarily under the influence of drink, or drugs, or delirium, but also by mental illness. Even as staunch a supporter of the freedom of patients as Thomas Szasz, who holds that 'mental illness' is in any case either not an illness at all or a 'brain illness' since the brain, not the mind, is the diseased organ, agrees that some brain illnesses or diseases, such as advanced Alzheimer's disease, leave a patient as incompetent as if they were actually unconscious, so that decisions have to be made on their behalf.[1] Szasz thinks such cases are a tiny percentage of the instances of (as he would say) so-called mental illness. But the evidence is that there are many others, where a person's delusional beliefs or emotional pressures make it impossible for them to make competent decisions: the failure of many anorexics to admit the harm they are doing to themselves is an example of the first; the inability of people in a deep clinical depression to make any decisions at all is an example of the second.

This also, though, illustrates the problem. To hold beliefs that are false and based on poor, or no, evidence, is not peculiar to the 'mentally ill' but statistically absolutely normal, as is having one's judgement distorted by one's emotions. Yet we not only distinguish these normal conditions from such things as delusion or depression, or phobia or addiction, but often the experts, and sometimes even we as laypeople, have no difficulty in deciding whether a person is normal or disturbed: only a few cases seem to appear as borderline. There are celebrated cases of misdiagnosis in both directions, involving both the lengthy detention of people who did not have a mental illness and the failure to detain people who were ill. But these cases often, perhaps always, involved a failure to consider the evidence. Sometimes this was a cynical and deliberate political move, as with the hospitalisation of political dissidents in the Soviet Union.[2] Sometimes it was the result of assuming that 'immoral' or anti-social behaviour of certain types was always a sign of mental illness, and investigating no further, as with the unmarried mothers who were 'put away', sometimes for years. Sometimes very few pieces of evidence were considered, as in the Rosenhan experiment, in which several mentally normal members of a university psychology department were admitted as mental patients solely because they complained of hearing voices.[3] Sometimes evidence was discounted for ideological reasons, as when followers of R.D. Laing (though perhaps not Laing himself) ignored what was said by a person's close family.[4] So the mere fact that mistakes have been made merely shows that decisions must be properly based on the evidence available.

Nevertheless, the problem remains. Not all cases are clear, and even in the clear cases, although there may be widespread agreement that a person is or is not competent, there still exists no clear and explicit definition of the distinction that is being operated. The problem is made somewhat easier with regard to compulsory admission, because the decision required is not simply whether a person is competent but whether their incompetence is likely to result in their injuring themselves or others. At this point we have to deal, once again, with an objection from Thomas Szasz. It is that this question is a moral and political one, and not a medical one at all. If people injure others, that is a matter for the law; if they injure themselves, that is their business. As to whether anyone should intervene merely because people are, supposedly, likely to injure themselves or others, this is a political issue. If one believes that freedom is the supreme political value, one will hold that there should be no intervention merely on the ground of what a person might do. If one has a different political and moral view, one may support intervention. But the question, according to Szasz, is one of values, not one of medical science.

This, however, is based on the belief that, except when a person is so affected by brain illness that they in effect cannot make decisions at all, their decisions are always competent – they may be wise or foolish, justifiable or wicked, but not 'well' or 'ill'. But the evidence is that even when someone does make a decision, that decision may be the result of, or be affected by, such things as a delusive belief or set of beliefs, a deep disturbance in the functioning of memory or perception, an emotional disturbance such as mania or depression, an inability to control acting on one's desires or fantasies, or an abnormal lack of conscience or concern for others. When this happens, and when, in addition, it is likely that their consequent actions, or failure to act, will do harm, it must be right to regard the person as having a mental illness, and also (which is by no means the same thing) as being a danger to themselves or others because their mental functioning is impaired. It is true that all these conditions have analogous states that are normal, in the sense of not preventing a person from being responsible for their actions, so that they may be stupid, or wicked, or both, but not 'ill'. But people in the disturbed conditions often in practice behave very differently from those in these analogous states, sometimes so much so that this is obvious to anyone, even a lay person, who deals with them, although they may not be able to define the difference in words.

So, to repeat, the problem is to identify those people who are likely to be a danger to themselves or others because of some failure in mental functioning: what causes these failures is a further question, but does not affect the question of whether it is or is not present. As has also been said, if the new legislation goes through, nurses will be more involved in these decisions, and the decisions will be less controlled by the law. This is because, as Gunn and Rodgers explain, the law will refer simply to 'mental disorder' in general terms and will not list specific disorders or even require that the disorder be treatable. The reason for this is the very practical one of closing the loophole that has resulted in some very dangerous people not being detained in hospital because their condition was a 'personality disorder': untreatable, and not on the list of disorders for which a person could be compulsorily detained. But the effect is likely to be that the judgements made by nurses about particular people are going to be crucial in determining whether they are or are not compulsorily detained in hospital, and that it will be harder than previously to challenge these judgements on any legal ground. So it becomes that much more important that the decisions be made in a way that is ethically as well as legally appropriate.

What, then, constitutes making these decisions ethically? First, that the decision to detain someone in hospital compulsorily is made only on the ground that there is good evidence that they have a mental disorder and are dangerous because of it, or in part because of it. It should not be made on punitive grounds, however unpleasant the person's behaviour; and this may require some self-awareness on the part of nurses, since this is the kind of motivation people will reject on the conscious level but can be influenced by without noticing it. Nor should it be made on the grounds of someone's convenience. Here, though, caution is needed, especially when the 'someone' is the family. On the one hand, there are people who have been 'put away', to use the phrase of an earlier time, when they did not have a mental illness but were merely an embarrassment. On the other hand, there are people who were seriously disturbed and yet allowed to make life intolerable for their families, to threaten their lives, and to end with murder or suicide because what the family kept saying was not taken seriously. So in saying that people should not be hospitalised because it suits their family, or anyone else, one should not deny that in deciding whether they are 'disturbed' and dangerous the evidence of the family, or generally of those in close contact with them, may well be crucial and should never be taken lightly.

Second, the decision should be made taking into account all the evidence, or as much as there is time to take into account. It is particularly this family evidence that in some quarters has got discounted for ideological reasons. But this is not the only example: what the person actually says may itself get discounted if it is already assumed that they have a mental illness. There is also the need to interpret words and behaviour correctly, which requires awareness of different ways of speaking and acting: forms of address and ways of behaving that are absolutely normal in one place have sometimes been marked as deviant or inappropriate by interviewers who come from somewhere else.

The other element in handling evidence is the converse: not allowing one sort of evidence to be too conclusive. Rosenhan (see above) is an example of this: people were diagnosed as having a mental illness on only one piece of evidence, that they heard voices – which was in fact a lie! In particular, the fact that a person in general resembles those with a type of mental disorder, or comes from a group in which a particular type of disorder is thought to be common, should not be in any way conclusive. Even someone's behaviour, without evidence of mental disturbance, direct or indirect, is probably not enough. If the behaviour appears bizarre, the person may have unusual tastes: we should be warned by the fact that it is not very long since homosexuality was classed as an illness. Even if the behaviour is cruel and destructive, this may indicate that the perpetrator is morally bad rather than 'sick'.

This, though, raises two further questions. What constitutes a mental disturbance, over and above behaviour that is inappropriate, or worse? And what constitutes evidence of its existence? The diagnosis of physical illness can be hard enough, let alone that of mental illness. As regards evidence, one might suggest that there are two kinds. One is what people say about their experiences, whether perceptual, emotional or both. It is important to note that those such as Szasz who oppose the whole concept of mental illness are wrong to assert that diagnosis is based simply on behaviour: it is very much based on what can be learned about a person's experiences. But one has to note that a person may lie, or exaggerate, or misinterpret: neither malingering (deliberately pretending to be ill) nor hypochondria (exaggerating the significance of symptoms) are confined to physical illness.

The other kind of evidence comes, roughly, from the style of behaviour. Thus to steal is not in itself a sign of mental illness: it may simply indicate dishonesty and lack of concern for others. But to steal objects of no use or value, or only objects of a very specific type, or to steal when one is bound to be caught, is evidence, though not always conclusive, of a mental problem. There are of course those who would regard the very existence of certain desires, such as a desire to torture, as itself a sickness. But if a person sees acting on the desires as wrong, and has a normal capacity to control them, it is not clear that they are ill, as opposed to acting correctly if they control themselves and wrongly or wickedly if they do not. Nevertheless, the question 'Mad or bad?', as it is sometimes phrased,[5] remains.

This brings us to the other question – what is mental illness, or mental disorder, and which conditions should be called by this name? Given the framing of the new legislation, which will refer simply to mental disorder, some kind of answer has to be given. We have seen that the argument that 'mental illness' (with which 'mental disorder' is more or less synonymous) is not a valid concept and does not stand up. But it is clear that it is a concept that can be abused, and applied to people who are not ill in any sense, and indeed in the past has been misused in this way. Moreover, it could be argued that, though valid, it is irredeemably value-laden, and cannot be used truly objectively, and moreover that this is particularly the case when one is considering not simply whether someone has a mental illness but whether their condition justifies compulsory admission or treatment.

The reason is this. What is being assessed is whether someone's judgement is impaired in such a way as to make them a danger to themselves or to others. But it might be objected that what is actually the case is that this person is judging values and priorities differently from the person assessing them and acting on these judgements. To say that their judgement is impaired and that what they are going to do is harmful (which is what 'being a danger' means) is, according to this view, simply to impose the different values of the assessor.

However, this is needlessly pessimistic. First of all, one can have a more objective notion of 'harm'. Anything that in general reduces a person's capacity for action may be said to harm them objectively, because whatever one thinks they ought to be doing and whatever aims one believes to be good and right, reducing their capacity for action will undermine the possibility of their pursuing these ends; and therefore whatever one's values, such interference will be undesirable. Death is the supreme example of something harmful in this sense; examples that can be mild or serious are injury, disease, being deceived, losing or being deprived of one's property, being imprisoned or tied up, and so on. Now any of these, even death, can under some circumstances be intelligibly endured for the sake of some good or to avoid something worse: it was rational, though arguably not right, for a man to cut off a finger to avoid military service. But when a person cannot see or admit that something reasonably serious of this sort is happening or going to happen, or simply likely to happen, to themselves or to others, unless they change their behaviour, or when a person is apparently indifferent to its happening, then they may quite appropriately be said to have a mental illness that makes them a danger to themselves or others, and to require compulsory admission to hospital.

One objection to this remains. It might be said that when the danger is to oneself then being unable to see it, or admit it, or consider it to be a danger, is indeed a kind of illness, as being an involuntary condition that interferes with proper mental functioning. But if the danger is to others, is the term 'illness' appropriate? That is, is it justifiable to bring in personality disorders as a type of mental disorder? The problem posed is not just that these are currently untreatable, but that they may be untreatable in principle. Loss of memory, distortions of perception, mania and depression, addiction, phobia might all fairly be called illnesses; but can lack of self-control and lack of a conscience be put in the same category? (Anthony Flew[6] is an example of a philosopher who raised this problem some years ago.)

There are three reasons why one might wish to make a distinction here. First, the conditions in the first list can all sometimes (admittedly not always) be fairly clearly distinguished from their 'normal' analogues, whereas to distinguish an involuntary mental disorder of having no self-control, or no conscience, or no empathy for others, from plain selfishness or wickedness, is appreciably harder: can one be sure one is not dealing with ordinary wrongdoing? Secondly, other illnesses are a danger to the person who has them, whereas these are dangers, in the first instance, to other people. Thirdly, are lack of a conscience and lack of self-control involuntary, as these other conditions are? (Addiction may be produced by voluntary self-indulgence, but is itself an involuntary state.)

As regards the first objection, one may say that it is harder but still not impossible. As regards the second and third, one may say that to apply the notion of 'illness' or 'disorder' to these cases is indeed to extend the concept, which has already been extended by being applied to mental illness. But there is nothing wrong with extending a concept, if there are good reasons for doing so: the fact that the concept of mental illness has been wrongly extended does not show that it cannot be rightly extended. So why in this case might it be right?

First, it is being extended to people who are dangerous. Secondly, they are dangerous because of a mental abnormality. To fail, sometimes, to control oneself, and to let one's own interests override those of others are, very regrettably, normal. But to be radically unable to control certain desires or emotions, or to be unable to see the point of morality at all (as opposed to having different moral ideas from one's own society), or to be unable to see that other people even matter, is abnormal. It is, indeed, radically abnormal, not simply statistically: a person in one of these conditions is cut off, to some extent, from normal human understanding and relationships, except insofar as they learn to conceal it.

It might still be objected that there are 'normal' people who are even more dangerous, and that there is the threat of the law to control both the normal and the abnormal, so that it cannot be right to lock up people who have committed no crime, on the ground that they might commit one. But this is an identifiable group (identification may be difficult, but is certainly possible and is made), particularly likely to be undeterred by the law: and it is highly desirable, to put it mildly, to prevent them committing, for example, assault or murder, rather than simply punishing or incarcerating them after the event. On balance, it seems better to stretch the notion of illness to include them, and to hope that treatments that help, whether physical or involving psychotherapy, can be found, rather than to accept, in the name of freedom, murders and assaults. But this does require resisting the temptation to sweep 'innocent' and 'normal' people into the net, in the interests of being on the safe side.

So we may finally summarise the ethical position regarding compulsory admission to hospital. The aim is that all and only those who are dangerous to themselves or others because of a mental disorder should be compulsorily admitted (if they will not go into hospital voluntarily). I have argued, against Szasz and others, that this aim is both intelligible and ethically sound, even if it includes those with a personality disorder. It follows from this that the proposed framing of the new law is in line with the aim, and is also ethically sound. But it must be ethically administered by nurses, and this requires two things. First, there must be awareness that, because the law is deliberately very general, there is a danger that, from the current situation in which too few people were admitted to hospital, we move back to the situation in which too many are admitted. Secondly, the decision to admit must be made solely on the grounds that the person in question has a mental disorder that renders them dangerous. Thirdly, this must be decided solely on the evidence, and using as much evidence as possible.

9.10 Compulsory treatment

As regards compulsory treatment, as opposed to compulsory admission, there are four main ethical issues. The first of these is once again the issue of competence: only if the patient or client is genuinely unable to decide issues concerning their treatment should it be imposed by compulsion, and the presumption should be that they are competent unless the evidence shows otherwise. What is involved in deciding whether someone is competent has already been discussed. But what is very important is to note that the fact that someone has been compulsorily admitted does not of itself show that they are incompetent as regards treatment. They might indeed have a mental disorder, and be a danger to themselves or others; but they might still be able to decide competently whether they should have treatment and how they should be treated. So the question of compulsion needs to be reconsidered; it is not settled by the fact that the admission was compulsory. (This issue has been very well explained in an excellent article by Simona Giordano.[7])

Secondly, any treatment prescribed must be in the 'best interests' of the patient: here ethics and law are in total agreement. 'Best interests' is a problematic term but, as Gunn and Rodgers explain at section 9.2.3, the law gives quite a lot of guidance as to how it is to be interpreted. From the point of view of ethics, what is particularly important is that 'best interests' is in effect defined, even by the law, not 'objectively' but with regard to the tastes and values of the patient, in so far as these can be discovered if the patient is not in a condition to be asked and to reply. It appears to mean, in effect, what they would choose if they were able to make the decision, and/or were free from the mental characteristics that are merely the result of their illness but in other respects were mentally as they are now. There can of course be problems in deciding what is a long-term value commitment of the client or patient and what is produced by the illness: but sometimes this may well be more of a problem in theory than in practice. Once again, certainty may be impossible, but the decision should at any rate be made on the evidence, if it is to be ethically sound.

Thirdly, respect for patients or clients needs to be maintained, whatever form the treatment takes, even if the patients do not accord the nurses the respect that they should in their turn provide: having a mental illness does not automatically absolve a person from all moral obligations, though it does of course sometimes make a person not responsible for their actions. In particular, this is not only a matter for individual nurses dealing with individual patients. It is also a matter of designing procedures that maintain respect for patients and are not geared only to staff convenience, and, perhaps even more importantly, of fostering a culture of respect, through such things as the education of new staff and the example set by senior staff. For the worst abuses seem to arise when a particular ward, or perhaps even an institution, develops a culture with no respect for the patients. It is particularly in this area that ethics requires, within reason, an appreciably higher standard of behaviour than is required by the letter of the law. It is worth noting, however, that one consequence of this may well be that, once patients feel respected, there is less 'trouble', and of a less serious sort, so that 'respectful' procedures are practically useful as well as ethically right.

Fourthly, there is a range of ethical issues regarding different types of treatment. The position of the law is explained in detail by Gunn and Rodgers. They note in particular, under section 9.1.2, that the law imposes no limits on the types of treatment that can be compulsorily imposed, provided they are for the mental disorder. They point out, correctly in my opinion, that there is a difficult legal issue of deciding what is or is not 'for the mental disorder', one judge holding that this could cover a compulsory Caesarean section if having a live baby was essential to the effectiveness of the treatment, another holding that this could not be construed as treatment for the mental disorder. Gunn and Rodgers support the second judge, but it is not clear that the argument of the first judge, whatever the original intent of Parliament, is unsound. For the issue is surely not what the legislators would have said at the time, but what they would now say when presented with the actual case. At the time, they might well say, 'We do not expect this to include compulsory Caesarean section.' Faced with a woman who because of her mental disorder was in danger of bringing into the world a brain-damaged or even dead child and thereby greatly aggravating that disorder, they might well take the opposite view.

This suggests that ethically and legally any treatment may be compulsorily imposed, provided there really is good evidence that it is in the best interests of the patient. But there is a general ethical issue as regards physical treatments: electro-convulsive therapy, administration of drugs, psychosurgery and the surgical implantation of hormones. The last two are much less common and in any case legally require the patient's consent, as Gunn and Rodgers point out. Nevertheless, ethical objections have been raised to physical treatment as such, even in its commonest form of the administration of drugs.

The first objection is that physical treatment can tackle only the symptoms – the depression, or the compulsive behaviour, or the phobia, to take three examples – and not the underlying social or psychological conditions (or the combination) that constitute the real problem. This may well often be true; but even to relieve the symptoms is to do some good, sometimes much good, and, even more importantly, the symptoms may have to be relieved before the person can begin to tackle the underlying problem. A clinically depressed person may well be depressed for very good reasons – no job, lousy accommodation, a violent partner – but the depression may still need to be lifted by medication or even ECT before they are able to do anything about its causes.

The second objection is that it is inherently wrong to try to alter a person's mental state by physical means rather than by rational argument. But the proper use of physical treatments (which can of course be misused, but no one is defending their misuse) is precisely to remove obstacles to rational thinking. These obstacles are themselves often either physical in origin or made worse by the physical state of the brain and nervous system. To use drugs to enable a person to stop hearing voices, or experiencing hallucinations, or having sudden frightening changes in perception, is to restore, not to remove, the opportunity to think and act rationally.

So there is no ethical problem with the physical treatment of mental illness, as such: it becomes unethical if it is forced on a competent patient, or if it is not in fact in the patient's best interests. Nor is there a problem with behaviourist therapy, as such: if the aim is to free a person from such things as compulsive gambling or alcoholism, then rationality is once again being increased, if the treatment works. There may well be objections to such things as the use of behaviourist methods to try to 'cure' homosexuality, but the objection here is to the whole purpose, not to the method.

Moreover, though psychotherapy and 'talking' methods of treatment are not, normally, issues for the law, they also raise problems for ethics. It is true that it is impossible, in one sense, to impose psychotherapy: a person can be forced to attend one-to-one or group sessions, but cannot be forced to let them have any effect. But there is still such a thing as unethical psychotherapy, mainly in the form of covert manipulation: lip-service to the idea that the therapist is non-directive and non-judgemental, but considerable pressure, from the therapist or the group, to adopt certain views and ideas. The extreme case of this is the creation of false memories: there is still a problem, regarding some supposed memories of being sexually abused as a child, of which 'memories' are genuine and which have been planted, not necessarily intentionally, in the client's mind and are in fact false. This all brings out a point that applies also to physical treatments: that they should be used honestly. Provided that the patient can understand their aim and their likely consequences, they must be informed as to what these are.

So we may conclude this section by saying that no treatments are by their nature ethical or unethical. For any of them to be administered ethically, there are four conditions, easy to state but not always easy to apply in practice. First, they must not be imposed compulsorily on competent patients. Secondly, patients who can understand the purpose and likely effects of the treatment must be told them. Thirdly, respect for patients must always be maintained, even if the treatment is compulsory. Fourthly, there must a genuine effort to ascertain, using all the available evidence, what is in the patient's best interests, and this includes, if reasonably possible, considering their tastes and values.

9.11 Seclusion, treatment in the community and other issues

Two somewhat contrasting ethical issues remain: these are the use of seclusion, discussed in section 9.5.1 by Gunn and Rodgers, and the use of supervised community treatment, discussed in section 9.6. As regards the ethics of seclusion, or 'supervised confinement', little on paper, though quite a bit in practice, needs to be added to the guidance given by the law, and in particular the Code of Practice attached to the law of 1999, as explained by Gunn and Rodgers. Seclusion is sometimes a regrettable necessity in dealing with violent or aggressive patients; it should nevertheless be a last resort, used for the shortest possible time; it should not be used as a punishment or for staff convenience; and measures must be taken to keep the patient safe (see section 9.5.1). The main points that should be added concern the need to maintain respect for patients in these very difficult situations, and the need to maintain all the elements already mentioned in the previous section in the paragraph about respect. Seclusion will only be genuinely a last resort, and carried out for the right reasons and with regard to patients' safety, if there are procedures for defusing situations of potential violence or conflict; if nurses are trained to use these procedures and to have an ethical attitude that thinks first about 'defusing' a situation and about the use of seclusion only if defusing fails; and if all wards develop this ethos among their staff.

As regards supervised community treatment, this, if it becomes law, will, unlike seclusion, be a new development, and one that may increase rather than decrease the freedom of patients since it will allow some people who might otherwise be compulsorily kept in hospital to live in the community, provided they continue to attend for treatment and to take prescribed medication. This treatment will in one sense not be compulsory, since it may not be given by force. But in another sense it is 'compulsory', since if the patient refuses it, and this is reported, they may be compulsorily admitted or returned to hospital. As Gunn and Rodgers indicate, the only new duty on the nurse will be to report the failure to accept medication, and I think they are right to say that normally there would be an ethical as well as a legal duty to do this, rather than risk the danger to the community that could arise if the patient were left there while refusing medication. There might be a possible situation in which a nurse felt that a patient presented so little danger to themselves or others, even without their prescribed medication, that it would be best and most helpful not to report them, despite the legal requirement. The nurse must then solve the ethical dilemma according to his or her conscience; but this situation is, mercifully, likely to be uncommon.

Also uncommon, one hopes, is the issue not discussed by Gunn and Rodgers, and which I have therefore left to the end, of the nurse who is convinced that a patient is being given treatment that is legal (they discuss the legal requirements at length) but not the correct or appropriate treatment for that patient. This presumably comes under section 8.3 of the NMC Code of Professional Conduct: 'Where you cannot remedy circumstances in the environment of care that could jeopardise standards of practice, you must report them to a senior person with sufficient authority to manage them.' The nurse obviously needs to be very sure about the situation before making such a report, for both moral and prudential reasons; but such situations do arise. The final decision has to rest with the individual; and the situation is not peculiar to mental health nursing.

As a final conclusion, one may say that the proposed changes in the law do not raise any special ethical dilemmas, but they do raise certain ethical dangers, mainly the danger of the excessive use of compulsion in admission to hospital and in treatment. The onus is on nurses to use the increase in their power in an ethical way – I have tried, as a lay person, to outline what this means but only the nurses themselves can fill in the detail – so that it is used to the benefit of patients and clients, and hence to the benefit of society as a whole. These benefits do not normally conflict, since it is not in fact to the patient's benefit to be allowed to harm others. But it can be a very difficult decision, at times, to decide when it is freedom that promotes them and when compulsion is required. One can only hope that this discussion of the ethical issues can be of some slight help.

9.12 Notes and references

1. Jonathan Miller, *States of Mind: Conversations with Psychological Investigators* (London, BBC, 1983).
2. Peter Reddaway and S. Bloch, *Soviet Psychiatric Abuse: The Shadow over World Psychiatry* (Barnes and Noble, 1985).
3. D.L. Rosenhan, On being sane in insane places, *Science*, **179** (1973), pp. 250–8.
4. Caroline Dunn, *Ethical Issues in Mental Illness* (Aldershot, Ashgate, 1998), pp. 43–59.
5. Michael Bavidge, *Mad or Bad?* (Bristol, Bristol Classical Press, 1989).
6. Anthony Flew, *Crime or Disease?* (London, Macmillan, 1973).
7. Simona Giordano, For the protection of others, *Health Care Ethics*, **8** (2000), pp. 309–19.

10 The Critically Ill Patient

A   The Legal Perspective

Linda Delany

This part of Chapter 10 examines the legal aspects of the dilemmas inherent in nursing critically ill patients. Caring for the patient whose life hangs in the balance or whose prognosis is very uncertain can test the limits of the negligence and consent principles discussed in earlier chapters and the impact of the Human Rights Act 1998, which incorporated the European Convention for the Protection of Human Rights and Fundamental Freedoms into English Law.[1] The stress for all involved in dealing with grave illness can provoke conflicts that highlight the need for careful adherence to court rulings, legislation and the guidance emanating from government departments, the Royal Colleges and professional bodies in this sphere of nursing.

To reflect the law's own approach to treatment decisions in critical illness cases, patients will, in this chapter, be divided into the following broad categories: babies and young children, teenagers, adults able to make their own decisions and adults unable to do so. The legal rules relating to each category will be examined separately, but some general points can be made at the outset.

First, nurses treating critically ill patients should be clear about the criminal implications of knowingly causing their death. Providing pain relief with drugs that, as a side effect, may shorten life, can be acceptable, but acts aimed primarily at hastening death are forbidden. Withdrawing treatment, in the knowledge that death will result, can be legitimate, and is discussed in more detail in sections 10.1.2, 10.3 and 10.4 below.

Secondly, English law has traditionally extended a large measure of professional freedom to doctors. The courts have felt unable to dictate to doctors and have refused to let patients do so. Coercive remedies against doctors have simply not been made available, on the grounds that doctors should not have to choose between their professional, clinical judgement and a court order (*Re J (a minor) (wardship: medical treatment)* (1990)). Where patients demand a treatment option deemed unsuitable by their doctor, the most the latter is obliged to do is to offer to arrange a second opinion (*The Queen on the application of Burke* v. *General Medical Council* (2005)) and to keep the management of the patient's condition under review (*Wyatt* v. *Portsmouth NHS Trust* (2005)). This dominance of professional opinion is often challenged by the relatives of critically ill patients. In two recent cases (*An NHS Trust* v. *A* (2005)); (*Wyatt* v. *Portsmouth NHS Trust* (2005)), the adult sons of an 86-year-old man suffering multiple organ failure and parents wanting a guarantee of aggressive medical intervention for their two-year-old daughter, respectively, tried to persuade the Court of Appeal to overrule decisions to limit treatment. Neither appeal succeeded. Article 2(1) of the European Convention under which 'Everyone's right shall be protected by law' did not assist the two families. Where a responsible clinical decision is made to withhold treatment on the grounds that it is not in the patient's best interests, the positive obligation to preserve life is deemed to have been discharged. Nurses may have to absorb the tensions that obviously arise on such occasions. On a more positive note, they may be able to mediate between the patients, their families and the doctors when disagreements about treatment options arise. They should not hesitate to draw on and share their own insights into a patient's requirements.

The third and final point concerns the limits to the courts' powers over the allocation of health care resources. While courts are allowed to vet how decisions are made, they must confine themselves to procedural points and ignore the benefits that patients might derive from receiving the resources they request. The cases have shown that no exception is made even for critically ill patients whose survival depends on treatment being funded.[2] Whether Article 2(1) of the European Convention demands a more robust judicial approach remains to be tested.

At local level, scarcity of resources should be monitored by nursing staff. Nurses have been reminded by the Nursing and Midwifery Council (NMC) that they infringe their Code of Professional Conduct if they fail to report their concerns about inadequate resources to an appropriate line manager.[3] The duty to report arises whenever patient care or welfare is at risk.

10.1 Babies and young children

10.1.1 The significance of parental responsibility

The importance attached by the law to a patient's ability to consent to medical procedures produces an obvious problem in the case of children. As children lack the legal capacity to give a valid consent, nurses who treat them are exposed to the risk of being sued for 'battery', the unauthorised physical contact with another person. They may also be regarded as infringing the child's bodily integrity under Article 8 of the European Convention on Human Rights. To overcome these difficulties the law allows consent to be given by proxy. In an extreme emergency, anyone looking after a child can offer or authorise medical treatment.[4] For example, if the condition of a child in hospital deteriorated suddenly then no consent to intervene on his or her behalf would be needed. If time permits, however, the consent of a person with parental responsibility for the child must be sought (*Gillick* v. *West Norfolk and Wisbech Area Health Authority* (1985); *Glass* v. *UK* (2004)).

Mothers acquire parental responsibility automatically. So do fathers if they are married to the mother of their child at the time of the birth. Unmarried fathers need to be pro-active: they may obtain parental responsibility by registering the child's birth jointly with the mother,[5] by applying for parental responsibility through the courts, or by entering into a parental responsibility agreement with the mother.[6] The form of such an agreement is prescribed by law, and to be valid the agreement must be recorded at the High Court.

An unmarried father's capacity to act as proxy for his children should be investigated before his instructions are complied with. If this seems officious or embarrassing, it may help to remember that schools too have to explore this issue before accepting a father's authority over a pupil.

10.1.2 Acting in the best interests of children

The proxy powers conferred by parental responsibility must by law be exercised in the best interests of the child. What is in the best interests of critically ill children has been explored by the Royal College of Paediatrics and Child Health, most recently in 2004. Their report, *Withholding or Withdrawing Life-saving Treatment in Children. A Framework for Practice*,[7] identified the following five situations in which palliation, rather than a continuation of life-saving treatment, 'might be considered':

(1) where brain-stem death has been diagnosed
(2) where the child has developed a permanent vegetative state
(3) where the child has 'such severe disease that life sustaining treatment simply delays death without significant alleviation of suffering'
(4) where survival with treatment is possible but will be accompanied by an intolerable degree of physical or mental impairment
(5) where 'in the face of progressive and irreversible illness further treatment is more than can be borne'.

The first and second categories are self-explanatory. The third category is exemplified by the 1998 case of *Re C (a minor) (medical treatment)* (1998), in which, incidentally, the court explicitly approved the report's approach to this type of case. C was a severely disabled and terminally ill little girl, aged 16 months at the time that her case went to court. She suffered from spinal muscular atrophy, type 1, weighed only 5.4 kg, and her condition was deteriorating. She nevertheless seemed to interact with her parents, appearing to recognise them and smiling at them. In the view of C's medical team, her interests demanded the withdrawal of ventilator support, non-resuscitation in the event of respiratory arrest, and palliative care till she died. C's parents, who were orthodox Jews, agreed that the withdrawal of supportive ventilation could be attempted but wished it to be restored if C could not breathe without it. In view of the disagreement, the health authority applied to the court, which authorised the doctors to ease C's suffering, and to permit her life to end peacefully and with dignity.

The situations that trouble all concerned most are undoubtedly those that make up category 4 and involve children who with medical intervention will survive indefinitely, but whose survival entails pain and distress due to their health deficits. Several such cases have come before the courts. One of the earliest and most controversial was that of *Re J (a minor) (wardship: medical treatment)* (1990). J had been born at 27 weeks of gestation, with very severe and permanent brain damage. The medical evidence, some four months after J's birth, suggested that he was probably blind and deaf, had epilepsy, would probably develop serious spastic quadriplegia, and was unlikely to develop speech. J was, however, judged to feel pain to the same extent as other babies. He had been oxygen-dependent for significant periods in his young life and suffered sudden collapses resulting in the need for artificial ventilation. The medical team proposed that they should not re-ventilate J the next time his breathing stopped. In assessing where J's best interests lay, the court considered the distress and hazardous nature of reventilation, the risk of further deterioration if J was subjected to it, and his extremely unfavourable general prognosis. Because J's disabilities seemed to make his life intolerable, the court was prepared to spare him further invasive medical intervention.

The judgment, and others like it, can be criticised for the importance that was attached to the medical opinions about the baby. Psychologists, physiotherapists, teachers and respite centre staff are among the professionals who could, better than doctors, illuminate whether a disabled child might learn to interact with others, or at least to derive some satisfaction from his or her life. But unless such professionals are already involved with the young patient, they are unlikely to have the opportunity to give evidence to the court. Potentially valuable insights are thus neglected, and the basis for the court's assessment of the child's future quality of life is incomplete.

The fifth type of situation identified by the Royal College of Paediatrics and Child Health as potentially sanctioning the cessation or withholding of life-sustaining treatment involves very painful and distressing interventions that will fail to reverse or even halt the illness from which the child is dying. In such circumstances, the College says, further treatment 'is more than can be borne', and the courts have endorsed this approach. Just recently, however, the 'intolerability' test has somewhat fallen out of favour. In *Wyatt* v. *Portsmouth NHS Trust* (2004), the first stage of the proceedings already referred to at the start of this chapter, the Trust sought a ruling that would allow its staff to discontinue the invasive and aggressive treatment of the then one-year-old Charlotte Wyatt. Although the High Court judge agreed that such treatment would be intolerable to Charlotte, he chose a more positive justification for permitting it to be withheld as being more compatible with a determination of what was in her best interests. Instead of dwelling on the disadvantages of the treatment the parents wanted, he in effect listed the advantages of avoiding aggressive intervention by highlighting the comfort she would be nursed in, the increased contact she would enjoy with her parents and the tranquil death that would follow (although he accepted that the moment of that death would be slightly advanced by this treatment regime). The Court of Appeal in 2005 supported this approach, declaring that judges should focus on the best interests of the child rather than the concept of intolerability, although the latter might be encompassed within the former.

The value of the intolerability test has been vigorously defended[8] and it seems likely that it will survive *Wyatt*,[9] albeit as a subordinate component of a wider investigation into the factors that contribute to a child patient's overall welfare. In any event, such an investigation should not be deemed complete without the evidence of those, including nurses, whose contact with the child is greatest. A poignant occasion for such consultation arose in *An NHS Trust v. MB* (2006). M, the patient at the centre of the case, was a little boy born in August 2004. Like C in the 1998 *Re C (a minor) (medical treatment)* case mentioned above, he suffered from spinal muscular atrophy, a degenerative and progressive condition, in its most severe form. At the time of the proceedings he could no longer use his muscles in an age-normal way although he was still capable of some barely perceptible movement of his eyebrows, corners of his mouth, thumbs and toes. He was, however, conscious, awake most of the day, aware of those around him and of music, TV and DVDs, preferring, so his mother said, *The Jungle Book* to *EastEnders*.

The medical evidence offered a bleaker assessment than that presented by M's parents, dwelling as it did on the recurring pain and/or discomfort associated with the physiotherapy needed to loosen secretions, the occasional localised infection around the site of his gastrostomy tube, blood tests, the insertion of intravenous lines or cannulae, the changing and regular suctioning of his endotracheal tube and deeper suctioning towards the lungs. M could not wriggle his limbs, change his position unaided or ask for suction when he felt secretions accumulate in his chest and was increasingly unable to show distress because of the growing inability to open his eyes, and the complete inability to produce sounds. Only the formation of tears and his fluctuating heart rate would remain as clues to what he was feeling. The nurses caring for him had mixed views about his future management, with those who had most experience of the condition least keen to see M's life prolonged.

After balancing all the factors, the judge determined that for the time being continuous pressure ventilation and its associated procedures should be maintained as being in M's best interests. More painful treatment was not to be undertaken. The court also accepted that when the benefits of ceasing treatment outweighed the benefits M's life still conferred on him, he should be allowed to die. Labelling his life 'intolerable' was said to be unhelpful; a careful assessment of where the balance of M's interests lay was what was needed.

Is it obligatory to involve the courts where family and professionals agree that treatment should be withheld from a child? The judges in *Re J* (1990) ruled it was not. However, in the later case of *Re C (a baby)* (1996) the High Court suggested that the issue of referral to court should be decided in the context of each specific situation. Such a selective approach may fail to meet the requirements imposed by Article 2 of the European Convention on Human Rights. As was explained at the start of this chapter, our domestic law is now expected emphatically and transparently to protect life. This surely must entail that the decision to let a child die rather than 'inflict' treatment should go to court for an assessment of where the child's best interests lie. Furthermore, explicit criteria will need to be devised, to guide decision-making where a child's life is at stake.

10.1.3 Family disputes about treatment

Where adults share parental responsibility for a child, does the consent of just one of them, acting independently, protect the team treating the child? The answer provided by the Children Act 1989 in section 2(7) is affirmative. Nevertheless, in 1999 the Court of Appeal ruled that there were some decisions that should not be acted upon unless everyone with parental responsibility agreed.[10] Examples given were sterilisation and circumcision, rather than any treatments likely to apply in the case of critically ill child patients. Caution suggests that for irreversible procedures, particularly controversial ones, the consent of all who share parental responsibility should be obtained.

Proceeding on the basis of just one consent where there is conflict may anyway seem so invidious that going to court becomes preferable. It is at least an option available to 'piggy-in-the-middle' professionals seeking to respect the position of the dissenting adult. The latter, under Article 8 of the European Convention, in any case has the right to participate in the decision.[11] Because medical treatment disputes are regarded as complex, they must be referred to the High Court (*Re R (a minor) (blood transfusion)* (1993)) rather than the Family Proceedings Court or County court.

10.1.4 Disagreement between the family and the professional carers

Where there is serious disagreement about how best to proceed, either the family or the health care team (backed by the relevant health authority) may ask the High Court to intervene. Alternatively, social services may invoke the court's jurisdiction. The court will take account of the views of all involved in caring for the child and of the child's legal representatives, before reaching its own independent assessment of the balance of advantages or disadvantages of the particular medical step under consideration (*Re T (a minor) (wardship: medical treatment)* (1996)). The views of the nursing team can and should be very influential (*Re C (a minor) (wardship: medical treatment)* (1989)).

Although the courts' intrusion into family life could amount to unjustified state interference, under article 8(2) of the European Convention it is usually deemed necessary 'for the protection of health or morals, or for the protection of the rights and freedom of others'. The aim of safeguarding a child's physical, psychological or emotional welfare is thus considered to be a legitimate basis for court intervention. Indeed, a failure on the part of an NHS Trust or health authority to refer a case involving disputed treatment to court is regarded as an infringement of the Article 8(1) right of child patients to respect for their private life and, in particular, their physical and psychological integrity. In *Glass* v. *UK* (2004) the European Court of Human Rights reviewed the Portsmouth Hospitals NHS Trust's management of a 12-year-old patient with severe mental and physical disabilities. A series of respiratory tract infections had led to repeated emergency hospitalisation. When, during one such stay, the patient's doctors concluded that he had entered a terminal phase of lung disease, they advised the administration of diamorphine. The child's mother disagreed with both the prognosis and the advice, but counter to her express wish a diamorphine infusion was commenced and a 'Do Not Resuscitate' notice was placed in her son's notes without her knowledge. The judges were not persuaded by the Trust's contention that there had been no time for an emergency application to the domestic courts and held the decision to overrule the mother without court backing to be a violation of Article 8.

Understandably, treatment decisions concerning critically ill children have frequently reached the courts. In Re D (wardship: medical treatment) (2000) the applicant NHS Trust cared for a 19-month-old little boy suffering from severe, worsening, irreversible lung disease, coupled with heart failure, hepatic dysfunction, renal disjunction and learning difficulties. The Trust wished to spare him artificial ventilation in the event of respiratory or cardiac failure, but his parents disagreed strongly with this approach. The High Court sided with the Trust in this case, finding the benefits of a probably short extension to lifespan outweighed by the distress intensive mechanical treatment would inflict. Similarly, in the 1998 case of baby C, discussed at 10.1.2 above, the High Court agreed with the health authority that ventilator support should be withdrawn from a terminally ill little girl, despite parental opposition. By contrast, in Re T (a minor) (wardship: medical treatment) (1997), it was the parents who objected to medical intervention. T at the time of the hearing was 17 months old. He suffered from the life-threatening liver defect biliary atresia, and the medical recommendation was a liver transplant. He had had an operation already, and his pain and distress at that time had persuaded his parents that he should not undergo major surgery. Of the three transplant teams consulted, one was prepared to respect the views of the parents, but one was determined that a transplant should go ahead. The parents, who were themselves trained health professionals experienced in the care of young, sick children, found that their opposition to the transplant was referred to social services, and from there to the High Court.

Although the High Court judge ruled that a transplant was in T's best interests, the Court of Appeal disagreed. The judges were not convinced that a short but happy life, ending in a peaceful death, was a worse option than 'a lifetime of drugs and the possibility of further invasive surgery'. Instead, they looked beyond T's purely medical interests to the 'broader considerations' that applied and concluded that the views of the parents could be allowed to determine T's future treatment. Although in Re T the 'broader considerations' were put forward by the parents, it will often fall to a child patient's nurses to alert others to relevant factors and concerns.

No doubt the most controversial case to feature conflict between parents and health care professionals was that involving the conjoined twins born in Manchester on 8 August 2000 (Re A (children) (2000)). The weaker twin only lived because her circulation was sustained by her stronger sister. Unless a separation was performed, the heart of the stronger twin would fail and both girls would die. The health authority sought permission to surgically separate the twins, which would allow the stronger one to survive but kill the weaker one immediately. The parents rejected this active encompassing of the death of one of their children and refused to sanction the strategy, but were overruled by the Court of Appeal. Although the judges stressed that their decision 'was authority for the unique circumstances of the case' only, they did in effect approve the active killing of the weaker twin, albeit out of concern for the best interests of her stronger sister. The ruling is difficult to reconcile with the protection for respect to life demanded from the state by Article 2 of the European Convention. It also highlights the elasticity of the best interests test, as applied to the weaker twin: out of the four judges (one High Court, three Court of Appeal) who considered her plight, two thought death would be in her best interests, given her poor prospects and increasingly painful life, while for the others her life reaching its natural end was the better option.

10.1.5 Neglecting the child's medical needs

Where the medical needs of children are neglected by those with parental responsibility, the latter forfeit their right to make treatment decisions. If time permits, the case should be referred to the High Court. If there is no time for this, the health care team should proceed to do what it thinks best for the child. This is the basis on which the children of Jehovah's Witnesses are given blood products against their parents' wishes. Nurses should be prepared for the difficulties inherent in these painful situations. They should, before any emergency arises, familiarise themselves with their employer's guidance on how to deal with the parents in such circumstances.

10.2 Teenagers

10.2.1 Capacity to consent

The provisions of section 8 of the Family Law Reform Act 1969 ensure that by 16 at the latest teenagers can give their own consent to medical treatment. Many will reach sufficient maturity to authorise specific procedures at an earlier point. Assessing that maturity is something the professional treating the teenager must do in the light of the guidance offered in the case of *Gillick* v. *West Norfolk and Wisbech Area Health Authority* (1985): the patient's capacity to understand all the issues surrounding the proposed treatment is the vital criterion.

When a teenager is judged competent to give a valid consent to treatment, involving his or her parents is recommended but not essential. If the patient insists on confidentiality, it must be maintained. This view, adopted by the government in the wake of the Gillick case, was challenged in *R (on the application of Axon)* v. *Secretary of State for Health* (2006) on the grounds that it undermined respect for family life, thereby infringing Article 8 of the European Convention on Human Rights. The Applicant further argued that if parents were to fulfil their responsibility for the physical, mental and moral welfare of their children, they needed all relevant information to help them do so. The court, while sympathetic to this last argument, felt bound to respect the autonomy of the mature young person. The judge went on to hold that the Article 8(1) right to family life owed to a parent (here, specifically, the right to be notified of the medical advice given to children) dwindles as the child matures and ceases when the child can make his or her own decisions.

The above rules do not prevent health authorities and social services, or even a relative, from referring a medical dilemma to court, using the wardship or inherent jurisdiction. Once this has been done, the decision of the court can overrule that of any young person, however competent, who has not yet reached the age of 18 (*Re W (a minor) (medical treatment)*) (1992).

Teenage consent to medical treatment has not proved controversial in the sphere of critical illness. Where medical advice is accepted and followed, no conflict arises for the health care team involved. The situation is, however, very different where a young person refuses vital treatment. This problem is considered in the next section.

10.2.2 Capacity to refuse treatment

Although the principle of 'Gillick competence' was clearly meant to apply to all medical treatment decisions rather than just to consent, the law will not allow teenagers to refuse essential treatment. The case of *Re W (a minor) (medical treatment: court's jurisdiction)* (1992) confirmed that children, whatever their age or maturity, lack power to override the consent that a person with parental responsibility gives in their best interests. Sixteen-year-old W's severe anorexia meant that she was close to death at the time of the legal proceedings. The local authority, which had parental responsibility for her, wished her to receive treatment at a clinic that W refused to attend. The Court of Appeal overruled her refusal, holding that neither section 8 of the Family Law Reform Act 1969 nor the concept of 'Gillick competence' applied to refusal of treatment. The judges, alive to the family conflicts that might ensue when teenagers and their parents disagree about treatment, did, however, suggest that health professionals should, as a matter of ethics, refer difficult cases to court. They also emphasised that the views of teenage patients must be explored and given due weight in accordance with their age and maturity.

The guidance given by the Court of Appeal in *Re W* was applied in *Re M (child: refusal of medical treatment)* (1999). M was a 15-year-old girl who suffered the sudden onset of heart failure. It became clear that her survival depended on her undergoing a heart transplant. Although M herself opposed the procedure, her parents agreed with the health care team that the transplant was in her best interests. There was thus sufficient legal consent for the proposed transplant to go ahead but in view of what had been said in *Re W* the health authority decided to refer the case to court. The urgency of the situation meant that a duty judge had to be contacted, and the decision made overnight. M's views were conveyed to the judge via her solicitor; although they were overridden, the judge prepared a careful record of his reasoning for M's benefit.

Decisions like *Re W* and *Re M* would have little effect if they could not be implemented. The courts have recognised that force may be needed if essential treatment is to be delivered to an unwilling young patient. Although orders authorising a minimum degree of force or restraint are issued sparingly and cautiously they are available on application to the court.[12] The Royal College of Nursing has issued guidance on the problems related to forcing young people to undergo treatment.[13]

10.2.3 Participating in decision-making

To nursing staff caring for teenage patients, the law may not seem sensitive enough to the principle of respect for autonomy. However, the rather limited scope that teenagers in the past had to affect treatment decisions acquired new potential for growth under the European Convention on Human Rights. Its emphasis on the significance of human life (Article 2), of due process (Article 6) and of family privacy (Article 8) is likely to result in new respect for a young person's point of view and right to participate in the decision-making process.

Attention should also be paid to the provisions of the Convention on Human Rights and Biomedicine 1997. A supplement to the European Convention on Human Rights, this second Convention resolves 'to take such measures as are necessary to safeguard human dignity and the fundamental rights and freedoms of the individual with regard to the application of biology and medicine'.[14] Article 6(2) insists that 'the opinion of a minor shall be taken into consideration as an increasing determining factor in proportion to his or her age and degree of maturity'. A violation of this Article, while not actionable by itself, could be challenged in proceedings brought to enforce a European Convention on Human Rights provision.

10.3 Adults able to make their own decisions

10.3.1 Refusal of treatment

Where adult patients are critically ill, the temptation to intervene on their behalf, regardless of their wishes, may be hard to resist. But even life-threatening conditions do not validate non-consensual treatment, as paragraph 3 of the NMC Code of Professional Conduct and case law make clear. Where patients do refuse treatment, it is important that nurses keep a summary of the discussions and decisions with the patient's records.[15]

The courts have repeatedly asserted the right of patients to reject medical procedures in any circumstances. However, faced with a refusal to consent to life-saving treatment, nurses, in common with other health care professionals, should give 'very careful and detailed consideration to the patient's capacity to decide' (*Re T (adult: refusal of treatment)* (1992)). The more serious the decision, the greater the capacity needed to make it.

Authoritative guidance on how patients should be approached was made available by the Court of Appeal in the case of *Re MB (medical treatment)* (1997).

Medical teams should start from the presumption that patients have the capacity to reach their own decisions, a principle now endorsed by the Mental Capacity Act 2005. Patients are entitled to make irrational or foolish choices. Scope for overriding their wishes arises only when there is evidence of impaired mental functioning. Pain, shock, medication, fatigue and drugs may induce temporary loss of competence. So may fear, if it destroys the ability to make decisions.

Where there are genuine reasons to doubt a patient's capacity, the safe course is to determine a treatment plan that is in the patient's best interests, and to invite the court to declare it lawful. Procedural safeguards to protect the patient in such a case were put in place by *Re MB*, and must be strictly complied with.

10.3.2 Maternal–fetal conflict

Where a pregnant woman wants her baby to be born alive and healthy, its safe birth will normally be in her best interests. But where the wishes of a competent mother rule out a safe birth then, according to *Re MB*, they must nevertheless be complied with. The issues raised in such a situation are more fully discussed in Chapter 7 on consent.

10.4 Adults unable to make their own decisions

10.4.1 General principles

The starting point is that adults who lack the legal capacity to make treatment decisions cannot give a valid consent to medical interventions; nor can anyone else do so on their behalf (*Re F (mental patient: sterilisation)* (1989)). It is, however, lawful to treat them provided that treatment is in accordance with the appropriate professional standard and is in the best interests of the patient concerned (*Re A* (1999)). Nurses have a key role to play in the process of determining what is in the patient's best interests. It is good practice to consult the patient's family, but, as the case of *An NHS Trust* v. *A* (2005) discussed at the start of this chapter clearly shows, the final say rests with the health care team. The courts can be asked to declare whether or not a proposed intervention is lawful. Once a referral has been made it is for the judge, guided by all the evidence, to assess where the patient's best interests lie (*Re SL (adult patient: medical treatment)* (2000)).

New legislation, not yet in force at the time of writing, extends the protection offered by the law to people unable to make their own decisions. The Mental Capacity Act 2005 provides a best interests checklist for people acting on behalf of others and the opportunity for adults to appoint an attorney who can consent to or refuse medical treatment on their behalf. The power, particularly relevant to critical illness cases, to decide on the administration, withdrawal or withholding of life-sustaining treatment is not conferred automatically by the appointment, and must be expressly conferred on the attorney,[16] who can be expected to provide evidence of it.

10.4.2 Advance directives

Patients increasingly prepare for the onset of their own mental incapacity by pro-ducing a set of instructions as to the treatment they would seek, or seek to avoid, at that point. Known as 'advance directives', such instructions may take a variety of forms ranging from signed, witnessed documents to a spoken wish. Statements requesting specific treatment options should normally be respected but cannot override professional judgements, as in law no one can dictate how health care teams should proceed. By contrast, cases including *Re C (adult: refusal of treatment)* (1994) and *Re AK (adult patient: medical treatment: consent)* (2001) confirm that state-ments that take the form of an advance refusal of treatment have full effect in law, provided that they are clearly articulated, with full understanding of their implications, and cover the circumstances that subsequently occur. The Mental Capacity Act adds the requirement that decisions about life-sustaining treatment must be in writing, signed and witnessed (section 25). Under the Act, evidence of a change of mind on the part of patients may invalidate their directive, and it may fall to nurses to alert others to such a change.

The case of *Re T (adult: refusal of treatment)* (1992) illustrates some of the prob-lems linked with advance refusals in an emergency. T was a young pregnant woman admitted to hospital after a road traffic accident. A decision was made to deliver her baby by Caesarean section, and the issue of administering blood was raised in this context. T, whose mother was a fervent Jehovah's Witness, asked whether there was a substitute treatment and was told that there was. She then signed a form of refusal of consent to blood transfusions. The form was not read out, nor explained, to her, nor was she advised of the risk to her own health and life that her refusal entailed. Following the Caesarean section (the baby was stillborn), T's condition deteriorated and she was transferred to intensive care. After she became unconscious, her father and boyfriend sought a declaration from the court that it would be lawful for the hospital to administer blood, despite T's prior refusal.

The Court of Appeal emphatically endorsed the right of adults to reject medical advice and treatment, if their decision is reached while they have the capacity to make it. The judges then explored T's capacity at the point at which she refused the transfusion. They found that her capacity had been undermined by the influence of her mother, the pain and confusion T was in, and by the failure to fully advise her of the potentially serious consequences of her decision. In the light of this finding, the proposed blood transfusion was declared lawful. The decision shows that advance refusals must be approached with some caution, and with attention to the circumstances in which they were made, if these are known.

10.4.3 Patients in, or close to, permanent vegetative state

Arguably patients in, or close to, a permanent vegetative state (PVS) are not critic-ally ill: the maintenance of nutrition and hydration may keep such patients alive for many years. It should, however, be recognised that the perceived futility of life in PVS presents dilemmas akin to some of those associated with critical illness.

Furthermore, the emergencies that arise during the nursing of PVS patients are often life-threatening.

In *Airedale NHS Trust* v. *Bland* (1993), the House of Lords upheld a declaration that the doctors' proposal to withdraw food and water from their patient was lawful. In the judgement of the medical team (and the family), keeping Anthony Bland alive had become futile because there was no hope that he would ever recover from the carefully diagnosed PVS he was in. The court accepted that this judgement was one that a respectable body of medical opinion shared, and agreed that the continuation of artificial nutrition and hydration was not in the best interests of the patient. The Law Lords did request that the moral, social and legal issues raised by the case should be reviewed by Parliament and, as an interim safeguard for patients, insisted that life-sustaining treatment should be withdrawn from adults in PVS only with the backing of a court declaration.

Since the decision in *Bland*, the clinical description of PVS has received much attention. In 1994 the House of Lords' Select Committee on Medical Ethics recommended the setting up of a working group to produce guidance on the diagnosis and management of PVS. A Working Party of the Royal College of Physicians responded to the challenge in 1996 with the publication of *The Permanent Vegetative State*,[17] which set out guidelines subsequently endorsed by both the BMA and the Official Solicitor. These have been superseded by fresh guidance issued in 2003.[18]

Nevertheless, diagnosis of PVS remains difficult, and ever since the decision in *Bland* courts have struggled to fit the clinical aspects of cases into the guidelines framework. In *Frenchay NHS Trust* v. *S* (1994) the Court of Appeal heard arguments questioning the PVS diagnosis of the 24-year-old male patient, who had suffered acute and extreme brain damage after taking a drug overdose. The nurses on the health care team were convinced that S seemed to suffer, and medical reports recorded what appeared to be voluntary and volitional behaviour. Attempts at rehabilitation had been made for two years, which called into question the confidence with which PVS had been diagnosed in the first place. Although there was no doubt among the judges that the decision to allow S to die promoted his best interests, it is clear from this case that PVS guidelines need not always be strictly adhered to. It is worth noting that the application to the court was triggered by the dislodging of S's feeding tube, a typical life-threatening emergency in the PVS context.

It now clear that the withholding of treatment from PVS patients is not deemed to infringe Article 2 of the European Convention on Human Rights, which protects people's right to life. In the cases of *NHS Trust A* v. *M* (2000) and *NHS Trust B* v. *H* (2000) the High Court ruled that treatment may cease where, as in PVS cases, there is no positive obligation to prolong life. The court issued declarations that artificial nutrition and hydration could lawfully be withdrawn from two female patients in PVS.

10.4.4 Borderline cases

Where there is evidence of a real possibility that meaningful life continues for the patient, cessation of treatment (which, according to *Bland*, includes artificial nutrition and hydration) would obviously be harder to justify than it is in the PVS cases. Health care teams and the courts would have to balance factors similar to those taken account of in children's cases at present (see section 10.1.2 above).

10.4.5 Emergency resuscitation

Where the emergencies that arise during the treatment of critically ill patients raise the question of whether resuscitation should be tried, decisions should be informed by the advice issued in the joint statement of the Royal College of Nursing, the Resuscitation Council (UK) and the British Medical Association[19] as well as that in GMC guidance.[20] The presumption is that cardio-pulmonary resuscitation should be attempted unless the patient has ruled it out. Advance decisions by the health care team that it should not be can, however, be justified by reference to the likely outcome of resuscitation, and the ascertainable wishes of the patient and of his or her family. Such 'Do Not Resuscitate' decisions must involve consultation with the patient's nurses, although responsibility for the decision would lie with the consultant in charge. Decisions should be recorded in the nursing notes as well as in the medical notes. If this professional guidance is adhered to, the legal duty of care to the patient will be discharged. A fundamental aspect of this duty is to keep patients alive but only for as long as this serves their best interests (*The Queen on the application of Burke* v. *General Medical Council* (2005)).

10.5 Conclusion

Legal problems commonly associated with the delivery of health care tend to present themselves in acute form during the management of critical illness. Assessing the patient's capacity to make treatment decisions and his or her best interests becomes more difficult than usual. The need for limits to the duty to maintain life and for court intervention at key points of uncertainty is highlighted. As this chapter has shown, the law's response has been to augment the basic framework of principles within which nurses are expected to work. Attention to legal developments and a sound understanding of legal requirements have become vital components of a professional approach to nursing critically ill patients.

10.6 Notes and references

1. As explained in Chapter 1.
2. See, for example, *R* v. *Central Birmingham Health Authority. Ex parte Walker* [1987] BMLR 32; *R* v. *Cambridge Health Authority. Ex parte B* [1995] 2 All ER 12 (CA).
3. Nursing and Midwifery Council, *The NMC Code of Professional Conduct: Standards for Conduct, Performance and Ethics* (London, Nursing and Midwifery Council, 2004), para. 8.3.

4. Children Act 1989, section 3(5).
5. Adoption and Children Act 2002, section 111.
6. Children Act 1989, section 4.
7. Royal College of Paediatrics and Child Health, *Withholding or Withdrawing Life-saving Treatment in Children: A Framework for Practice* (London, Royal College of Paediatrics and Child Health, 2004).
8. C. Foster, Burke: a tale of unhappy endings, *Journal of Personal Injury Law*, **4** (2005), pp. 293–303.
9. Despite what was said about intolerability in *An NHS Trust* v. *MB* and *Wyatt*, the Nuffield Council on Bioethics in a 2006 report called *Critical Care Decisions in fetal and neonatal medicine: ethical issues* refers to 'intolerable' lives.
10. *Re J (Specific Issue Orders: Child's Religious Upbringing and Circumcision)* [2000] 1FLR 571 at 577 (d).
11. *W* v. *United Kingdom*, July 8, 1987. Series A, No. 121; 10 EHRR 29.
12. See *Re S (a minor) (consent to medical treatment)* [1994] 2 FLR 1065, and *Re C (detention: medical treatment)* [1997] 2 FLR 180.
13. Royal College of Nursing, *Restraining, Holding Still and Containing Children: Guidance for Good Practice* (London, Royal College of Nursing, 1999).
14. Preamble to the Convention on Human Rights and Biomedicine, 4 April 1997.
15. Para. 3.5.
16. Mental Capacity Act, section 9.
17. Royal College of Physicians, The permanent vegetative state, *Journal of the Royal College of Physicians*, **30** (1996), pp. 119–21.
18. Royal College of Physicians, *The Vegetative State: Guidance on Diagnosis and Management* (London, Royal College of Physicians, 2003).
19. British Medical Association, Resuscitation Council (UK), Royal College of Nursing, *Decisions Relating to Cardio-pulmonary Resuscitation: A Joint Statement* (London, BMA, 2001).
20. General Medical Council, *Withholding and Withdrawing Life-prolonging Treatments: Good Practice in Decision-making* (London, GMC, 2002).

B   Ethical Issues

Robert Campbell

10.7 Introduction

How should we treat those who are seriously ill and who might well be dying? Patients with a strong chance of recovery and a clearly indicated and effective treatment present us with few ethical issues. What challenges us are cases where it is unclear what treatment will be effective or, indeed, if any treatment would be. Unfortunately, it is often in those very cases where we need to communicate clearly and sensitively with patients that we find that they are too ill, frightened or bewildered to hear and understand what is being said. Sometimes this can be compounded by the patient's situation; the very young, the very old and those with communication or learning difficulties all pose particular challenges for those whose responsibility it is to care for them.

As has rightly been noted, the responsibility of care can also create legal liability, and nurses and other related professionals have a duty of care for their patients, which legally – and, arguably, morally – goes far beyond what we normally owe each other as a matter of course. This means we can find ourselves liable for consequences far beyond anything we ever imagined. What an ethical perspective can provide us with is some help in seeing what, in the circumstances, is the best we can do. In the unhappy event that the best is not good enough, it can also help give us the defences and explanations we may need.

10.8 Consent

Consent is absolutely basic to all medical care. This is because in law to touch someone without their consent is a battery, and medical treatment, especially in critical situations, will normally involve physical contact at the least. For everyday treatments, such as having a tooth filled or an eye examination, consent is both presumed and implicit in the patient's simply being there. For more complex, unusual or potentially dangerous interventions, more formal procedures are needed to establish consent. This is because both the law and morality (and common sense) assume that consent involves more than just saying yes. To consent in any real sense you must know what you are consenting to, and your consent must be genuine, that is unforced. The previous section has looked at the case of *Re T (adult: refusal of treatment)* (1992). T had signed a form of refusal of consent to blood transfusions (on religious grounds). She had been told there was an alternative to a blood transfusion, but the form was not read out to her; nor was there any discussion of the possible consequences of her refusal. The court held that this refusal of consent could not be relied on when subsequently T lost consciousness in intensive care and needed a transfusion in order to survive. It could not be relied upon because the evidence that T really understood what she was refusing was not convincing.

If I were to get you to sign the bottom of a blank sheet of paper on which I then type a deed of gift that transfers all your worldly wealth to me, then no one would suppose that this constituted a genuine agreement. You did not realise that you were agreeing to anything, let alone that you were agreeing to that. In the same way, a patient must understand the nature of the treatment proposed if any verbal or written declarations are to count as genuine consent. What counts as 'understanding the nature of the treatment' is more complicated, but courts have held, quite reasonably, that it involves more than simply being told what will be done. In particular, it also involves having some understanding of the likely consequences – both good and bad – and of how likely they are.

Consent to treatment is problematic for critically ill patients for two reasons: first, because their condition may make it hard for them to express consent, or it may mean that they are not able to give consent at all (because they are unconscious, or no longer capable of full consent – see section 10.9.1 below); and secondly, because the difficulty of deciding on an appropriate course of treatment may not be wholly a matter of medical science. Sometimes a particular procedure becomes less and less effective each time it is performed, and the benefit to the patient declines correspondingly. This can be especially true of palliative or symptomatic care that does nothing to arrest an underlying condition. At some stage a judgement must be made that the benefits are now too negligible, or too heavily outweighed by the discomfort of the treatment or its possible side effects. Equally, a treatment may be uncertain, and although the degree of uncertainty may be a matter of medical science, the question of whether the risk is worth taking is not. For a patient with advanced cancer there can be a difficult decision as to whether an outside chance of aggressive chemotherapy securing a remission is worth the severe discomfort the treatment will certainly cause. Some might think that, when it is a matter of life or death, any chance, however remote, is worth taking. Others, who might be more temperamentally risk-averse, could see it as a gamble not worth taking.

10.8.1 Why does consent matter?

The job of the therapeutic team is to do their best for the patient, given the resources at their disposal. Indeed, this is more than their job; it is their legal and moral duty once the patient has been accepted as a patient. And it is hard to see how the patient, unless in some way deranged, can object to this. After all, is it not one of our informal tests for how sensible and rational someone is that they should want the best for themselves? Why should we also need their consent? There are four major reasons why we do.

The first is related to the issue raised at the end of the previous section and has to do with expertise and the authority that goes with it. Most would agree that, normally, medically trained staff are more likely to know what the probable prognosis is of a given intervention or treatment. That knowledge gives them an authority that may be unfashionable but is none the less real for that. However, judgements to do with how much risk is worth taking or how much pain or discomfort may be discounted against future benefit lie outside that area of expertise.

The expertise in these matters, and hence the authority, lies with the person who has to take the decision. (See also the fourth reason below.)

The second is located in the idea of a *person*. Most human beings are persons and most persons are human beings, but the terms do not have the same meaning.[1] A human being is a member of a particular biological species; a person is a moral agent who has plans and purposes and the capacity for free choice. From the point of view of personhood, all persons are morally equal in as much as there is no inherent reason for preferring one person's plans and purposes to another's. It is not possible for everyone to realise each one of their plans. What I want may conflict with what you want, and may even make it impossible for you to get what you want. This is why we need mediation, compromise, negotiation and, eventually, law. But such procedures do not ignore a person's moral agency. On the contrary, they only make sense when they are addressed to a person as someone capable of making choices and acting on them.

Disregarding a patient's right to consent to or refuse treatment ignores the fact that the patient is an agent and assumes that your plan to treat a patient in a particular way is the only plan that matters. It is, in Kantian terminology, to treat the patient as a means to an end and not as an end-in-herself.[2] It therefore fails to accord that patient the respect and dignity due to a person whose moral importance is as great as your own. And if you believe that your plans and choices are important, you must allow that other people's are equally important. To fail to do so is illogical as well as insensitive.

The third reason why consent matters has to do with human psychology rather than logic or morality. A patient whose agreement to treatment has been sought and obtained will feel empowered in a number of ways. First, they will *own* the treatment as an equal member of the team that has decided on it. They will be acting, rather than acted on. Secondly, they will be less apprehensive about what will happen since, if the agreement is real and not just stage-managed, they will understand what is involved and its implications. And thirdly, they will have retained control over their situation, and in situations where people are profoundly vulnerable and probably distressed, this is clearly, and in some cases literally, vital. They will feel, and will be, *autonomous*. It is also important to see that this process of empowerment will go on whether the patient agrees with the proposed course of treatment or whether they refuse it.

The fourth reason why consent matters has to do with human fallibility. People can be wrong, and in particular they can be wrong about what is good for another person. The medical team is composed of experts in various fields, but the only person who is an expert on what is good for me is me. Fallibility can come in here too, admittedly: I can be wrong about what is in my own best interests. We all know that can happen. But I am less likely to be wrong about it than someone else is because I'm an expert on me, and I have, as well, an incentive to get it right that no one else does. I will bear the consequences – good or bad.[3] It is therefore vitally important that when decisions need to be taken about what will be good for me, I am the one who takes them, even though I may need expert advice from others. What this means, in practice, is that I must have the opportunity to decide whether to accept the treatment offered even though others may feel that I am wrong in the decision I come to.

10.9 Refusing treatment

It is clear that, in English and American law,[4] I have the right to refuse treatment, however unreasonable this may seem to someone else. Treatment carried out against my wishes would, in theory, ground an action for battery. What is less clear is how far I have the right to decline treatment when such treatment is, or is likely to be, life-saving; for, in practice, the refusal of life-saving treatment is often regarded as *prima facie* evidence of an inability to give or withhold consent on a rational basis.[5]

This is not entirely unreasonable. Declining to have dental treatment or a hip replacement is not only, as I have argued, your business, but it also leaves you around afterwards to change your mind. Declining life-saving treatment does not. This is not just a practical issue, for if the moral importance of consent has to do with autonomy – that is, self-determination – then choosing a course of action that you know is highly likely to result in your death seems inconsistent with this. Self-determination disappears when there is no self left to determine. Perhaps we can merely pass over this as a puzzling oddity since there are many other examples of it that we accept quite readily: people who risk their lives, and lose them, in the attempt to help others; people who choose death rather than the violation of a principle or value that seems to them more important that their own lives; and people who rationally choose to commit suicide. Counselling this latter category does, however, raise some practical difficulties also thrown up in dealing with those who refuse life-saving treatment, for the general principle that people should make their own decisions and learn from their own mistakes cuts a little too deeply here. If choosing suicide or refusing treatment turns out to have been a mistake, then it is, in the nature of things, too late to learn anything from that. Just as consent can only be genuine if the patient fully understands what she is consenting to, so equally the decision to refuse life-saving treatment should only be respected if there is no doubt at all that the patient fully understands that and what she is refusing. (See the discussion of *Re T (adult: refusal of treatment)* (1992) above and in the previous chapter.)

10.9.1 Capacity

This last point is related to both knowledge and understanding. Clearly I cannot be said to have consented to something if I am kept in ignorance of, misled about or simply fail to understand its nature. Doctors, like any other group with specialist knowledge, are perfectly capable of explaining something in such a way that no non-specialist could hope to understand it. This is rarer than it used to be and most doctors at least understand that it is something they should strive to avoid. Nonetheless, it is not always easy to explain a complicated matter in terms that are perfectly clear to the layperson and, at the same time, both accurate and complete. Nor are patients always very good at admitting that they have not completely understood and would like it explained again. It is *always* possible, in other words, for anyone to give apparent consent, which is undermined by lack of knowledge or genuine understanding.

There are, however, classes of people for whom consent is problematic not in specific cases but in general. These are people who, in legal terminology, lack the *capacity* to give consent, not because they *don't* understand, but because they *can't* and can't be brought to understand. Small children are an obvious example. It isn't that they cannot make choices, but that they do not understand the world well enough to realise what their choices might imply. Their developing knowledge means that they are gradually better able to understand, and therefore more and more able to give consent that is real and informed. Capacity is, in other words, not something that either exists or does not exist. It is a gradual thing. Children can be in a position to be told or consulted about what may happen without being ready to take the final decision for themselves (see previous chapter). Or else they may be ready to take decisions in some areas but not in others. In practice, the law's willingness to allow young people aged under 18 to make treatment decisions will rest on the seriousness of those decisions (see previous chapter). Equally with adults it can be true that capacity can be diminished or partial.

For example, there is the case of T, where the court decided that a refusal of treatment was made under the undue influence of the patient's mother and that there was reason to believe that the patient did not fully understand its implications. There might be enormous difficulty in determining this kind of issue. In the American case of Mary C. Northern,[6] the patient was described by the guardian appointed for her by the court as '. . . 72 years of age . . . [and] in possession of a good memory and recall, responds accurately to questions asked her, is coherent and intelligent in her conversation and is of sound mind'. She was suffering from gangrene in both feet consequent upon frostbite and burns, but refused to have the feet amputated, as her surgeons were urging her to. Though otherwise apparently entirely rational, it emerged in conversation that she very much wanted to live *and* very much wanted to save her feet. She did not seem able to grasp that there was only a one in ten chance that both things could happen and resolutely refused to consider, except as abstract hypotheses, that she would have to choose between them. The court decided to authorise surgery, apparently accepting the view that an otherwise apparently competent adult might, nonetheless, be incompetent in the matter of one specific decision. In the light of the transcripts, which are too lengthy to quote here, this would seem to have been the right decision. Mary Northern seems to have combined a general rational competence with a pathological block with regard to the condition of her feet, which she believed had got better and about which her physicians were lying or mistaken.

Consider this imaginary case:

Carla, aged 30 and pregnant, has been admitted to hospital with ruptured membranes and in spontaneous labour. If natural labour is allowed to continue, there is a grave risk of rupture of the uterus owing to the position of the fetus. The life of the fetus is also in danger and the medical team wish to perform a section immediately. Carla, who is in great pain and very worried about losing her baby, nevertheless refuses the caesarean on religious grounds. Carla is an evangelical Christian, but not a Christian Scientist or a Jehovah's Witness, and none of the chaplaincy team are aware of any other Christian sect that might object to this procedure.

Is this a rational refusal of consent to treatment? May we characterise Carla as an otherwise rational patient with a pathological block about caesarean sections? We might wish to argue that she is not irrational, but simply has beliefs that the rest of us do not share but cannot disprove. Mary Northern's irrationality, in the end, came down to her refusal to give up a belief about the condition of her feet that no one was able to prove to her was false. There is no easy answer to the question of what makes belief irrational. It may help resolve the problem of distinguishing non-standard religious beliefs from those of people like Mary Northern that Mary Northern's came from nowhere; that they were ungrounded by anything apart from what seems to be a desperate attempt to wish the circumstances other than they actually were. Most religious beliefs do form a system; they are shared by large numbers of people and they are culturally transmitted – they have rational validation even if not that of those who do not share them. This is hardly conclusive, but it is persuasive.

10.9.2 Balancing rights and duties

There is another factor here, however, that is disquieting. The mother's refusal of treatment did not just involve herself, but also her unborn baby. The case of *Re S*[7] raises the issue of how far a person's refusal of treatment can be allowed to impact on a third party, for it is clear that the judgement arrived at in that case (where a full-term fetus in a transverse lie threatened the life of both fetus and mother) turned on consideration of the welfare of the fetus as well as the rationality of the mother's decision. Whatever the legal position, this cannot be ducked. The fetus was at term. The law may not recognise the rights of an unborn child, but morally it would be curious to assert that a fetus at term is in any significant way different from a newborn baby. What might be arguable is whether its life may be saved at the cost of what has been called 'a massive intrusion into a person's body',[8] that is, a caesarean section. In a parallel American case, that of Angela Carder, the original decision to permit the caesarean section was overturned on appeal and Angela Carder's parents won undisclosed damages from the hospital in a separate action for medical malpractice, wrongful death and violation of civil rights. In that case neither the mother nor the child survived the operation. Though the mother was suffering widespread and irreversible cancer of the bone and lungs, the death certificate listed the caesarean as a contributing factor.[9]

A caesarean section is a major surgical intervention, with all the risks and dangers that involves. It would seem unreasonable to *require* someone to take those risks in order to benefit someone else. In an American case, the courts ruled that someone cannot be forced to donate bone marrow (a procedure considerably less risky than a caesarean section) even where failure to do so would result in the death of a third party (because only one person could be found who was tissue-type compatible).[10] But it does not follow that the person had no *moral* obligation to be a bone-marrow donor, nor that we may not think badly of him for ducking it. Nor is there an exact carry-over from that case to *Re S* or section 10.3.1. Those who willingly become pregnant have, in doing so, already accepted a degree of responsibility for the welfare of the child they carry. And a caesarean section is not so dangerous or unusual an intervention that it is obvious that no one could be expected to risk it. Nor are the declared grounds for refusal as coherent as they may seem. The couple in *Re S* were reported as believing that a caesarean was against their principles as born-again Christians. According to *The Guardian*, most evangelical Christians would not share the view that a caesarean section was impermissible and would, indeed, advocate one if the child's life was at risk, and Jehovah's Witnesses do not object to caesareans as long as they do not involve blood transfusions.[11]

Here there is clearly a balance to be struck between anyone's right to refuse life-saving treatment and the rights of the unborn child (which must have some moral force even if not normally recognised in English law). There must also be a question mark, though perhaps not more than that, over the coherence of the reasons given. These considerations ought to affect what happens when treatment is refused, or indications given that it will be, for a refusal in the circumstances of section 10.3.1 or *Re S* will not be accepted at face value. Efforts will and should be made to explain the consequences of the refusal and to persuade the patient to reconsider. It would be desirable, in such a case, to ask for the patient's spiritual adviser to offer counselling. If the patient is simply mistaken about what his or her religious beliefs require then the situation could be resolved at this stage without resort to law.

Such a reaction to a refusal of treatment can only be properly understood in terms of our moral disquiet about the decision taken and/or the reasons for it. But though there are good moral reasons for wishing to oppose such a decision, it may well be that there are equally good policy reasons for not giving that opposition legal force. We may, in other words, disagree, perhaps profoundly, with the decision without thinking that it would be right to enforce another course of action on the patient. And, clearly, there are excellent reasons for thinking that a general policy of enforcing caesarean sections on unwilling women would be an extremely bad thing.

10.10 Advance directives

As mentioned above, it can happen that patients are no longer capable of consenting to treatment. This may be because of mental or physical deterioration, or both. In such cases treatment becomes a matter of what the health care team consider to be in the patient's best interests (see sections 10.1.2 and 10.4, above). Ordinarily it might be thought that such a situation would be eased if there exists what has come to be called an 'advance directive'. This could take the form of anything from a simple statement ('if it comes to it, I don't want to be kept alive as a vegetable') to the much more formal 'living will' comparatively common in the US. A living will can be of two kinds. There is the simpler formal declaration of the circumstances in which you would no longer wish further treatment, for example. There is also a durable power of health care attorney which, effectively, nominates a proxy to take decisions on your behalf should you no longer be able to yourself.[12]

A simple living will can be problematic. First of all, it is invariably hypothetical ('this is what I want *if* the following circumstances apply . . .') and also general rather than specific. This is inevitable, since in writing a living will we are trying to anticipate what might happen rather than dealing with an actual situation. What it means, however, is that it may still be difficult to determine how the will was meant to apply since the circumstances will necessarily not be precisely those envisaged. This is especially true if the will maker is not – and most of us are not – medically qualified or knowledgeable. There is also a problem of timescale, and for two quite different reasons. The first is perhaps the most obvious one, and it is that treatments may change in the interval between drawing up the will and it coming into operation. Someone who anticipates that they would rather be allowed to die rather than undergo a particular kind of treatment might well have opted differently had they known the extent to which that treatment had improved. The second has to do with change in personal identity over time. To what extent it is reasonable for a younger version of me to legislate on what will be in the best interests of an older me? I might, by the time it is necessary, come to have taken an entirely different attitude to risk-taking, for example. Or I might have become an entirely different person.

Dworkin[13] cites the case of Margo, someone with Alzheimer's dementia who 'despite her illness, or maybe somehow because of it, [. . .] is undeniably one of the happiest people I have known. There is something graceful about the degeneration her mind is undergoing, leaving her carefree, always cheerful.'[14] This is an unusual consequence of Alzheimer's disease which, more often, leaves people anxious, confused and profoundly disoriented. But that is the point. Had Margo considered the prospect of dementia and executed an advance directive, she might well have decided that she would not wish to receive treatment for any other life-threatening illness once she was suffering from Alzheimer's. Had she done so, and the relevant situation had arisen, would it be better to respect the autonomy of the person Margo had once been and comply with the wishes set out in the advance directive? Or would it be better to address the best interests of the person Margo now is, and treat her for any adventitious, life-threatening illnesses unless and until the Alzheimer's deteriorated much further?[15]

10.11 Withdrawing treatment

Consent to or refusal of treatment is not the only problem in this area. There can be patients from whom treatment can be withdrawn, on the grounds that they are in fact dying and it would be considered neither proper nor humane simply to prolong the dying process. Both the American and British Medical Associations endorse this view, as do the Catholic and Anglican churches, and it is, for the GMC, clearly a part of good medical practice:

> Life has a natural end, and doctors and others caring for a patient need to recognise that the point may come in the progression of a patient's condition where death is drawing near. In these circumstances doctors should not strive to prolong the dying process with no regard to the patient's wishes, where known, or an up to date assessment of the benefits and burdens of treatment or non-treatment.[16]

The cessation of the employment of extraordinary means to prolong the life of the body when there is irrefutable evidence that biological death is imminent is the decision of the patient and/or his immediate family.[17]

In its narrow current sense, euthanasia implies killing, and it is misleading to extend it to cover decisions not to preserve life by artificial means when it would be better for the patient to be allowed to die. Such decisions coupled with a determination to give the patient as good a death as possible, may be quite legitimate.[18]

[N]ormally one is held to use only ordinary means . . . that is to say, means that do not involve any grave burden for oneself or another . . . Consequently, if it appears that the attempt at resuscitation constitutes such a burden for the family that one cannot in all conscience impose it upon them, they can lawfully insist that the doctor should discontinue those attempts and the doctor can lawfully comply.[19]

The distinction between deliberate killing and the administration of painkilling drugs or the withdrawal of treatment such as to have the effect of shortening life, though sometimes a very fine one in practice, must remain a guiding principle.[20]

It is widely believed that this position involves drawing a moral distinction between active and passive euthanasia. Many people seem to think, if they think that euthanasia can be justified at all, that it can be more readily justified if it is passive rather than active. Many people also seem to think that, whereas English law strictly forbids active euthanasia, it does sometimes allow that passive euthanasia may be permissible. Both doctors and lawyers talk as if they believe that this is so. For example:

A Down's syndrome child is born with an intestinal obstruction. If the obstruction is not removed, the child will die. Here . . . the surgeon might say 'As this child is a mongol . . . I do not propose to operate; I shall allow nature to take its course.' No one could say that the surgeon was committing an act of murder by declining to take a course which would save the child.

A severely handicapped child, who is not otherwise going to die, is given a drug is such amounts that the drug itself will cause death. If the doctor acts intentionally then it would be open to the jury to say: yes, he was killing, he was murdering that child.

There is an important difference between allowing a child to die and taking action to kill it.[21]

No paediatrician takes life; but we accept that allowing babies to die – and I know the distinction is narrow, but we all feel it tremendously profoundly – is in the baby's interests at times.[22]

This is potentially most misleading, and should not be taken at face value. I am not a lawyer, and the law in this area is complicated, but it is perfectly clear that being passively responsible for someone's death is, *in itself*, no defence in law to a charge of either murder or manslaughter. *Bonnyman* was a doctor who realised that his wife was exhibiting all the symptoms of diabetes, and he refrained from telling her. Thinking that she merely had a particularly bad bout of influenza, she did not seek treatment and died. Dr Bonnyman was found guilty of manslaughter by criminal negligence.[23] There are many other such cases.

Pitwood was a level-crossing keeper who failed to close the gate when a train was approaching and was held to be responsible for the deaths that ensued;[24] *Gibbins and Proctor* were found criminally responsible for the death of their children, whom they had failed to feed;[25] *Stone and Dobinson* were convicted of manslaughter for the neglect of a dependent relative who died in their care.[26]

English law holds that murder and manslaughter, specifically, are crimes that can be committed either by act or by omission. Of course, where a death is caused by someone's action it is usually relatively easy to identify the responsible agent. He or she is the one who performed the action in question. But who is responsible when someone dies as a result of a failure to act? The responsible agent here is anyone who failed to act *when they had a legal duty to act*. According to one authority,[27] this duty can arise either through a contract, a special relationship (such as parent and child or doctor and patient) or where a person has voluntarily undertaken the care of another. But in a famous case – *Donoghue* v. *Stevenson*[28] – Lord Atkin held that I owe a duty of care to '. . . persons who are so closely and directly affected by my act that I ought reasonably to have them in contemplation as being so affected when I am directing my mind to the acts or omissions which are called in question'. This definition of the duty of care is so much more comprehensive that it is perhaps fortunate that it is only applicable in civil – tort – cases. Either way, it is clear that health care teams owe a duty of care to their patients and that wanton or reckless neglect of that duty that results in death can result in a criminal prosecution for murder or manslaughter. Why, then, did the House of Lords, in the case of *Bland*,[29] authorise the non-treatment of the patient when it was known that it would lead to his death?

Tony Bland was a victim of the Hillsborough football disaster. As a result of his injuries he was comatose and remained in what is known as a persistent vegetative state until 1993, when his parents applied through the courts for permission for artificial nutrition and hydration to be withdrawn. The courts held that artificial nutrition and hydration was a form of treatment. They also held that, in view of the extreme unlikelihood of Mr Bland's ever regaining consciousness, the treatment was of no benefit to him and withdrawing it would take the form of a legal omission rather than commission, that is, the medical team had no duty to continue to treat Mr Bland.

The arguments were:

(1) A doctor is under no duty to continue to treat a patient where such treatment confers no benefit on the patient.
(2) Being in a persistent vegetative state with no prospect of recovery was regarded by informed medical opinion as not being a benefit to a patient.
(3) The principle of the sanctity of life was not absolute, for example:
    – where a patient expressly refuses treatment, even though death may well be a consequence of that refusal,
    – where a prisoner on hunger strike refuses food and may not be forcibly fed,
    – where a patient is terminally ill, death is imminent and treatment will only prolong suffering.
(4) Artificial hydration and nutrition required medical intervention for its application and was widely regarded by the medical profession as medical treatment.

The governing principle here was not that it was permissible to let a patient die so long as he or she was not actually *killed*. It was rather that *caring* for a patient (in cases where cure was not possible and recovery was extremely unlikely) did not require medical interventions that were of no benefit to the patient. But it is also clear that the treatment in question was not a *disbenefit* to Bland. If it did him no good, it also did him no harm. If doctors were under no duty to continue to treat Bland, they were also under no duty not to. But there was a benefit – to Bland's relatives and friends, especially his parents, who were to be spared the grief of continuing to see their son in this exceptionally distressing condition and would, finally, be able to mourn the loss they had suffered two years before. That is not a negligible benefit, by any means, and if, whatever happened, nothing more could be done to harm or benefit Bland himself, it seems right to let the choice of outcome be decided by what would most benefit those closest to him.

But it is interesting to compare the case of Tony Bland with that of *Cox*. Dr Nigel Cox was found guilty of attempted murder in 1992 for administering a lethal dose of potassium chloride to a patient, Lilian Boyes, who, dying and in acute pain, had pleaded with him to help her die. It is indeed, hard to see how, on the face of it, this case is to be distinguished from that of *Bland*, without invoking the distinction between active and passive euthanasia. The remarks of Lady Butler-Sloss in the Court of Appeal hearing of *Bland* would seem to do just that:

> The position of Dr Nigel Cox, who injected a lethal dose designed to cause death, was different since it was an external and intrusive act and was not in accordance with his duty of care as a doctor. The distinction between Mr Bland's doctors and Dr Cox was between an act or omission which allowed causes already present in the body to operate and the introduction of an external agency of death.[30]

The *Guardian*'s leader writer called that position a 'philosophical nonsense' (20/11/92), and maybe it is if taken at face value. What is not true is that there is no other morally relevant distinction to be drawn between the two cases. What follows should not be seen as implying any criticism of Dr Cox who, it would seem, was placed in an extremely difficult situation and, in all good faith, was probably doing what he believed was the only thing he could do to help Ms Boyes. But whether Cox's decision was the right one in the circumstances (and I, inevitably not knowing all the relevant information, am inclined to think it was), the explanation for its rightness must be different from the explanation of the rightness of withdrawing treatment from Tony Bland.

The source of this distinction is an old notion, thought by many to be now discredited, called 'the principle of double effect'. It should, I think, be seen not as a rule for resolving moral problems but as a guide that can clarify what is at issue in particular cases. It relies on a distinction between what one intends and what one merely foresees as a result of one's actions. The principle suggests that whereas one is fully responsible for what one intends to do, one is not responsible for foreseen but intended effects of one's actions, provided that:

(1) What is done must be, at the least, morally permissible.
(2) What is intended must include only the good and not the bad effects of what is done.

(3) The bad effects must not be the *means* whereby the good is brought about.

(4) There must be *proportionality* between the good and bad effects of what is done.

Whereas Dr Cox must have intended Lilian Boyes's death as the only way, as he saw it, of sparing her further pain and suffering, the medical team treating Tony Bland intended to spare him further suffering (or at least to spare his relatives, given that Tony Bland himself may have been aware of nothing at all) while foreseeing that this would probably lead to his death. This distinction may have no practical consequences in those two actual cases, given that both led to the death of the patients concerned. It matters, nonetheless, in so far as they are treated as precedents for action in future cases, which may be similar but will be never be precisely the same.

I do not believe that passive euthanasia is permissible because it is merely a matter of allowing a patient to die rather than acting in order to bring about their death. But I do believe that in cases where the patient's death is imminent, or where treatment is painful and offers only a very remote chance of success, it is justifiable, if the patient and/or his or her relatives consent, to cease to continue treatment.

Moral responsibility for an event is not determined by whether it came about because one acted or failed to act; it is determined by one's intentions and duties. If there is no duty to treat, and also persuasive reasons for not doing so, it must normally be entirely permissible to withdraw treatment, even if to do so results in the death of the patient.

So what about Dr Cox? Clearly he cannot be excused on these grounds, for they do not apply to his case. What can be said is that it is possible to imagine circumstances where the suffering of the patient is so great and the possibility of immediate remedy so small that killing the patient is the only available means of preventing the pain. In national disasters or wars such circumstances may arise, or in parts of the world where medical resources are extremely limited. In those circumstances it is possible that acting so as to bring about the death of the patient as easily and quickly as might be would not be wrong. It may be that those were the circumstances in which Nigel Cox found himself. Without being a part of the situation it is impossible to say. It must be a matter of judgement, and it involves a kind of judgement that I hope never to have to exercise. For that reason it cannot be said conclusively that what Cox did was wrong, but also for that reason it is a matter that the law, on policy grounds, can never permit.

10.12 Notes and references

1. For example, it has been doubted whether babies, fetuses, or those who, while still biologically alive, lack any response to the world around them are persons in the strict sense of the term. (See Robert F. Weir, *Abating Treatment with Critically Ill Patients* (New York, Oxford University Press, 1989), pp. 70–71 and 405–12.) It can also be argued that higher apes and cetaceans (dolphins, porpoises and whales) might conceivably be persons in the required sense. (See Peter Singer, *Practical Ethics* (Cambridge, Cambridge University Press, 1979) *passim.*) A useful source on the whole debate is H. Kuhse and P. Singer (eds), *Bioethics* (Oxford, Blackwell, 1999), Part IV.

2. But see E. Matthews, Autonomy and the psychiatric patient, in *Journal of Applied Philosophy*, **17** (2000), no.1. He sees this as a misinterpretation of Kant and would prefer to ground the point on Mill's argument. (See footnote 3 below.)

3. For a more complete, and classic, exposition of this view, see John Stuart Mill, *On Liberty*. (There are many editions of this, but a good recent one, which includes critical essays, is edited by John Gray and G.W. Smith, *J.S. Mill On Liberty In Focus* (London, Routledge, 1991).)

4. This is also heavily stressed in many professional codes of conduct. See, for example, the Nursing and Midwifery Council, *The NMC Code Of Professional Conduct: Standards for Conduct, Performance and Ethics* (London, NMC, 2002).

5. See Margaret Brazier, *Medicine, Patients and the Law*, 3rd edn (Harmondsworth, Penguin, 2003), pp. 449–50.

6. *State of Tennessee Dept of Human Services* v. *Mary C. Northern*, C.A. Tennessee, Middle Section, Feb.7, 1978; cited in John Arras and Nancy Rhoden (eds), *Ethical Issues in Modern Medicine*, 3rd edn (McGraw-Hill, 1989), pp. 72–9. (1989)

7. See *The Guardian* (14/10/92 and 20/10/92).

8. Judge John Terry, in the case of Angela Carder (district of Columbia Court of Appeals, 1990), the American case cited in evidence in *Re S*. (*The Guardian*, 20/10/92). Compare his remarks with the argument put by Judith Jarvis Thompson, A defense of abortion, *Philosophy and Public Affairs*, **1** (1971), no1: a pregnant woman is no more *necessarily* responsible for the welfare of the fetus she is carrying that she is for anyone else's welfare. She may owe it a duty of care if she is responsible for its being there, but that duty has limits and she is not obliged morally to risk her life for it.

9. See *The Guardian*, 20/10/92, p. 23.

10. See the *Montreal Gazette*, 27/7/78; the case is discussed in R. Campbell and D. Collinson, *Ending Lives* (Oxford, Blackwell, 1988), pp. 174–5.

11. See *The Guardian*, 14/10/93, p. 3.

12. Above, section 10.4.1; see also the Mental Capacity Act 2005, section 9, and Margaret Brazier, *Medicine, Patients and the Law*, 3rd edn (Harmondsworth, Penguin, 2003), pp. 457–8.

13. R. Dworkin, *Life's Dominion: An Argument about Abortion, Euthanasia, and Individual Freedom* (Vintage Books, 1994), pp. 218–19.

14. A.D. Firlik, Margo's logo, *Journal of the American Medical Association* (1991), pp. 265, 201. Quoted by R. Dworkin, *Life's Dominion: An Argument about Abortion, Euthanasia, and Individual Freedom* (Vintage Books, 1994).

15. See also R. Dresser, Dworkin on dementia: elegant theory, questionable policy, *Hastings Center Report*, **25** (1995), p. 6, and D. Degrazia, Advance directives, dementia, and 'the someone else problem, *Bioethics*, **13** (1999), no. 5, pp. 373–91.

16. General Medical Council (2002) *Withholding and Withdrawing Life-Prolonging Treatment: Good Practice in Decision-making*, para. 12.

17. *Journal of the American Medical Association* (1974), p. 227.

18. Church of England National Assembly (Board for Social Responsibility), *On Dying Well*, Church Information Office (1975), p. 10, and *The Guardian* (20/11/92), leading article.

19. Pope Pius XII, *The Pope Speaks*, **4**, no. 4, p. 396.

20. Principles endorsed by the House of Bishops of the Church of England in October 1992, as cited by David Sheppard in a letter to *The Guardian*, 27/10/92.

21. *Obiter dicta* in the case of *Arthur* (1981), taken from trial transcripts cited by H. Kuhse, A modern myth . . . , *Journal of Applied Philosophy*, **1**, 1.

22. Expert testimony from consultant paediatricians in the case of *Arthur*, cited in D. and M. Braham, The Arthur case, *Journal of Medical Ethics*, **9** (1981), pp. 12–15.

23. (1942) 28 Cr App 131.

24. (1902) 19 TLR 37.
25. (1919) 13 Cr App Rep.
26. [1977] QB 354, [1977] 2 All ER 341.
27. Card, Cross and Jones, *Introduction to Criminal Law*, 17th edn (Oxford, Oxford University Press, 2006), p. 32.
28. [1932] A.C. 562.
29. (1993) 2 WLR 316.
30. Court of Appeal: *Airedale NHS Trust* v. *Bland*, 9 December, 1992.

11 Clinical Governance

A   The Legal Perspective

Vanessa L. Mayatt

11.1 The advent of clinical governance

Several decades ago the corporate world on both sides of the Atlantic had to contend with a series of organisational developments that ranged from embarrassing to disastrous. These developments called into question how well companies manage their financial affairs and their businesses in general. Thus the organisational problems encountered at Polly Peck, Maxwell, Enron and others not unexpectedly fuelled the drive for a more rigorous approach to organisational management. This lead to the current requirements for governance that are now an integral part of the day-to-day running of large private organisations on both sides of the Atlantic.

In response to this corporate turbulence, a series of reviews were undertaken with the intention of identifying what steps organisations should take to implement good practice in corporate governance. Each successive review built upon the principles of the previous one, so that collectively they helped shape the current approach to corporate governance and the requirements for internal control. These requirements are set out in the Combined Code[1] that companies listed on the London Stock Exchange seek to comply with.

The Combined Code is concerned with the establishment of corporate objectives, identification of the risks to the achievement of those objectives and a system of internal control to ensure that business failure does not happen. It is therefore concerned with the management of risk and the integration of risk management into the day-to-day running of businesses. In simple terms corporate governance is about moving away from firefighting to a more proactive approach to managing risk. While compliance with the Combined Code is voluntary, the pressure on companies to make positive statements in their published annual reports on their arrangements for governance and internal control is sharply felt. The arrangements are subject to close scrutiny by internal and external auditors as well as by company risk management groups that are usually led by a board member.

To a large extent the developments in corporate governance in the private sector have been mirrored in the public sector. The health care sector has, like the corporate world, experienced a series of high-profile incidents that have called into question how well hospitals, Trusts and other health care providers are managed and how well clinicians are treating and providing care to patients. The circumstances surrounding the death of hundreds of Harold Shipman's patients, the multiple deaths of babies at Bristol Royal Infirmary and the failures in the cervical cancer screening services at Kent and Canterbury hospitals are all evidence of the failure both of individuals and of the health care system in which they work. The lessons from these major incidents, set out in official Inquiry Reports, have in conjunction with other incidents shaped the current expectations for clinical governance and the management of risk. These expectations are not unlike those relating to private companies.

The public sector has its own 'Combined Code', in the shape of HM Treasury's Orange Book, *Management of Risk: Principles and Concepts*.[2] The Treasury document recognises the link between the management of risk, the successful delivery of business objectives and meeting the needs of stakeholders. Audit committees in public sector organisations, including the health care sector, use the Orange Book to determine their strategy for managing risk and develop their arrangements for internal control. External auditors, such as the NAO (National Audit Office), also use the Treasury guidance to judge how well public sector organisations are governed.

In the health care sector, governance includes the arrangements for clinical governance. The guidance *Clinical Governance in the New NHS*,[3] published in 1999, defined clinical governance as 'a framework through which NHS organisations are accountable for continuously improving the quality of their services and safeguarding high standards of care by creating an environment in which excellence in clinical care will flourish'. Clinical governance had been described as akin to organisational conscience and the 'beating heart' of care, encapsulating an organisation's responsibility for the delivery of safe, high-quality patient care.[4]

11.2 The development of clinical governance

In the early 1990s, following the formation of NHS Trusts, the concept of clinical risk management was taken forward in the UK health care sector. The evidence for the nature and extent of clinical risk came from clinical negligence claims, complaints about clinical experience and patient outcomes, and improving arrangements for clinical incident reporting in NHS Trusts. In a typical Trust at that time, reported clinical incidents demonstrated the magnitude of drug errors, the multitude of ways that drug errors arose, and poor clinical decision-making and clinical practice, all leading to unacceptable patient outcomes. It was clearly the case that while the vast majority of patients were well served by the health care sector and the dedicated staff it employs, there was clear evidence of some fundamental organisational problems concerning the quality of patient care provision. This evidence fuelled the drive for better quality and clinical governance.

In the late 1990s, the consultation document *A First Class Service: Quality in the New NHS*[5] set out the arrangements for improving the quality of health care provision. The main elements of the document concerned:

- national standards for services and treatments
- local delivery of high quality health care
- effective monitoring of progress by the newly established Commission for Health Improvement (CHI)
- a national survey of patient and user experience.

This development was a part of the agenda to modernise the NHS and clinical governance was viewed as a central part of this strategy. Clinical governance was synonymous with the drive for improved quality in health care. The document stated that the principles of clinical governance were applicable to all involved in the provision or management of NHS patient care. It also set out the accountability of Trust chief executives for assuring the quality of service provision on behalf of Trust boards.

In 1999 this consultative document[5] was followed by the introduction of a statutory duty for the quality of health care provision under the Health Act. Under the legislation Trust chief executives became ultimately responsible for assuring the quality of health care provision. In the following year an independent inquiry was established in the light of the Harold Shipman case. Part of the inquiry's remit was to consider what changes were necessary to existing systems to safeguard patients in the future. This lead, in 2003, to the General Medical Council requirement for the periodic revalidation of doctors.

11.3 Clinical governance now

In the 1990s, NHS Trusts and other health care organisations almost universally developed separate arrangements to manage clinical and other areas of risk. While this enabled individuals within organisations with relevant expertise to come together to analyse specific areas of risk and make informed decisions about what improvements were necessary, it lead to a fragmentation of approach to managing risk and to some duplication of effort. The current expectation is quite rightly for integrated governance, so that areas of risk are no longer dealt with in silos and governance arrangements are streamlined as a result.

In 1999 a five-year vision for clinical governance was set out in *Clinical Governance in the New NHS*.[3] This included an expectation that there would be cultural change, a shared commitment to quality, participative working with stakeholders, multidisciplinary team-working and leadership at board level. The guidance set a number of targets for Trusts, health authorities and primary care groups. During 1999/2000 these bodies were expected to:

- identify lead clinicians for clinical governance and establish appropriate structures for overseeing clinical governance
- agree a process and timescale for conducting a baseline assessment of capability and capacity for implementing clinical governance and thereafter produce an action plan
- report clinical governance arrangements within their Annual Reports.

These expectations were underpinned by the requirement for a comprehensive programme of quality improvement, which for Trusts included the participation of hospital doctors in audit programmes, routine application of evidence-based practice and CPD (continuing professional development) programmes. These are currently some of the main components of clinical governance.

The National Audit Office has recently summarised the key principals of clinical governance as:

- a coherent approach to quality improvement
- clear lines of accountability for clinical quality systems, and
- effective processes for identifying and managing risk and addressing poor performance.

The NAO envisages that this involves putting into place arrangements and systems so that there is early identification and analysis of problems and action is promptly taken to prevent repetition.[6]

In 2004 the Department of Health (DH) introduced integrated governance as a means of developing a more integrated approach to the management of all risks while combining the principles of clinical, management, financial and corporate accountability. This was followed in 2006 by the publication of the DH's *Integrated Governance Handbook*.[7] The guidance defines integrated governance as 'systems, processes and behaviours by which Trusts lead, direct and control their functions in order to achieve organisational objectives, safety and quality of service and in which they relate to patients and carers, the wider community and partner organisations'. Integrated governance is therefore concerned with managing risk so that organisational objectives can be delivered and the needs of stakeholders can be met. While the words are not the same, the meaning is no different from HM Treasury's requirements for managing risk or indeed the requirements of the Combined Code. The DH guidance contains an expectation that all health care organisations will have best practice arrangements in place for integrated governance and that these arrangements will function across all health care communities and clinical networks.

A key aspect of the integrated governance agenda is the requirement for co-ordinated information collection and inspection within the health care sector. These two points relate directly to the current remit of the Healthcare Commission and the National Patient Safety Agency explored next in this chapter.

11.4 The role of external bodies in clinical governance

There are a number of organisations who work in conjunction with the health care sector in connection with clinical governance. They each have related and in some instances overlapping roles. The following provides a summary of the remit and functioning of the main external bodies in clinical governance, which include:

- Healthcare Commission
- National Patients Safety Agency
- National Institute for Health and Clinical Excellence
- NHSLA.

11.4.1 Healthcare Commission

The Healthcare Commission (HC) (statutory name: the Commission for Healthcare Audit and Inspection (CHAI)) replaced an earlier body, the Commission for Health Improvement (CHI), which had a role in relation to clinical governance. CHI established a programme for clinical governance reviews and undertook investigations into serious incidents within the health care sector. These functions have now been taken on board by the Healthcare Commission. The HC was established under the 2003 Health and Social Care (Community Health and Standards) Act, under which it has a number of statutory responsibilities, which include:

- conducting reviews and investigations into the provision of health care
- carrying out studies focused on improving economy, efficiency and effectiveness in the NHS
- publishing information on health care provision from both the NHS and private health care sector, including the findings from national clinical audits
- reviewing the quality of data relating to health and health care.

The HC aims to assess the health care sector from a stakeholder perspective: this means from a patient, service user and general public perspective. While the organisation reports to government, it is independent of it. The NHS and its composite parts are scrutinised by a wide range of external bodies that each conduct inspections, audits and reviews. One of the aims of the HC is to reduce the inspection load on the NHS. It has attempted to do this by introducing an Inspection Concordat to which bodies such as the Health and Safety Executive (HSE) and the National Patients Safety Agency (NPSA) are signatories. The Concordat provides for the sharing of performance information between the signatory organisations in order to reduce duplication of effort. It follows on from a joint statement, agreed by review organisations in the days of CHI, to work together in a more coordinated fashion. The more recent Concordat may support the drive for integrated governance by encouraging the removal of the silo arrangements for reviewing the management of risk in the inspection bodies.

The HC clinical governance review programme is a part of its statutory review function. Healthcare Commission Clinical Governance Reviews (CGRs) are normally conducted by a team of individuals lead by an HC project manager. The team importantly includes lay representation. The role of the review team is to assess how well clinical governance is being handled within a Trust. The review methodology, set out in its review manual,[8] includes assessment at corporate and directorate levels and among clinical teams. The reviews focus on nine related areas, the first seven of which the HC regards as key components of clinical governance:

(1) patient, carer, service user and public involvement
(2) risk management
(3) clinical audit
(4) clinical effectiveness
(5) staffing and staff management
(6) education, training and CPD
(7) use of information
(8) strategic capacity
(9) the patient experience.

The Healthcare Commission performs a number of additional functions in England, which include reviewing the performance of each local NHS organisation and awarding an annual performance rating. This was known colloquially as the 'star rating system', which ran until 2005. The HC have now introduced a new approach (the annual health check) to assessing organisational performance.[9] This approach was introduced after a period of public consultation. The health check focuses on two elements: first, 'the basics' – core standards, existing targets and the use of resources; and secondly, 'making and sustaining progress' – new national targets and improvement reviews. The core standards are split into seven domains:

- safety
- clinical and cost effectiveness
- governance
- patient focus
- accessible and responsive care
- care environment and amenities
- public health.

Clearly these domains fall within the scope of clinical governance. Aside from the independent scrutiny by the HC, boards of Trusts are required to make public declarations on the extent to which their organisation meets the core standards. The likely vehicle for this will be their published annual reports. The declarations will, however, be subject to checking by the HC. The HC publishes, on its website, performance information on health care organisations it has reviewed. This in itself may prove to be a useful driver to better clinical governance.

11.4.2 The National Patient Safety Agency

In 2002, the chairman of the NPSA, in the wake of the Kennedy Report on the public inquiry into children's heart surgery at Bristol Royal Infirmary, stated that the Agency had been created to revolutionise patient safety in the NHS.[10] He described the arrangements for collecting information about problems, learning from them and putting in place measures that save lives and prevent adverse events happening again. As such the NPSA has a key role to play in clinical governance.

The NPSA was established in 2001 following the publication of a report, in 2000, lead by the Chief Medical Officer for England.[11] *An Organisation with a Memory* (OWAM) addressed the problems associated with reporting incidents and potential incidents involving patients, and the inadequacy of arrangements to learn lessons and prevent incidents happening again. At that time it was estimated that each year there were 900,000 incidents that either harmed or could have harmed patients in NHS hospitals. The scale of clinical errors and the scope for improving patient safety was becoming increasingly apparent.

One of the first tasks for the NPSA was to set up a national patient incident recording system. The NPSA aims to change the culture within the NHS that acts as a barrier to full incident-reporting and to making improvements to patient care provision. It has therefore focused on the need to remove the blame culture within the NHS and create a culture of openness and learning. As a central body, it claims to be able to facilitate learning across health care organisations and the sharing of experience.

11.4.3 NICE

The National Institute for Health and Clinical Excellence is also a part of the clinical governance arena. NICE was set up in 2004 and preceded an earlier organisation, with the same acronym but a slightly different remit, that came into being in 1999. NICE is currently responsible for producing national guidance aimed at promoting good health and both preventing and treating ill health. It produces guidance in three main areas:

- public health
- health technologies
- clinical practice.

While guidance produced in all of these areas impacts upon clinical governance, it is the clinical practice guidelines that are especially relevant. NICE clinical practice guidelines confirm the treatment that is appropriate for particular conditions and are based upon best available evidence. While the purpose of the guidelines is not to override clinical decision-making, they are intended to be used as a guide to best practice. Following clinical guidelines is therefore likely to lead to the avoidance of clinical risk and to good clinical governance.

After clinical guidelines are published, health organisations are expected to review their practice of managing clinical conditions against the requirements of the NICE guidelines. This review is expected to include consideration of the resources needed to implement the guidelines and the system that will be necessary for successful implementation. In situations where clinical practice is markedly different from NICE guidelines, there is likely to be a more significant need for investment, both in time and money, to effect the necessary changes.

Aside from the expectation that NICE guidelines will be complied with, the activity of NICE is associated with two further areas of encouragement for health care organisations to improve. First, since January 2002 NHS organisations in England and Wales have been required to provide funding for medicines and treatments recommended by NICE in its technology appraisals. The usual expectation is that within three months of the date of publication of the appraisal, NHS organisations need to meet the cost of medicines and treatments recommended by NICE. Additional funding is not normally made available for this and the money has to be found from existing budgets. Clearly, when technology appraisals concern expensive drugs or the use of expensive equipment this can pose significant problems for health care providers. The second source of encouragement is from patients, and their connections, who increasingly source NICE guidelines with a view to challenging the appropriateness of treatment and care that is being offered.

11.4.4 NHSLA

The NHS Litigation Authority is responsible for dealing with claims for clinical negligence in connection with NHS Trusts and other health care organisations. The NHSLA manages the Clinical Negligence Scheme for Trusts (CNST). This scheme, introduced in 1994, was the first major initiative to be introduced in England to tackle clinical risk. The CNST is essentially a risk-pooling scheme where member organisations pay an annual contribution. Contribution levels are determined by past claims experience, the extent of high risk health care activity, such as obstetrics, and performance against a number of clinical risk standards. Associated with the CNST is the *General Risk Management Manual*,[12] which details the standards to which Trusts need to comply and the various compliance levels. To progress up through the compliance levels, CNST members need to be able to demonstrate more complex and robust arrangements for managing clinical risk. Compliance with the standards by CNST members needs to be taken forward within their clinical governance arrangements. As most Trust members have not yet attained compliance level 3 and the vast majority remain at level 1, there is still much that needs to be done to improve the management of clinical risk and hence clinical governance.

As part of the drive for integrated governance, the CNST general clinical risk management standards were replaced at the end of March 2006 by the NHSLA Risk Management Standards for Acute Trusts. It is therefore necessary for Trusts to have an eye to both residual CNST and newer NHSLA standards in order to identify what they need to do in order to perform well against these standards.

11.5 Revalidation and fitness to practice

At the centre of many of the recent health care disasters has been the question of the competence of the clinicians involved. Comparisons have been drawn with other industries and their arrangements for ensuring the continued competence of professional staff. Outside of health care, auditing performance, being supervised, checking working procedures, re-training and implementation of documented guidelines are an integral part of daily working activity in many organisations. These arrangements elsewhere and the poor quality of health care provision have sharpened the focus on the adequacy of the arrangements to train clinicians.

The most significant change to the regulation of doctors since 1858, when the General Medical Council (GMC) was created, is the revalidation of doctors. Since the late 1990s, it has been argued, and indeed all too clearly demonstrated by the activity of doctors such as Harold Shipman, that the continued registration of doctors based upon past qualifications was no longer sufficient. From 2005 doctors need to demonstrate to the GMC, their governing body, that their clinical practice remains up to date and that they are fit to practice.[13] There are around 200,000 doctors registered with the GMC, each of whom is now required to supply evidence on their fitness to practice in order to secure continued registration with the GMC.

The GMC's *Maintaining Good Medical Practice*,[14] was published in 1998, at a time when major change was underway in the whole area of quality of patient care provision. In this document, the GMC stated:

> In the NHS . . . employers are setting up local 'clinical governance' – formal arrangements to maintain the quality of patient care . . . Along with this, the medical profession and management need to work to set up effective local arrangements for medical regulation . . . Good medical practice and sound local clinical governance are keys to the way forward.

Revalidation is therefore a key part of clinical governance.

Doctors need to continually accumulate a portfolio of evidence to demonstrate that their clinical skills are up to date and that they remain fit to practice. The evidence, together with the views of colleagues, is scrutinised regularly as a part of the local appraisal process. The evidence also has to be submitted to the GMC. In July 2004 the GMC set out its plans for the issuing of licences to practice, which doctors will need to hold in order to practice medicine in the UK. Doctors who fail or refuse to participate in revalidation will lose their licence. Decisions by the GMC, for example from investigations into clinical practice, to limit an individual's practice are now accessible by the public and confirmed on their licence.

11.6 The context for clinical governance

The arrangements for clinical governance in the health care sector need to be taken forward against the backdrop of both managing risk (in the broadest sense) and complying with health and safety legal requirements. It is therefore important to understand the relationship between risk management, health and safety legal compliance and clinical governance.

11.6.1 Risk management

All organisations exist for a purpose, whether that purpose is to make a profit and deliver value to shareholders or to provide a service to the public. Additionally, all organisations need to meet the expectations of their stakeholders, whether they are shareholders, partners, purchasers of services, employees or members of the public. In delivering organisational objectives, organisations encounter risks to the delivery of those objectives. Risk management is concerned with the identification of those risks, assessing both their likelihood of arising and impact upon the organisation and making decisions about how to control them so that the delivery of organisational objectives is not jeopardised.

Organisations control the risks that they face in a number of ways:

- risk avoidance (ceasing or not engaging in the activity giving rise to the risk)
- risk tolerance (doing nothing more)
- risk treatment (implementing measures to reduce the chance of risk arising and its outcome)
- risk transfer (to another organisation such as an insurer or joint venture partner).

Healthcare organisations control risk in all four of these ways as illustrated by the following examples:

- referring patients to health care providers with appropriate clinical expertise – this equates to risk avoidance by the referring organisation
- judging existing arrangements to control (but not remove) risk to be adequate – risk tolerance
- introducing arrangements to increase the competence of staff to undertake a particular clinical procedure and ensuring the presence of experienced staff to supervise the activities – risk treatment
- paying contributions to the NHSLA in connection with the CNST – risk transfer.

The links between clinical governance and risk management will be clear from these examples.

It is not possible for organisations to completely manage out all risk, nor is it desirable for them to do so. Risk management is based upon practical considerations of available resources and the residual level of risk that the organisation is prepared to accept following risk treatment. Running an organisation is an inherently risky process; the nature and extent of that risk depends upon the business of the organisation and its operating parameters. Private sector organisations tend, by definition, to be less risk averse that those operating in the public sector, as entrepreneurial spirit inherently involves the willingness to take risks. This has been exploited by the current government in the Private Finance Initiative (PFI) arrangements that have been established to build new schools, roads and hospitals. PFI deals intrinsically recognise the private sector's greater ability and willingness to accept risk.

Health care organisations have to contend with a diverse range of risks to the delivery of their organisational objectives. These can be categorised into external, operational and those associated with change.[2] The health care sector is beset by significant external risk associated with changes in government expectations, performance targets and the need to function within set budgets. In the main, the sector has no control over these risks but it can take a number of steps to mitigate the associated risks. Operational risks will arise, for example, from the delay in the completion of a new hospital building, inability to attract and retain key staff and the reputation the organisation has with stakeholders. Operational risks will include those that arise from clinical service provision. Change can create risk, for example when a Trust merges with one or more other Trusts and when clinical service provision is reallocated between neighbouring health care providers. All of these examples have the potential to block the achievement of organisational objectives to a greater or lesser extent.

11.6.2 Health and safety legal requirements

Despite the drive for integrated governance, it normally comes as a surprise to health care organisations that poor clinical practice can result in criminal prosecution for breaches of health and safety legislation. The requirements of this legislation, and in particular the duty to protect patients under section 3 of the 1974 Health and Safety at Work etc. Act, are not normally uppermost in the corporate mind of health care organisations or of individual clinicians. However, there have now been a number of successful prosecutions following clinical incidents that have lead to patients dying. The following cases brought under section 3 illustrate this development:

- Norfolk and Norwich NHS Trust prosecuted for the death of a patient during a cardiac angiogram: fine including costs £58,000[15]
- a University Hospital prosecuted following the death of two patients in unrelated incidents during anaesthesia: fine including costs circa £30,000[15]
- a Scottish Trust prosecuted in connection with a patient suicide: fine £10,000[15]
- a University Hospital prosecuted following the death of a patient whose operation was not completed owing to poorly maintained equipment: fine including costs £50,000[16]
- Southampton University Hospitals NHS Trust prosecuted for failing to manage two doctors who failed to diagnose toxic shock syndrome resulting in a patient's death: fine including costs £110,000.[17]

The last case was preceded by the conviction of the two junior doctors involved in the care of the deceased patient for gross negligence manslaughter. Each doctor received an 18-month prison sentence suspended for two years. The criminal case against the Trust under health and safety legislation concerned their failure to adequately supervise the junior doctors, and it was alleged that this lead to the patient's death. The Trust pleaded guilty and was fined accordingly. Ineffective clinical governance arrangements can therefore lead to legal sanction against both health care organisations and individuals.

11.7 Clinical governance in practice: a summary

It will be clear from this chapter that the clinical governance arena is both crowded and fairly complex, with a number of organisations allied to health care having remits to set standards, to guide, to check working practice and to penalise both organisations and individuals when arrangements do not match up to current requirements.

For clinical governance to be taken forward appropriately in a health care organisation there has to be demonstrable commitment from the top of the organisation. This means at board and senior executive levels. The board of any organisation should concern itself with the arrangements for managing risk and for effective governance. Organisations normally do this by ensuring that an appropriately constituted committee reporting to the board has responsibility for governance and risk management. Healthcare organisations may therefore choose to take forward clinical governance within a broad governance agenda or to establish a separate committee to deal specifically with clinical governance. In either case, these high-level committees will be responsible for determining strategy and the necessary organisational arrangements and reporting regularly on progress to the board. Verification of how well clinical governance arrangements are working in practice is normally addressed within the organisation by its audit committee and externally by the Healthcare Commission and other bodies.

Supporting the high-level committees, clinical governance needs to be a part of the responsibility of all those who impact upon patients. This includes not just doctors and nurses, but also allied health care providers, pharmacists and clinical support services. To practice good clinical governance, these individuals and teams will need to be actively engaged in the following activities:

- CPD
- performance appraisal
- clinical audit
- incident and adverse event reporting
- learning lessons from mistakes
- implementing best clinical practice
- commitment to high-quality health care provision.

Healthcare organisations benefit from having in place good arrangements for clinical governance by:

- reduced CNST contributions
- positive HC annual health checks
- enhanced quality of patient care
- reduced levels of clinical risk
- better outcomes for patients
- trained and competent staff.

In contrast, in the worst case scenarios health care organisations that do not have good arrangements in place for clinical governance can face adverse national and local media attention, missed targets, critical reports that are published, and financial penalty by way of the CNST and prosecution in the criminal courts. Patients pay the ultimate price for poor clinical governance by loss of life or poor quality of life following clinical intervention. This on its own should be a sufficient driver for excellence in clinical governance.

11.8 Notes and references

1. The Combined Code and Cadbury, Greenbury and Hampel Reports can be accessed at: www.ecgi.org/codes/country_pages/codes_uk.htm
2. HM Treasury, the 'Orange Book', *Management of Risk Principles and Concepts* (London, The Stationery Office, October 2004).
3. NHS Executive, *Clinical Governance in the New NHS*, HSC 1999/065 (Department of Health, 1999).
4. Clinical governance: assuming the sacred duty of trust to patients, Professor Aiden Halligan, 2005.
5. NHS Executive, *A First Class Service: Quality in the New NHS*, HSC 1999/32 (London, Department of Health, 1998).
6. National Audit Office, *Achieving Improvements in Clinical Governance: A Progress Report on Implementation by NHS Trusts*, HC 1055, 2002–03 (London, The Stationery Office, 2003).
7. Department of Health, *Integrated Governance Handbook 2006: A Handbook for Executives and Non-Executives In Health Care Organisations* (London, Department of Health, 2006).
8. Healthcare Commission, Manual of Clinical Governance Review/Inspection Practices, 4th edn (London, Healthcare Commission, 2004).
9. Healthcare Commission, *Assessment for Improvement: The Annual Health Check* (London, Healthcare Commission, 2004).
10. NPSA Board statement, 18 January 2002.
11. Department of Health, An Organisation with a Memory: Report of an Expert Group on Learning from Adverse Events in the NHS, 2000.
12. NHSLA, *Clinical Negligence Scheme for Trusts: Risk Management Standards*, August 2003.
13. General Medical Council, The Policy Framework for Revalidation: A Position Paper, July 2004.
14. General Medical Council, *Maintaining Good Medical Practice*, 1998.
15. Vanessa L. Mayatt (ed.), *Tolley's Managing Risk in Healthcare: Law and Practice*, 2nd edn, (London, Lexis Nexis, 2004).
16. http://news.bbc.co.uk/1/hi/england/staffordshire
17. Vanessa L. Mayatt, Health and safety prosecutions following harm to patients, *Health Care Risk Report*, **12** (2006), p. 9.

Key websites

www.hm-treasury.gov.uk
www.dh.gov.uk
www.npsa.nhs.uk
www.healthcarecommission.org.uk
www.nice.org.uk
www.gmc-uk.org
www.hse.gov.uk

B   Clinical Governance: An Ethical Perspective

Lucy Frith

Clinical governance has been a central part of health care policy since the late 1990s. The main aim of clinical governance is to improve the quality of care provided by the NHS. At first sight this seems a common sense message – we should aim to provide the best health care that we can and always seek to improve the quality of that care. Surely, this is what health care providers have always done? There are several aspects of clinical governance that differentiate it from previous practice. First, clinical governance makes health organisations legally responsible for the quality of the health care they deliver and creates a statutory duty on them to improve the quality of health care. With this legal responsibility comes greater accountability. Secondly, health care practice is more closely and systematically monitored, and finally, there are more structured and clearly defined ways of implementing changes in practice.

Clinical governance can be defined as: 'A framework through which NHS organisations are accountable for continuously improving the quality of their services and safeguarding high standards of clinical care by creating an environment in which clinical care will flourish.'[1]

There are three main components of clinical governance:

(1) *Setting standards* – bodies such as the National Institute for Health and Clinical Excellence (NICE) and the National Service Frameworks (NSF) set standards and aim to ensure equality of access and standardisation of health provision through out the NHS.
(2) *Putting these standards into practice* – measures such as care pathways and clinical guidelines will be used to implement these standards and recommendations for care. Clinical governance aims to create a more open environment where professionals will share good practice and participate in life-long professional learning. The Clinical Governance Support Team (CGST) was set up in 1999 to support the implementation of clinical governance through out the NHS by providing information about governance, running training schemes and disseminating good practice examples.
(3) *Monitoring these measures* – the Healthcare Commission (HC), which replaced the Commission for Health Improvement in 2004, conducts reviews and audits on health care provision and will publish information on the performance of Trusts in terms of three dimensions of quality: effectiveness (health outcomes), equity (access to their services), and humanity (patients' and carers' views).
(4) *Incorporating patients' views* – the Health and Social Care Act 2003 made it a statutory duty for NHS bodies to involve and consult the public to fulfil the aim of making the NHS 'patient centred'.[2]

I will now consider these four elements in turn, focusing on the ethical implications of these components of clinical governance.

11.9 Setting standards

Various bodies have been established to set standards and policies for the NHS. NICE produces evidence-based clinical guidelines and information on good practice. A key function is the systematic appraisal of medical interventions. For example, in June 2006 NICE issued guidance on the management of hypertension in adults in primary care.[3] This guidance includes sections on how to diagnose hypertension, assessment of risk factors for the condition and recommendations for drug treatments based on the latest clinical evidence. Under this guidance beta blockers are no longer the first or second line of treatment for hypertension, thus changing previous standard practice. The National Service Frameworks (NSFs) have the overall aim of ensuring equity of access and standardisation of care for all patients in the NHS and link related policies to formulate an integrated national policy. For example, the long-term (neurological) conditions NSF, launched in March 2005,[4] sets out standards of care for patients with long-term conditions and links this to other policy areas such as transport, housing and education. These frameworks bring together the best evidence of clinical and cost-effectiveness with the views of users, to determine the best ways of providing a particular service.

The overall aim of standard-setting is to improve the quality of health care provided by the NHS, and in order to do this we need to have some notion of what we mean by quality in this context. Although quality of health care provision is something we all want, the term 'quality' is very hard to define. As Professor Campbell notes, 'The term "quality enhancement" is used, as though its meaning were self-evident. But in the absence of specification, the term is as empty as "quantity" – it refers merely to a dimension for measurement.'[5] 'Quality' is a value judgement; it is an expression that the intervention provides us with certain outcomes that we think are desirable. 'Quality' is not a scientific term, but our opinion of the outcomes data. It is our judgement of whether the intervention is appropriate or helpful for the condition we want to treat and an expression of how we compare it to other treatments. So rather than assuming that by employing the term 'quality' we can answer the questions of what we should be doing with certainty, we need to remember that there could be disagreement over the definition of quality that there will not be one 'right' way of defining or interpreting the term. Hence, questions of what should we be doing will require us to make important value judgements and these should be made explicit so that they can be subject to justification.

The aim of setting standards in clinical governance is to determine the 'best' treatment or approach to a condition and implement these findings across the whole of the NHS, thus improving the quality of health care provision. These standards will be set by considering the medical evidence and by employing a rigorous methodology to determine the best treatment scientifically. There is an implicit assumption that by establishing the quality of a treatment in this way it will be done without recourse to values or personal opinion. I want to consider the view that this method will tell us which treatments are 'better' scientifically and argue that, although medical science can make an important contribution to treatment decisions, value judgements still come into quality assessments and that these should be explicitly recognised.

It could be argued that by using such a scientific methodology to set standards values can be eradicated completely from this whole process. There is an implicit strand running through the literature that by using such tools in setting standards decisions will be made on a more objective basis. Book titles such as *The Scientific Basis of the Health Service*[6] conjure up images of a value-free utopia. It is easy to suppose that as the evidence of effectiveness is improving, we are increasing our knowledge base and thus decreasing the need for values. Medicine in both clinical practice and research is concerned with establishing the facts of the matter and scientific method is often thought to be defined by impartiality and objectivity. 'It is the objective nature by which the evidence based medicine paradigm approaches the question of "what are we doing" and "how can we do better" that causes health care providers and funding agencies to increasingly adopt this paradigm as a primary principle.'[7]

Underlying the position that by employing the tools of evidence-based medicine (EBM) values can be eradicated from the standard-setting process are two assumptions: the improvement in medical evidence gives us a more accurate picture of which treatments work, and the use of systematic reviews can provide us with mechanisms that enable us to gain accurate knowledge of these findings. These findings are then implemented in clinical practice; because the findings are thought to be objective it is inferred that the decision is objective too – values have no role to play. Given this understanding, by using high-quality evidence standard-setting decisions can be made on a 'scientific' basis and are therefore are supposedly open to less interpretation. As Klein *et al.* note, this appears to allow decision makers 'the prospect of less pain, [and] less responsibility for taking difficult decisions'.[8]

So can bodies aiming to set national standards of service provision decide, by the application of the methodology of EBM, what is the best treatment without recourse to any value judgements? I will argue that this is not possible for two reasons. First, the very term 'effectiveness' is a subjective one in that incorporates important value judgements. Secondly, even if what is the best treatment could be proven scientifically and objectively we would still need to use value judgements to help tell us how to use that information. I will deal with these points in turn.

11.9.1 Effectiveness and value judgements

To say a treatment is effective, and hence of better quality, incorporates a non-objective value judgement, namely a judgement of what is a good outcome. It is generally argued that clinical trials are designed to find out certain effects of a drug, for example the lowering of plasma cholesterol levels; these effects are capable of being measured by a piece of laboratory equipment. The findings that this equipment produces will be independent of the experimenters' perceptions and hence can be said to objective. This point is accepted. However, in what follows I argue that the significance given to the effect – whether that effect is to be termed a good outcome – are factors inherent not in the data but in the values we ourselves impose on the data.

Randomised control trials (RCT) are designed to produce data on the effectiveness of a treatment. These trials can be organised in two ways: first, by comparing the new treatment with a placebo; and secondly, by comparing it with an existing treatment. The clinical trial, which seeks to provide information on the comparison between a new treatment and/or a placebo and an existing treatment, is a practical technique to enable clinicians to make working comparisons between different treatments. These trials are often called intention-to-treat trials as they are designed to establish the clinical effect of the drug or treatment.

The purpose of intention-to-treat trials is to assess whether a drug works, not how it works. They provide information on which treatment is *better* than another or more *effective* than a placebo. It is in this assessment of what makes a treatment better than another that trials incorporate evaluative elements. The researcher makes a value judgement as to whether a particular effect is good or bad and hence whether the treatment is effective. Effectiveness, good outcomes, quality, a 'better' treatment are not pre-existing facts waiting to be discovered by medical science: they are value-laden assessments of the weight given to a particular effect of the treatment. Thus, to say a treatment is effective is summing up one's opinion on the data.

For example, a clinical trial may produce data that says that treatment has a 48% success rate in treating a given condition. Such data do not automatically tell us whether this treatment is an effective treatment for our given condition and whether we should recommend it to our patients. Our assessment of how good the 48% success rate is cannot be objectively determined, but is dependent on a number of factors. First is the severity of the condition being treated. If a condition is life-threatening, a 48% chance of success would be very good and the treatment would be judged to be very effective. Secondly, the acceptable level of side effects of this treatment will depend on the type of condition that is treated. If the condition is life-threatening we will bear very bad side effects to achieve this 48% success rate (e.g. the side effects of chemotherapy are very severe but are held to be acceptable). However, for a minor complaint we would not see such side effects as acceptable and would not class the treatment as an effective one. Thirdly, the existence of other treatments and how the new treatment compares will influence how effective we judge our treatment to be. If there is another treatment Y with a 60% success rate and comparable side effects, our treatment will not be seen as effective. If treatment Y has much worse side effects than our treatment X, determining which treatment is most effective will be a matter of individual clinical judgement and will depend on the goals and preferences of the standard-setting authority.

It could be said that it is not important that the results produced by clinical trials incorporate a particular view of what defines a good outcome. If we can formulate a general consensus over what constitutes a good outcome this can provide an adequate foundation for non-subjective agreement over outcomes. I would respond to this argument by raising two points. In the first place, it is very hard to gain consensus over what constitutes a good outcome. Even basic imperatives like preserving life can be contentious in certain situations. For instance patients in persistent vegetative states, if correctly diagnosed, will never recover from the coma and it has been argued that simply preserving their life is unwarranted. Secondly, even if a consensus can be reached it is still important to recognise that this is a particular view of a good outcome and it is possible that in different times (or places) a different view of a good outcome could prevail.

11.9.2   How we employ the data in practice

To turn to the second argument, if we agree that clinical trials produce generally accepted factual data about the interaction of particular drugs or therapies, how can these facts establish which course of action should follow from them? 'The evidence itself will not automatically dictate patient care but will provide the factual basis on which decisions can be made.'[9] No matter how good one's evidence is, it will not automatically determine which course of treatment should be recommended. The evidence of effectiveness may form the basis of a very good reason for pursuing a particular course of action, but value judgements are needed to tell us whether we *should* take that course of action.

EBM claims that by using evidence that is of a higher quality, more scientific and more objective it can make clinical decision-making more objective. This is, to my mind, a confusion between two different things: the quality of evidence and the decision. While a decision that is made on the basis of good evidence will be of a higher quality, it will not be more objective in the sense that it will be independent of value judgements or our perceptions and priorities. The evidence may be more objective but the decision is not, as it necessarily incorporates the values of those making the decision. This confusion leads to the belief that the evidence will indicate the course of action to be taken and that it is possible to locate the *best* treatment for a condition. As Muir Gray says in *Evidence Based Health Care*, 'Decisions about groups of patients or populations are made by combining three factors: 1. evidence; 2. values; 3. resources.'[10]

A central area where values shape how we should use the data and scientific evidence is that of priority setting. When bodies such as NICE decide on which health care interventions to recommend they have to balance two possibly competing claims: do we promote the interests of individual patients as paramount and focus on the effectiveness of the treatment? Or should this individual ethic make way for concerns over the collective good, a population-based ethic, and focus on the cost-effectiveness of the treatment? I think this is one of the key value judgements that has to be made by all health care systems and it is not a dilemma that can be solved by appealing to scientific evidence. It is a dilemma that can only be solved by deciding what kind of values we wish to see drive health care.

Alan Maynard argues that EBM focuses on finding out which treatments are most effective and is therefore grounded in the individual ethic.[11] EBM is concerned with finding out what is the most effective treatment for a particular patient. However, the treatment that is the most effective might not also be the most cost-effective. A physician who adopted the population-based ethic would be more concerned with recommending a treatment that was cost-effective and in the interests of society as a whole rather than just the interests of the individual patient. Maynard illustrates this tension between the individual and population-health ethic with an example.

A purchaser is choosing between two treatments, A and B: therapy A produces five health years (HY) and therapy B produces ten HY. Leaving aside the problem of how to define health years, we can say treatment B is the more effective treatment and should be purchased. This would be purchasing according to the individual ethic, to do the best for the individual patient and provide the most effective treatment.

However, therapy A produces a HY for £300 and therapy B produces a HY for £700. Given a fixed budget of £70,000, therapy A will produce over 130 more HY than therapy B. So if one adopted the population ethic and was concerned with maximising the number of health years gained with a specific budget, then therapy A should be purchased. Hence when making decisions as to what care pathways to recommend a value judgement has to be made as to whether the relevant evidence is that of effectiveness or that of cost-effectiveness. As Maynard's example indicates, with different value judgements different treatments will be purchased.

A further tension between the good of the individual and the good of the population is illustrated by an example cited by Wendy Rogers. Guidance on the use of antibiotics for sore throats issued in Scotland in 1999 stated, 'Antibiotics should not be used to secure symptomatic relief in acute sore throat.'[12] Although the evidence for this claim was scant, the main concern of the guidance writers in not recommending antibiotics for sore throats was that their over use could mean they became ineffective for patients with more serious illnesses. As Rogers states, 'If antibiotics offer only slight benefits to people with sore throats, then it may be justifiable to limit their use to prevent the more serious problem of resistance. But if this is the case, it is misleading to claim that the recommendation to withhold antibiotics is based upon evidence about lack of clinical effectiveness, rather than this other consideration.'[12] Therefore it is for the general good that antibiotics are not over-prescribed, and if this is the reason for not recommending their routine use then the employment of this population-based ethic should be made explicit.

NICE has as its remit the appraisal of health care technologies on grounds not just of clinical effectiveness but of cost-effectiveness as well, and this gives an often controversial slant to their appraisal decisions. While the public are more accepting of the supposed objective nature of clinical effectiveness, a denial of a treatment on the grounds of cost-effectiveness is often seen to be a form of health care rationing, denying treatment options purely on the grounds of lack of funding. However in a review of the decisions NICE made between 1999 and 2005, Raftery noted that one fifth of guidances rejected the use of the intervention and the remainder recommended use with restrictions.[13]

There have been a number of cases where NICE has come into conflict with patient groups over its decisions not to provide particular treatments on the NHS. A recent example is the reversal of previous guidance on drugs used for the treatment of Alzheimer's. Guidance on drugs for the treatment of Alzheimer's issued by NICE in 2001 recommended the use of donepezil, galantamine and rivastigmine for all patients, with treatment stopping when these no longer had any effect. This guidance was reviewed in March 2005 and it was recommended that the drugs should no longer be available to all patients. This recommendation was highly contested by groups such as the Alzheimer's Society who issued an appeal against the decision arguing, 'The Society believed that NICE's work must reflect the value placed on the drug's impact on the disease by people with dementia themselves and their carers. Their evidence has not been given enough weight in these latest recommendations and the benefits for the quality of life for both patients and carers have not been fully taken into account.'[14] In response to such pressure NICE is now reconsidering the guidance and has launched further consultations. This example illustrates two important points. First, patients and patient groups, in this case the Alzheimer's Society, could have different definitions of an effective treatment than the standard-setting agency. Second, cost is a factor in weighing up what treatments should be recommended. In this case it was claimed that the outlay to the NHS was not justified by the benefit it produces for the recipients, whereas the Alzheimer's Society argued that NICE's cost-effectiveness assessment was too narrowly focused and did not take into account the fact that the cost of caring for sufferers was largely borne by their families.[14] In such a deliberation there is no scientific way of answering the question of what the treatment is worth. It is a matter for society to decide what values and priorities are important.

11.10 Putting clinical governance into practice

One of the main ways that quality will be managed under clinical governance is through the employment of care pathways and clinical guidelines. In this section I argue that such guidelines could adversely affect the interests of the individual patient. I first give a brief outline of the rationale behind the introduction of clinical guidelines and then consider how these guidelines can affect patient care.

Part of the process of clinical governance is to systematically assess current practice and formulate clinical guidelines that represent best practice. Since April 1994 all Trusts have to show that they have started to develop clinical guidelines. The NHS Executive stated that 'on the advice of the Clinical Outcomes Group, [they have] begun to commend a selected number of high quality guidelines.'[15] The rationale behind guidelines is an attempt to both increase the quality of care and reduce the inequalities in access to health care. The regional variations in service delivery and health outcomes have been seen as a central problem for the NHS. For example, the number of hip replacements in people aged over 65 years varies from 10 to 51 per 10,000 of the population. In Manchester the death rate from coronary heart disease in people aged less than 65 years is nearly three times higher than in West Surrey.[16] In 2004 NICE recommended that, where clinically indicated, couples should be provided with three cycles of IVF to end what was perceived as a 'postcode lottery' in the provision of infertility treatment.[17]

There can be ethical dilemmas raised by implementing guidelines in practice. Treatments that produce the desired effect can differ from person to person. Even patients with identical manifestations of a particular disease could give different weight to various outcomes depending on personal taste, social and family situations, life priorities and so on. When used to promote greater quality of health care, guidelines can incorporate an assessment of quality that is held to be the same for all patients. This could come into conflict with an individual's particular conception of desirable benefit and their own personal quality assessment.

Many authors have drawn attention to the importance of recognising that good outcomes must be seen as relative to the patient. Hopkins and Solomon illustrate this point with the example of the management of stroke patients.[18] They say that the course of the treatment and the outcomes of rehabilitation cannot be predetermined because each person's disability is unique. Hence the therapist has to concentrate on the goals and needs of the particular patient. This illustrates that effectiveness is usually seen as a relative concept, relative to the individual who receives the treatment. This is an implicit recognition of the role values play in the definition of effectiveness.

However, supporters of clinical guidelines might argue against this view of the treatment process. They might argue that there are enough similarities between patients suffering from the same condition for them to be seen as members of the same patient group (in statistical language, forming part of the same reference class of patient). Therefore all that needs to be established is which group the patient belongs to, and then the appropriate clinical guideline can be followed. Patrick Suppes, for example, has argued that a decision regarding the individual patient can be extrapolated from other cases.

> Even though patients may vary in many respects (age, wealth, etc.), the direct medical consequences and the direct financial cost of a given method of treatment are the most important consequences, and these can be evaluated by summing across the patients and ignoring more individual features.[19]

Suppes is right in one respect: it may be possible to construct broad generalisations about patients' preferences for certain medical consequences. However, these would have to remain at a very broad level as many of the individual factors affecting these consequences are ignored. For example, financial cost may not be an issue for someone very wealthy, whereas for others even the cost of a simple prescription could be prohibitive. Others may value their life in so far as they are able to look after their children. Although it might be possible to ascertain the types of consequences that are, on the whole, most important, it is impossible to predetermine their respective value objectively.

Guidelines rely on patient homogeneity – that is, patients being very similar. In stroke rehabilitation, where patient variation is high, it is difficult to write a precisely defined clinical guideline. There are, on the other hand, areas of health care where patient variation is much lower – the removal of wisdom teeth, for example. When this is the case guidelines can be useful. 'In conditions such as day case surgery, a single patient record is easy to introduce. In an intensive care setting, where variations are more common, a pathway together with freehand documentation may be more suitable.'[20] There may be areas where guidelines are more applicable; however, this should not be extended to areas of health care provision where guidelines may be inappropriate. Even when patients are suffering from the same condition guidelines should not be applied unthinkingly. Room should be made for the needs and wants of the patient to be accommodated. It could be argued that owing to the individual nature of many treatment decisions it could be difficult to produce guidelines that reflected each patient's treatment preferences. This drive to write standardised care pathways for patients could conflict with the other drive of current health care policy to be more patient centred.

However, guidelines can be used in a positive way and could increase patients' autonomy by involving them in the very formulation of guidelines and setting standards. Patients often have very different perspectives from the health care professionals, and soliciting their views on their health care provision could be invaluable. The National Service Frameworks are charged with bringing together the views of service users to determine the best way to provide particular services.[21] As part of the monitoring process, National Patient and User Surveys are regularly conducted to determine user perspectives. For example, in 2005 three surveys were conducted on Primary Care Trusts, mental health services and inpatients.[22] An example of involving the public in the creation of guidelines is the GMC's use of a citizens' jury as part of the process of drafting GMC policy on children's confidentiality.[23]

Guidelines can also be distributed to patients, enabling them to be better informed. When patients enter hospital they can be given a copy of the clinical guidelines and this can indicate what should be happening during the course of their treatment. It will give them an informed basis on which to question and challenge their treatment provision. This model has been adopted by a Liverpool hospital. The guideline is explained to the patient and they usually have access to it during their stay in hospital.[24] Patients therefore have a document that they can refer back to at any stage and so do not have to take in all the information at the beginning of their treatment. Used in this way, guidelines can be a useful aid to communication between patient and health carer. This will ensure that the consent the patient gives is based on a full understanding of what the treatment involves. Clinical risk management (CRM) schemes are designed to eliminate complaints, and by giving the patient a greater understanding and hence control over the treatment, complaints and dissatisfaction could be reduced.

11.11 Monitoring

I shall now consider how the implementation of clinical governance schemes is to be monitored. Standards of care are assessed by audit, inspection, appraisal and risk management. The HC aims to support organisations and conducts rolling reviews of all Trusts and Primary Care Trusts. One of the main ways that the provision of health care is monitored in practice is through the adoption of clinical risk management programmes (CRM).[21] It is the responsibility of the health care professional to promote the welfare of individual patients and ensure that they receive the best care. In this section I examine how such schemes can be used to create an environment that makes it easier for professionals to carry out their ethical duties in practice, looking at the issues of near-miss reporting and professional competence.

11.11.1 Near miss reporting: an ethical environment

One aspect of CRM that can be used as an important measure for preventing harm to patients is near-miss reporting and notification of adverse events. Such events are a common problem for the NHS. For example, 10% of hospital inpatient admissions may result in an adverse event and 18% of patients reported being a victim of medication error in the previous two years.[25] Every year 28,000 written complaints are made about aspects of hospital treatment; £400 million has been paid out in settlement of clinical negligence claims; 15% of hospital infections may be avoidable and cost the NHS nearly £1 billion.[26] To rectify such problems, 'The

NHS needs to develop: a unified mechanism for reporting and analysis when things go wrong [and] a more open culture, in which errors or service failures can be reported and discussed.'[26] This could be used to create a working environment that helps the professional to practice ethically. The hospital appoints a risk manager to compile information on accidents or possible accidents, which forms the basis of changes designed to protect the patient from further incidents. This mechanism can improve patient care and is a means by which CRM can promote ethical practice. As Professor Jones says, 'It cannot be ethical to continue with a method of providing health care that exposes patients to unacceptable risks of having an adverse outcome.'[27] This move by the medical profession to examine why medical accidents have occurred is a very positive trend.

Clearly any reduction in processes leading to patient harm, incidents of staff incompetence and general bad practice are to be applauded. However, there could be a potential difficulty with this approach when one considers the context in which it operates. Janet Lyon has argued that, in order for an adequate system of near miss reporting to operate, the staff must be able to trust their employer to use the information responsibly.[28] Various cases demonstrate this might not be the case. Dr Stephen Bolin, a consultant anaesthetist at Bristol Royal Infirmary, spent five years trying to draw attention to the problems with the paediatric cardiac surgery delivery. In light of such concerns the 1998 Public Interest Disclosure Act was passed to enable employees to raise concerns about dangerous or poor practice without endangering their careers, protecting whistle-blowers from sacking or victimisation.

Even with legal safeguards in place, staff members could feel threatened by having to report mistakes and accidents to the risk manager. (See Wu for a discussion of the practicalities of talking about mistakes.[29]) The NHS Executive has stated that 'the results of the risk management process should not be used for punitive or disciplinary purposes.'[30] It also states that the information given should be kept confidential and that the informant should remain anonymous. Such confidentiality could ensure that the near-miss reporting scheme could effectively carry out the stated aims. This would be beneficial to both staff and patients and ensure that the ethical aims of CRM schemes could be realised. As long as the possible fears of the staff are borne in mind by employers, a culture of trust could be fostered and non-punitive mechanisms developed for addressing the concerns of employees. An example of creating an environment where incident reporting is supported and encouraged is the Queens Medical Centre in Nottingham. Staff had felt reluctant to report incidents for fear of being blamed and/or disciplined. An incident-reporting manual was written and launched by providing workshops in which a low-blame non-punitive approach to such reporting was stressed. Since the introduction of the scheme there has been a 200% increase in the number of clinical incidents reported.[31]

11.11.2 The bad doctor

A specific problem clearly arises when a health carer is reporting a colleague who is allegedly incompetent. This issue has been brought to the fore of public debate by the events at the Bristol Royal Infirmary and the consequent inquiry. The GMC's longest running disciplinary hearing recorded verdicts of professional misconduct against three senior doctors.

The General Medical Council stipulates that it is a doctor's duty to inform the appropriate authority about a colleague whose performance is questionable: 'Where there are serious concerns about a colleague's performance, health or conduct, it is essential that steps are taken without delay to investigate these concerns, to establish whether they are well-founded, and to protect patients.'[32] The Nursing and Midwifery Council also has such requirements in their code: 'You must act quickly to protect patients and clients from risk if you have good reason to believe that you or a colleague, from your own or another profession, may not be fit to practise for reasons of conduct, health or competence.'[33]

The appropriate response to an allegation of incompetence clearly depends on the type of accident or incompetence that is reported. Serious misconduct or wilfully disregarding the welfare of the patient should merit disciplinary action. The issue that is of more concern here is a genuine accident or mistake that the practitioner did not wilfully cause. Whether the accident was caused by a lack of skill or an inadequate process, these factors should be able to be addressed without the practitioner facing any form of disciplinary procedure.

One mechanism introduced by clinical governance schemes to improve and monitor health care professionals is continuing professional development and life-long learning. This is seen in the White Paper *A First Class Service* to be an essential component of clinical governance and a way of setting and monitoring standards. Harold Shipman's serial killings have put even greater emphasis on ascertaining that doctors are still fit to practise, and the Fifth Report of the subsequent inquiry considered this issue in great detail.[34] The GMC is proposing that registered doctors will have to revalidate periodically. 'This means they will have to prove to us, every five years, that they are up to date and fit to practise; and they have been practising in line with our core ethical guidance.'[35] This, along with NHS appraisal systems, should ensure that doctors are encouraged both to continually update their skills and to monitor any unacceptable practise.

11.12 Involving patients

There are various ways in which patients are to be involved in commenting on and deciding what services should be provided. Patient surveys will be conducted, ranging from the national surveys carried out by the HC and annual patient surveys conducted by local Trusts and PCTs, to small-scale surveys conducted at ward level. Patient and Public Involvement Forums (PPIF) have been established in every NHS Trust and PCT area. Although patient surveys were always a part of clinical governance from its inception, there is now a greater focus on patient involvement in actual decision-making, with patients being consulted as to what range of options should be offered in the NHS rather than just what they think about existing services. This is, in principle, a positive move. Giving patients the opportunity of influencing the range of options and how those options will be delivered extends the notion of informed consent.

However, in a discussion document the Patients Forum, a coalition of voluntary patient health organisations, highlights how, with the changes in the structure of NHS provision, it might be harder than before for patient groups to influence decisions:

> The lack of stability and coherence in policy on patient and public involvement has made it difficult to create a climate of constructive dialogue with the Government and Department of Health . . . The range of regulatory bodies and next step agencies have contributed to a highly complex environment for health policy . . . Radical policies emerge and by the time the implications are understood it is too late too influence them.[36]

This lack of stability in policies on patient involvement can be illustrated by the case of the Commission for Patient and Public Involvement in Health. This was established in 2003 to be responsible for appointing and supporting the PPIFs. However, a year later it was announced that a DH review was recommending that it should be abolished.[37] The government's policies on public/patient involvement need to be implemented in a way that really gives people an opportunity to effect change, otherwise public/patient involvement will simply be a meaningless bit of rhetoric designed to give the impression of an NHS governed by consensus.

11.13 Conclusion

Clinical governance can be seen as a positive move by the government to ensure that both Trusts and individual practitioners are held to be more accountable and responsible for the quality of the care they deliver. However, although quality of health care provision is something we all want, the term 'quality' is very hard to define. Once it is recognised that questions of what we should be doing have important ethical dimensions, these ethical and value judgements can be debated. Where possible, value judgements should be formulated by general agreement. These debates can, hopefully, allow those who use the service to have a say in what kind of NHS they wish to see.

11.14 References

1. G. Scally & L. Donaldson, Clinical governance and the drive for quality improvement in the new NHS in England, *British Medical Journal*, **317** (1998), pp. 61–5.
2. Department of Health, *Creating a Patient-led NHS: Delivering the NHS Improvement Plan* (London, DH, 2005).
3. National Institute for Health and Clinical Eexcellence, *Hypertension: Management of Hypertension of Adults in Primary Care* (London, NICE, 2006).
4. National Service Framework, *Long-term neurological conditions NSF* (2005), http://[www.dh.gov.uk/PolicyAndGuidance/HealthAndSocialCareTopics/LongTermCoditions/fs/en]
5. A. Campbell, Clinical governance: watchword or buzzword?, *Journal of Medical Ethics*, **27**, suppl. I (2001), i54–i56.

6. M. Peckham & R. Smith (eds), *The Scientific Basis of the Health Services* (London, BMJ Publishing Group, 1996).
7. A.B. Cooper *et al.*, Pulmonary artery catheters in the critically ill: an overview of using the methodology of EBM, *Critical Care Clinician*, **12**:4 (1996), pp. 777–94.
8. R. Klein, P. Day, & S. Redmayne, *Managing Scarcity: Priority-setting and Rationing in the NHS* (Buckingham, Open University Press, 1996).
9. W. Rosenberg & A. Donald, Evidence-based medicine: an approach to clinical problem solving, *BMJ*, **310** (1995), pp. 1122–6, http://www.nice.org.uk/page.aspx?o=CG34
10. J. Muir Gray, *Evidence-based Health Care: How to Make Health Policy and Management Decisions* (Churchill Livingstone, London, 1997).
11. A. Maynard, Evidence-based medicine: an incomplete method for informing treatment choices, *The Lancet*, **349** (1997), pp. 126–8.
12. W. Rogers, Is there a tension between doctors' duty of care and evidence-based-medicine, *Health Care Analysis*, **10** (2002), pp. 277–87.
13. J. Raftery, Review of NICE's recommendations 1999–2005, *British Medical Journal*, **332**, (2006), pp. 1266–8.
14. Alzheimer's Society, *Drugs for the Treatment of Alzheimer's Disease: A Summary of the Alzheimer's Society's Response to Draft Guidance from NICE* (London, Alzheimer's Society, 2005).
15. NHS Executive, *Promoting Clinical Effectiveness* (London, HMSO, 1996).
16. Secretary of State for Health, *The New NHS: Modern, Dependable* (London, HMSO, London, 1997).
17. NICE (2004) *Fertility: Assessment and Treatment for People with Fertility Problems*, http://www.nice.org.uk/page.aspx?o=CG011
18. Hopkins, A. & Solomon, J.K., Can contacts drive clinical care?, *British Medical Journal*, **313** (1996), pp. 477–8.
19. P. Suppes, The logic of clinical judgement: Bayesian and other approaches. In H.T. Engelhardt *et al.* (eds), *Clinical Judgment: A Critical Appraisal* (D. Reidel Publishing Company, 1979).
20. D. Kitchiner & P. Bundred, Integrated care pathways, *Archives in Disease in Childhood*, **75** (1996), pp. 166–8.
21. Secretary of State for Health, *A First Class Service: Quality in the New NHS* (London, NHS Executive, 1998).
22. Health Care Commission, *National NHS Patient Survey Programme 2005*, www.healthcarecommission.org.uk
23. General Medical Council 'First GMC citizens' jury supports professional judgment on children's' confidentiality', Press Release (5 November 2005).
24. D. Kitchiner *et al.*, Integrated care pathways, *Journal of Evaluation in Clinical Practice*, **2**:1 (1996), pp. 65–9.
25. Chief Medical Officer, *Making Amends: A Consultation Paper Setting Out Proposals for Reforming the Approach to Clinical Negligence in the NHS* (London, DH, 2003).
26. Department of Health, *An Organisation with a Memory: Report of an Expert Group on Learning from Adverse Events in the NHS* (London, DH, 2000).
27. M. Jones, *Clinical Risk Management* (Liverpool, IMLAB Publications, 1997).
28. J. Lyon, *The Trojan Horse: Problems of CRM* (MSc dissertation, University of Liverpool, 1996).
29. A. Wu, Medical error: the second victim, *British Medical Journal*, **320** (2000), pp. 726–727.
30. NHS Executive, *Risk Management in the NHS* (London, HMSO, 1994).
31. Royal College of Nursing, *Clinical Governance: An RCN Resource Guide* (London, RCN, 2003).

32. General Medical Council, *Duties of a doctor* (London, General Medical Council, London, 1998).
33. Nursing and Midwifery Council, *The NMC Professional Code of Conduct: Standards of Conduct, Performance and Ethics* (London, NMC, 2004).
34. Catto, G. (2005) GMC and the future of revalidation, *British Medical Journal*, 330, 1205–1207.
35. General Medical Council, *Licensing and Revalidation Fact Sheet* (GMC, 2005), http://www.gmc-uk.org/doctors/licensing/archive/factsheet_2005_08.asp
36. Patients Forum, *Options for the Future* (London, The Patients Forum, 2006).
37. Department of Health, (2004) *Patient And Public Involvement: A Brief Overview*, www.dh.gov.uk/PolicyAndGuidance/OrganisationPolicy/PatientAndPublicInvolvement

12 Clinical Research and Patients

A The Legal Perspective

Marie Fox

The issue of clinical research on human patients poses complex bioethical and legal dilemmas for nurses. Over the last 20 years nurses have steadily assumed a greater role in the conduct of clinical research, largely because of the increasing emphasis on evidence-based medicine, but also because involvement in research may help to validate their professional status. Nevertheless, it has been argued that there are still too few nurse researchers and that most nurses in practice are not sufficiently research aware.[1] In an attempt to remedy this, the most recent national strategy for nursing, midwifery and health visiting is committed to developing 'a strategy to influence the research and development agenda, to strengthen the capacity to undertake nursing, midwifery and health visiting research, and to use research to support nursing, midwifery and health visiting practice'.[2] Such initiatives make it imperative for nurses to have a clear understanding of the ethical and legal implications of engaging in clinical research.

The fundamental ethico-legal issue raised by clinical research involves a balancing exercise, between on the one hand the interests of the health professional carrying out research and of medical science itself, and on the other the welfare of those human patients or volunteers who are the subject of research.[3] Against that backdrop, the aim of this chapter is to explore the legal framework within which clinical research may be conducted. It should be noted that nurses have the same ethical and legal obligations as any other health professional,[4] although the particular position of the nurse and her relationship to her patients may present specific problems in some cases. However, as recent RCN guidance stresses, 'In ethical terms . . . nurses have no more right than any other health professional to hide behind notions of subordination, compliance and obedience to justify avoiding personal responsibility for what they do as part of a research study'.[5]

It is worth noting that there is a relative absence of clear legal rules regulating research, although legislative intervention in this area is now growing and there is a proliferation of professional guidance. Thus although the Animals (Scientific Procedures) Act 1986 and the Human Fertilisation and Embryology Act 1990 created statutory bodies to regulate and license research that may lawfully be carried out on animals[6] and human embryos,[7] there has never been a statutory regime that licenses research on human patients in a comparable way. Equally, the common law in this area is marked by the absence of case law pertaining specifically to medical research. Thus, historically, the legal framework governing research has drawn heavily upon the principles laid down in relation to consent to conventional medical treatment and upon guidance for health professionals derived mainly from international declarations, which in turn have influenced codes of practice promulgated by professional bodies. However, in the past five years there have been significant legal developments in this area. In the first place, concerns about clinical trials have prompted the Department of Health to intro- duce a framework for clinical governance, while the introduction of a European Union Directive on the conduct of clinical trials, designed to harmonise the regulation of such trials throughout the EU has required the United Kingdom to produce new regulations to govern certain types of clinical research, which have been in force since 2004.

12.1 Definition of clinical research

Clinical research is traditionally classified in a number of ways. It is first dis- tinguished from conventional treatment that uses approved methods and tech- niques for therapeutic purposes. It is then subdivided into two broad classes of research. The first consists of those that do not involve any direct interference with the subject – for example, those involving psychological observation,[8] and the use of personal medical records or tissue samples. It can be difficult to draw distinctions between this and the second category – invasive research – which gives rise to much greater concern, as it involves direct physical or psychological interference with the subject. My focus in this chapter is on the issue of invasive research on human beings, but in the light of recent concerns and consequent legislation the issue of research using personal information and tissue samples is discussed (briefly) below. Invasive research on human subjects is conventionally further divided into two types:

(1) Therapeutic research is performed on a patient, and the use of new methods and techniques carries prospects of direct benefit to the individual patient.
(2) Non-therapeutic research involves the use of new procedures or drugs for purely or mainly scientific purposes that are unlikely to benefit the individual participant. While it may herald some collective benefit, the aim of the trial is

the acquisition of scientific knowledge, and it is often carried out on healthy volunteers.[9]

It is worth noting that this therapeutic/non-therapeutic dichotomy, which has generated much bioethical scholarship, has recently been subject to attack. Commentators have suggested that it is a problematic distinction for the following reasons. First, in some cases therapeutic research may be more hazardous than non-therapeutic research. Secondly, it is often difficult to distinguish between research and innovative therapy. For instance, it is unclear whether a new surgical technique, such as keyhole surgery, should be subject to special regulation, as the introduction of a new drug procedure would be.[10] Thirdly, in response to the lobbying of organised health pressure groups, such as AIDS patients, high-quality clinical care and responsible research have come to be recognised as a continuum rather than a dichotomy.[11] Priscilla Alderson has argued that ' "[t]herapeutic" is an oddly fuzzy, unscientific word; it expresses possibly unfounded hopes for the future as if they were present realities, it confuses the aim of research with the activity . . . scientific rigour would assess research in terms of outcome, effectiveness and efficiency'.[12]

Notwithstanding the validity of these points, there may be good reason to retain the therapeutic/non-therapeutic distinction, given that advances attributed to research that is clearly non-therapeutic have been obtained at the cost of many blighted lives. In this regard, it is significant that historically these costs have been disproportionately borne by members of oppressed groups in society.[13] A major advantage of the distinction is that it enables commentators to argue that there should be a greater obligation to disclose risks in the context of non-therapeutic research.[14] Consequently, considerable controversy has been generated by the most recent revision of the Declaration of Helsinki – the pre-eminent international agreement governing research – which in 2000 abandoned the distinction between therapeutic and non-therapeutic research. As some commentators have noted, an implied distinction between therapeutic and non-therapeutic research continues to underpin much of the guidance on research ethics promulgated by national professional bodies.[15] Moreover, issues arising from the catastrophic collapse of six healthy volunteers who participated in a Phase I trial of a drug compound – TGN1412 – designed to mitigate auto-immune and immunodeficiency diseases at Northwick Park Hospital in London in 2006 has indicated that the therapeutic/ non-therapeutic distinction may continue to have ethical purchase. Certainly the Northwick Park trial poses questions regarding the efficacy of the regulatory framework in general, which will be addressed below. These pertain to the validity of information about risks disclosed to the participants, the amount of money offered as an inducement (each participant was paid £2000), the complex way in which newer drugs function compared with the simpler compounds on which trials have traditionally focused, the reliability of prior animal testing, the failure to seek expert information from overseas sources, the absence of 'staggered dosing' in administering the compound, and the decision to administer the drug to healthy volunteers rather than to cancer patients who would have been less susceptible to toxicity (but more difficult and time-consuming to recruit). Latterly the adequacy of insurance cover has also been raised.[16]

12.2 Regulation of clinical research

12.2.1 International declarations

The Declaration of Helsinki was promulgated largely as a result of the involvement of health professionals in medical experimentation amounting to torture on stigmatised social and ethnic groups in Nazi Germany. Indeed many ethico-legal concerns raised by clinical research have their roots in the Nazi era. The aftermath of the Nuremberg trials of Nazi war criminals witnessed the promulgation of the Nuremberg Code, which in 1964 was revised and expanded by the World Health Organization's Helsinki Declaration. It has subsequently been amended in 1975, 1983, 1989, 1996 and 2000.[17]

While the Nazi-era experiments exemplify the most appalling abuses of research, numerous subsequent examples highlight the continuing need for international regulation.[18] Particular concern has been prompted by medical research on subjects in the economic south, where standards may be lower and subjects less likely to benefit from expensive drugs marketed in the 'developed' world. Trials of AIDS drugs and vaccines, in particular, have courted controversy.[19]

Domestically, all nursing research carried out in the UK should comply with the fundamental principles enshrined in the Helsinki Declaration. This stresses that the first responsibility of the health professional is to his or her patient, and that considerations related to the well-being of the human subject should take precedence over the interests of science and society (para. 5). Risks to the patient should be carefully evaluated and researchers should be confident that they can be managed satisfactorily, and that subjects are fully informed of them (para. 17). Furthermore, biomedical research must conform to generally accepted scientific procedures and be approved by an appropriate ethical review committee, carried out by those who are scientifically qualified and supervised by a clinically competent medical professional (paras 13–15). The 1975 revision of the Helsinki Declaration recommended codes of practice for researchers, and this has resulted in guidelines promulgated by national bodies, of which the most prominent are those produced by the Royal College of Physicians[20] and the Royal College of Nursing,[21] as well as the guidelines that the Central Office for Research Ethics Committees (COREC) has issued on *Governance Arrangements for NHS Research Ethics Committees* (hereafter the GAfREC guidance).[22] Each of these sets of guidelines is underpinned by principles similar to those contained in the Helsinki Declaration. More recently, the Council of Europe's Convention on Human Rights and Biomedicine (1997) and its additional protocol on Biomedical Research (2005) have reaffirmed these principles.[23]

Although such guidelines are useful in stipulating patient rights and stressing the ethical obligations of researchers, they are not directly enforceable in law, and indeed the UK has yet to sign the Convention on Human Rights and Biomedicine. Moreover, guidance is inevitably framed in broad terms that leave considerable discretion to the researcher, particularly in assessing physical, psychological and emotional harm.

12.2.2 The criminal law

Notwithstanding the discretion thus entrusted to the scientific researcher, it should be noted that all activities undertaken by health professionals are circumscribed by the criminal law. English criminal law provides that undue harm may not be inflicted on an individual even if they are prepared to consent to the infliction of such harm (*R* v. *Brown* (1993)). In a consultation paper, *Consent in the Criminal Law*, the Law Commission (the body that deals with law reform issues in England and Wales) addressed the issue of what harm a person may legitimately consent to. It provisionally suggested that:

> a person should not be guilty of an offence if she causes injury to another, of whatever degree of seriousness, if such injury is caused during the course of properly approved medical research (i.e. approved by a Local Research Ethics Committee) and with the consent of the other person.[24]

This is consistent with the Law Commission's general stance regarding medical treatment, which is that legitimate clinical procedures may be undertaken regardless of the degree of harm that may result. However, the Commission did not address the key question of how 'acceptable risk' may be defined. This leaves open the issue of whether a high-risk trial may be undertaken if the patient is prepared to accept that risk – a matter considered below in the context of xenotransplantation. Certainly, failure to obtain the consent of an individual before she is included in a clinical trial may give rise to a criminal prosecution for battery. There is a remote possibility that a prosecution could be brought for manslaughter if a research subject died while participating in a high-risk trial. For instance, given the ethical concerns voiced about the Northwick Park trial above, it is possible that such a trial could have given rise to homicide charges had any of the subjects died. In 2001 similar concerns about the adequacy of risk and safety analysis were raised by the death of Ellen Roche – a 25-year-old lab technician – who had been enrolled as a healthy volunteer in an asthma trial at Johns Hopkins University Baltimore. Critics claimed that subjects were exposed to unacceptable risks because of lax oversight at federal, institutional and investigative levels.[25]

12.2.3 The civil law

As well as potentially constituting a criminal offence, battery/trespass to the person is also a civil wrong entitling the patient to sue for compensation. Thus, where any research involves examining, operating on or injecting the patient, consent must be obtained in advance for it to be carried out lawfully; unauthorised contact entitles the patient to damages. Consequently, obtaining adequate consent to participation is the key legal requirement in relation to nursing research, since authority to carry out research on a competent adult human subject derives from that person's consent.[26] Effectively, English law imposes responsibility on the individual research subject to protect herself from abuse by giving or withholding consent.[27] The upshot, as Berg has noted, is that in the past virtually all documented cases of abusive medical experimentation have been those that failed to employ satisfactory informed consent procedures.[28] Therefore, it is not surprising that the key principle enshrined in the Helsinki declaration is that:

> each potential subject must be adequately informed of the aims, methods, sources of funding, any possible conflicts of interest, institutional affiliations of the researcher, the anticipated benefits and potential risks of the study and the discomfort it may entail. The subject should be informed of the right to abstain from participation in the study or to withdraw consent to participate at any time without reprisal. After ensuring that the subject has understood the information, the physician should then obtain the subject's freely-given consent, preferably in writing. If the consent cannot be obtained in writing, the non-written consent must be formally documented and witnessed.' (para. 22)

Similarly, in a nursing context, the Nursing and Midwifery Council's Code of Professional Conduct provides, *inter alia*:

> All patients . . . have a right to receive information about their condition . . . Information should be accurate, truthful and presented in such a way as to make it easily understood . . . You must adhere to the laws of the country in which you are practising.[29]

Hence, a major issue in relation to consent to nursing research is how to ensure that the consent is 'freely-given' and 'informed'. As we saw in Chapter 7A, in relation to medical treatment, the courts have stated that so long as a patient gives a very general consent to treatment, the health professional will not be liable in the tort of battery (*Chatterton* v. *Gerson* (1981)). Although in *Sidaway* v. *Bethlem* (1985) the House of Lords rejected the view that the doctrine of informed consent forms part of English law in the context of medical treatment, it is clear in the post-Sidaway case law that the courts are increasingly prepared to call doctors to account, and reject the view that a responsible body of medical opinion is decisive in determining what should be disclosed to the patient. Cases, such as *Pearce* v. *United Bristol Healthcare NHS Trust* have highlighted the importance of disclosing risks that would have affected the reasonable person's decision as to whether to consent to treatment, in order to avoid a finding of negligence. Moreover, although there have been no decided English cases on the duty of disclosure pertaining to clinical research, it is generally accepted by legal commentators that, in the context of research, law would impose stronger duties of disclosure.[30] Thus, someone who volunteers for research is entitled to a fuller explanation of the nature of the trial and the risks it carries than would be the case in relation to conventional medical treatment. It is highly probable that English law would follow Canadian law[31] in adopting an objective test requiring a researcher to disclose all relevant facts that a reasonable subject would wish to know, and to provide the opportunity for questions, to which full and honest answers would be given.[32] The General Medical Council frames this requirement in the following terms:

> You must ensure that any individuals whom you invite to take part in research are given the information which they want or ought to know, and that it is presented in terms and a form that they can understand. You must bear in

mind that it may be difficult for participants to identify and assess the risks involved. Giving the information will usually include an initial discussion supported by a leaflet or sound recording, where possible taking into account any particular communication or language needs of the participants. You must give participants an opportunity to ask questions and to express any concerns they may have.[33]

However, given that researchers themselves may lack adequate information about the risks of a proposed new drug or course of treatment, some commentators query whether informed consent is truly possible in the context of clinical research.[34] Certainly it is questionable whether the intended experimental subject can validly consent to procedures the results of which are uncertain, of dubious benefit or clearly harmful[35] – issues that are canvassed below in relation to xeno-transplantation. It is thus not surprising that in those few court cases where judges have addressed the issue of consent to research, they have tended to limit their role to ensuring that fully informed, voluntary consent has been given. Yet, as Tobias has pointed out, notwithstanding the legal emphasis on informed consent 'neither lawyers, ethicists, nor medical scientists have so far agreed precisely what this term actually means'.[36] In this regard, Jackson highlights the existence of various grey areas. For instance, should a researcher disclose details of the funding of the trial, including any personal or financial benefit that she hopes to obtain, or the fact that she has been paid to carry out the trial?[37] Furthermore, McNeil has contended that, notwithstanding the emphasis that courts have traditionally placed on obtaining consent, consent alone is an inadequate basis on which to regulate experimentation on human subjects. In his view, the focus on consent fails to fully address issues such as the weighting of the risks and benefits of experimentation for the subject and society, and enables courts to avoid issues such as whether they should endorse guidelines for researchers.[38]

Following the tragic consequences of thalidomide, which was marketed as a remedy for morning sickness during pregnancy and caused severe limb deformities in children, legislation was introduced to regulate the introduction of new pharmaceuticals. The Medicines Act 1968 introduced a new system for licensing and monitoring of new drugs overseen by the Medicines Control Agency, which in 2003 merged with the Medical Devices Agency to form the Medical and Healthcare Products Regulatory Agency (MHRA). In 2001 a Directive was issued by the European Parliament on the approximation of the laws regulating clinical trials of medicinal products, with the aim of ensuring that good clinical practice is observed in the design, conduct, recording and reporting of clinical trials on human subjects throughout the European Union.[39] The outcome in the UK has been the enactment of the Medicines for Human Use (Clinical Trials) Regulations 2004 (hereafter referred to as the Clinical Trials Regulations). Under this legislation, an authorisation must be sought from the MHRA before new medicines can be tested in clinical trials. The 1968 Act and 2004 regulations have established a complex reporting system to monitor the impact of the drug in question. Any unexpected or adverse outcomes during treatment with the drug must be reported to the MHRA.[40] The so-called 'yellow card' scheme enables nurses, midwives and health visitors as well as GPs and patients themselves to report any adverse drug reactions, following research indicating that GPs were failing to report adequately.[41]

12.2.4 The relationship between the investigator and the research subject

A further factor that impacts on the process of obtaining consent is the sometimes problematic nature of the relationship between the research subject and the health care professional engaged in research. As McNeil argues, the history of human experimentation is one of imbalance in favour of the interests of the researcher.[42] It has been extensively documented how in the research context the role of the health care professional has changed from that of a physician (or more recently a nurse) to that of a scientific investigator, to become, in Jay Katz's term, a 'physician-investigator' (or 'nurse-investigator'). Not only does this entail a potential conflict of loyalties to patients, employers and research aims, as a result of her multiple priorities as teacher, researcher, health professional and administrator;[43] it also means that the researcher is likely to be seen in a more ambivalent light by the subject. Kennedy has suggested that a health professional's primary duty to care for her patient is inevitably compromised by her duty to carry out clinical trials with due scientific rigour.[44] The researcher's commitment to such rigour leaves the patient in an even more disempowered position than is normally the case in engagement with health professionals, since scientific ideology generally requires the researcher to view the subject with dispassion and detachment.[45] As Katz points out, it follows that 'the commitment to objectivity invites the investigator's thought processes to become objectified and, in turn, to transform the human beings who are the subjects of research into data points to be plotted on a chart that will prove or disprove a research hypothesis'.[46]

Such power imbalances are especially likely to arise where the research subject is differentiated from the investigator by factors such as gender, class, race and ethnicity, which may pose communication difficulties. Given these disparities in power, researchers should bear in mind Morehouse's claim that '[t]here are many ways of introducing a research project to a patient which fall short of pressurising the patients, but certainly do not conform to total objectivity'. [47] This may particularly apply in the case of vulnerable groups of patients, discussed below. The Declaration of Helsinki provides that:

> [w]hen obtaining informed consent for the research project the physician should be particularly cautious if the subject is in a dependent relationship with the physician or may consent under duress. In that case the informed consent should be obtained by a well-informed physician who is not engaged in the investigation and who is completely independent of this relationship. (para. 23)

In common with many legal documents, the Helsinki declaration focuses on the role of doctors. However, the tension between scientific objectivity and concern for the patient is likely to be particularly disconcerting for nurses. Not only can it be argued that nursing is more firmly grounded in notions of care and nurturance than other health professions,[48] but in practice nurses tend to have closer relationships with their patients than do doctors. It may follow that nurses are viewed as better placed to explain the consequences of enrolment in a trial to a patient and to obtain their consent. Certainly, if a nurse finds herself in the position of seeking consent, guidelines promulgated by bodies such as the Medical Research Council (MRC) and General Medical Council (GMC) stress the need for explanations to be given in clear and easily comprehensible language. Any special communication or language needs of the participants should be taken into account.

As highlighted by the Griffiths Review into the conduct of research trials involving children at North Staffordshire Hospital during the 1990s, it is important to appreciate the difficulty of understanding and giving a valid consent at a time of severe physical, psychological or emotional stress.[49] The GMC guidance states that effective communication is key to obtaining valid consent and stresses that '[o]btaining consent is a process involving open and helpful dialogue, and is essential in clarifying objectives and understanding between doctors and research participants'. Potential subjects should also be given written information and adequate time to reflect on it. The guidance stipulates that patients or volunteers are entitled to an explanation about why they have been asked to participate, which should include an accurate description of the patient's clinical condition.[50] The MRC suggests that it is useful, as well as good practice, to seek advice from consumers or lay persons in drafting information for potential subjects.[51] As noted above, subjects should also be clearly informed of their right to withdraw from participation at any time without reprisal.[52] Additionally, they must be given an explanation of how personal information will be stored, transmitted and published. In terms of the form of consent, we saw in Chapter 7A that written consent is generally only evidence of consent, but the Clinical Trials Regulations 2004 require that the decision must be 'given freely after [the participant] is informed of the nature, significance, implications and risks of the trial' and either must be in writing or 'if the person is unable to sign or mark a document so as to indicate his consent, is given orally in the presence of at least one witness and recorded in writing' (para. 3(1), Part 1, Schedule 1).

12.2.5 Consent to randomised controlled trials

Particular problems arise in the context of consent to randomised controlled trials (RCTs). RCTs, which aim to compare treatments or approaches in two or more groups of subjects who are allocated randomly to those groups,[53] have been promoted as the most scientifically valid method of evaluating procedures.[54] Those who endorse randomisation (which aims to rule out a purely psychological reaction to new drugs) argue that if drugs are not investigated using randomisation and blinding of both researchers and subjects to the process then there is a strong possibility that bias will enter the study and affect the results. However, other commentators have suggested that RCTs may adversely affect the health professional–patient relationship by harming the bond of trust and mutual respect that is the ideal of medical practice, and run counter to the health professional's duty to decide what treatment is best for the individual patient.[55]

Oakley suggests that RCTs are ethically problematic since chance allocation may be antithetical to good ethical practice. In particular, she expresses concern at how 'the tension between the scientific aims of research and the humane treatment of individuals . . . is expressed in the very strategy of designing an experiment so as to restrict people's freedom to discuss with one another the commonality of the process in which they are engaged'.[56] What is certain is that the weighing up of risks and how they are presented to potential participants is crucial with RCTs. Fletcher *et al.* suggest that the fundamental issue is the purpose for which the research is being carried out, and that generally a trial should only proceed 'if the likely benefits to the individual taking part in the research and/or to society as a whole far outweigh the risks of participation'.[57] Additionally, the Declaration of Helsinki provides that '[p]hysicians should cease any investigation if the risks are found to outweigh the potential benefits or if there is conclusive proof of positive and beneficial results' (para. 17).

Given the uncertainties until such a point is reached, RCTs pose considerable problems for the law on informed consent since the technique of randomisation makes it more difficult for the researcher to fully explain the risks to an individual patient. As Oakley notes, 'What people understand may not be what researchers think they do; "informed consent" is a shifting, complex process, rather than a discrete cognitive event.'[58] Certainly, the crucial issue in obtaining consent will be how the risks and benefits of the proposed research are presented to the research subject. Tobias has pointed to the practical difficulties of gaining informed consent in such trials, especially given the potential for misconception and anxiety if the consequences of randomisation are fully explained to the patient. He argues that, instead, we should trust health professionals to engage in randomisation without explicit consent.[59] However, the consensus among legal commentators endorses Kennedy's view that with RCTs it is particularly important that the materiality of risk should be defined according to what the particular patient would want to know.[60]

The Griffiths Review into events at North Staffordshire in the 1990s highlighted numerous problems with the process for obtaining such consent.[61] Nurses were centrally involved and the review panel found that the nursing sister assigned to a project focusing on the treatment of respiratory problems in premature newborn babies did not appear to have been provided with a protocol or system for ensuring adequate documentation for all patients. It concluded that, in general, the nursing staff lacked adequate research experience for the tasks that they were asked to do, yet were not offered any training. Inadequate supervision by the researchers, coupled with a lack of support from the Trust nursing management, contributed to problems in documenting whether consent forms had been completed.[62] There were particular concerns about the adequacy of information given to parents who were asked to enter their children in a trial in which a new technique – continuous negative extrathoracic pressure (CNEP) – was compared with the conventional treatment of positive pressure ventilation, given that some of the children subsequently suffered brain damage or died. Hopefully the introduction of more detailed guidance on research governance (see below) will obviate these problems. However, nurses who are concerned by the conduct of trials or their qualifications for conducting them should be prepared to 'whistle blow' where necessary.[63] What is clear is that participants must be fully aware on enrolling in an RCT that they will have no choice as to which treatment is given, and will not know what treatment they have been given until the end of the trial.

Additional problems are posed by RCTs involving placebos. A 2002 clarification to para. 29 of the Helsinki Declaration urges that 'extreme care must be taken in making use of a placebo-controlled trial and . . . in general this methodology should only be used in the absence of existing proven therapy'.[64] However, it has been queried whether such caution is justified, given the scientific value of placebo trials. Miller and Brody argue that 'it can be ethical to use placebo controls in scientifically valuable RCTs that involve withholding proven effective medical treatment, provided that the risks are not excessive and participants give informed consent'.[65] Guideline 11 of the revised guidance issued by the Council for International Organizations of Medical Sciences (CIOMS) provides that 'as a general rule, research subjects in the control group of a trial . . . should receive an established effective intervention'. However, the guidelines sanction the use of placebos where there is no established effective intervention, or when such established intervention would not yield scientifically reliable results and using a placebo would not add any risk or serious or irreversible harm to the subjects.[66]

12.2.6 Research using personal information or human tissue

Many significant medical advances have resulted not from research trials involving human subjects but from the use of personal health information or human tissue samples retained following post mortem examinations. For instance, such research has improved understanding of suspected health hazards, facilitated recognition of the epidemiology of new diseases (such as new variant CJD and its relation to the BSE epidemic) and led to advice on reducing cot deaths. For many years such research was seen as less ethically problematic than research on human subjects, especially as well-coordinated use of such material can reduce the research demands on patients and the need for animal research.

However, more recently such research has become hugely contentious. In particular, public outcry over unauthorised retention of children's organs at both Bristol Royal Infirmary and Alder Hey Hospital in Liverpool led to the establishment of public inquiries in the late 1990s,[67] and subsequently to the passage of the Human Tissue Act 2004. This legislation introduces a new regime to regulate use of human tissue, and once again the concept of consent is enshrined as the cornerstone. When the Human Tissue Bill was originally promulgated it contained requirements for specific consent[68] but in the course of the passage of the legislation through Parliament this was watered down (though see below). Thus, although section 1 of the 2004 Act stipulates that 'appropriate consent' must have been obtained before human tissue or organs may be removed for the purposes of research, the notion of 'consent' is not further defined in the act itself. Section 3 does, however, specify three ways in which consent may be obtained for the use of cadaveric organs or tissue. First, the donor can stipulate her consent or lack of consent prior to death, either in writing (or by joining the organ donor register) or making her views clear to friends or relatives. Secondly, under section 4 of the Act she may appoint a person to represent her wishes after death for the purposes of giving or withholding consent to the removal of tissue or organs. Thirdly, where no wishes have been indicated and no representative appointed, the consent of a person in a 'qualifying relationship' to the donor must be sought. Section 27(4) of the Human Tissue Act defines and ranks qualifying relationships, providing that the consent of a spouse or partner should be sought first, followed by that of a parent or child, and so on to the consent of a friend of long standing. Section 2(7) provides that a competent minor can consent to organ or tissue donation for research; and that where the child is not competent the person with parental responsibility for her is authorised to consent or, in cases where no person has parental responsibility immediately prior to death, consent may be given by a person in a qualifying relationship to the child.[69] Where a living person wants to donate human organs or tissue for research purposes, according to section 3(2) of the Human Tissue Act 'appropriate consent' simply means the donor's consent, which is not further defined.

However, one of the Codes of Practice recently promulgated under the Act by the Human Tissue Authority established by the Act provides detailed guidance on obtaining consent for activities covered by the Act, which includes research on tissues donated by the living and taken from the deceased.[70] The code stresses the consent should be viewed as a continuous process involving dialogue rather than a single act (para. 68), that consent should be sought by a health professional who has been suitably trained (paras 59, 71) and that patients or their proxies must understand what is proposed and be told of 'material' or 'significant' risks, and informed of the implications of certain uses of samples, such as for genetic testing (para. 78). Although, as we have seen, this requirement was absent from the final Act, the Code of Practice does specify that patients should be asked whether the consent they give is 'generic' (i.e. for any future project approved by an REC) or specific, and they should be told if any samples will be put to commercial use (paras 79, 80). It is good practice for the consent to be in writing, although this is not a specific requirement for research under the HTA. Paragraph 92 summarises key points:

> Seeking consent is a process which involves listening, discussing, and questioning so as to arrive at a shared understanding – a signed form is not necessarily an indication that such an understanding has been reached. For consent to be valid it must be given voluntarily, by an appropriately informed person who has the capacity to agree to the activity in question. If these elements have not been satisfied, a signature on a form will not make the consent valid.

12.3 Ethical review

12.3.1 Research ethics committees

For most other forms of clinical research aside from that on tissues, the regulatory focus has, to some extent, now shifted from an emphasis on obtaining consent to ensuring compliance with codes of research practice, following the introduction of ethical review. Since 1968 official NHS policy has been that local research ethics committees (LRECs) should be established to oversee clinical research within the NHS. Under the EU Clinical Trials Directive ethics committee approval is now mandatory before any clinical trial can commence. Research Ethics Committees (RECs) were governed by Department of Health guidelines issued in 1991, which have now been revised under the research governance arrangements put in place in 2001.[71]

RECs have traditionally been envisaged as independent bodies, comprising both health professionals and lay persons, who are charged with the responsibility of protecting the rights and well-being of human subjects involved in a trial. They have until recently been self-regulating. However, since 1 May 2004 RECs that oversee clinical trials that come within the remit of the EU Clinical Trials Directive and the Clinical Trials Regulations 2004 that implement them (see page 280 above) are legally accountable to a new government body – the UK Ethics Committee Authority – which essentially comprises the secretaries of state for health for England, Wales, Scotland and Northern Ireland. Although in theory this new Authority should overcome lots of the problems inherent in self regulation – such as lack of transparency and accountability, and inadequate provision for monitoring and sanctions[72] – concerns have been expressed about subjecting research ethics to direct political control.[73] Equally controversial has been the recommendation by the Department of Health's Ad Hoc Advisory Group on the Operation of NHS Research Ethics Committees that the UK should move towards a fully professionalised REC workforce.[74] The consequence would be a reduction in the number of RECs, from around 200 currently to as few as 30, on the grounds of efficiency and reducing variation in decision-making.[75]

According to GAfREC guidance, the key function of RECs is defined as 'the ethical review of research proposals and their supporting documents, with special attention given to the nature of any intervention and its safety for participants, to the informed consent process, documentation, and to the suitability and feasibility of the protocol' (para. 9.7). The Department of Health's Ad Hoc Advisory Group has confirmed that the key question for RECs to address is the ethical acceptability of the protocol, with appropriate specialists judging the scientific merit prior to the REC assessment of whether it satisfies appropriate ethical standards,[76] although this view has been criticised for its failure to demarcate scientific and ethical review.[77] The GAfREC guidance stipulates that 'protocols submitted for ethical review should already have been reviewed by experts in the relevant research methodology, who should also comment on the originality of the research'. It thus takes the view that it is not the task of a REC to undertake additional scientific review. However, the REC should satisfy itself that the review already undertaken is adequate for the nature of the proposal under consideration. Before giving a favourable opinion, the committee must certainly be satisfied about various other matters, including the safety implications of the project for the research subject, the health and social care provision during and after the project, the qualifications of the researcher, and plans for publication of the research.[78] The new regulatory structure has increased the workload of RECs significantly, since all research proposals must now be reviewed by the full committee. Moreover, article 6 of the Clinical Trials Regulations 2004 requires RECs to notify the applicant of its opinion within 60 days of receipt of a valid application in most cases, prompting concerns that workload and time pressures may remove the space for negotiation between institutions and RECs and impact adversely on the quality of decision-making.[79]

12.3.2 The limitations of research ethics committees

Although the existence of ethics committees is clearly desirable, various concerns have in the past been voiced about their effectiveness as a mechanism for scrutinising and monitoring clinical research, and it remains to be seen how the new regulatory regime under the 2004 regulations will work in practice. The limitations of the self-regulatory system became strikingly apparent during the investigation into research on children at North Staffordshire Hospital. The Griffiths Inquiry found that, although the North Staffordshire REC generally operated in accordance with Department of Health Guidelines then in force, the level of detail in their minutes compared unsatisfactorily with minutes provided by a selection of other RECs to the review. Additionally, the computer-held register of research projects failed to include all the details required by the guidelines. The Inquiry also noted a lack of clarity in respect of how and when variations to a research project were to be reported.[80] Moreover, the LREC was criticised for doing little to ascertain whether its opinion was well informed or bore any relation to what other ethical review committees did or might have done in similar circumstances – increasingly this is regarded as a component of good practice (para. 9.2.2). A further concern related to the lack of training for members, with the Griffiths Inquiry finding that many members of the ethics committee had never been offered training.

These criticisms highlight the increasingly onerous duties entailed by membership of such committees. Thus, providing appropriate training for the members of RECs is a central plank of the current research governance framework for RECs. Para. 4.10 of the GAfREC guidance states that 'members have a need for initial and continuing education and training regarding research ethics, research methodology and research governance'. The North Staffordshire Inquiry also stressed that appointment of members should be an open process, compatible with Nolan standards and requiring public advertisement in the media as well as through professional networks, and the submission of CVs. On the composition of RECs, it proposed that among the recommended 12 to 18 members there should be a balanced age and gender distribution, while efforts should be made to recruit ethnic minorities and those with disabilities. Such proposals seek to address past criticism concerning the under-representation of lay people, and the fact that one British study found that women and ethnic minority groups were poorly reprsented.[81] The GAfREC guidance now stipulates that there should be a maximum of 18 members, of whom at least one third are lay members, but that it should have a 'sufficiently broad range of experience and expertise, so that the scientific, clinical and methodological aspects of a research proposal can be reconciled with the welfare of research participants, and with broader ethical implications'. It also specifies that the REC should be balanced in terms of gender and age, and make 'every effort' to recruit members from black and ethic minority backgrounds. The expert members should offer, *inter alia*, methodological and ethical expertise in clinical and non-clinical research, research methods applicable to health services, social science and social care research, statistics and pharmacy.[82]

Nurses who are members of RECs should also be aware of the possibility of legal action being taken against the decisions of RECs. Decisions may be judicially reviewed by the courts, and if RECs are found to have acted *ultra vires* or to have reached decisions irrationally or contrary to the rules of natural justice then decisions may be referred back to the committee or struck down.[83] No negligence action has been brought against an REC, and in the past they have been deemed not to have a legal personality distinct from their members (in the way a company has legal personality), so it was thought likely that any action would lie against individual members, who are under a legal duty to act with due care in decision-making (although strategic health authorities do offer indemnity when members are appointed to RECs provided they act in good faith).[84] McHale suggests that since RECs have been placed on a statutory footing under the Clinical Trials Regulations, there may now be the possibility of a finding in negligence against the REC itself.[85] However, as Jackson notes, in practice any persons harmed as a result of an REC decision are more likely to proceed against potential defendants with greater resources, such as the pharmaceutical company sponsoring the trial.[86]

Prior to the Griffiths Review and the new research governance framework, there had long been disquiet over variations in the practices of ethics committees, such as those exposed at North Staffordshire. Such variations resulted in part from the way in which trials tended to be scrutinised on a local rather than national basis. In 1996 the Department of Health recommended that regional bodies – multicentre research ethics committees (MRECs) – should be established to scrutinise research protocols that proposed to undertake a number of trials at different locations throughout the country. While this certainly has reduced variation in local rates of approval, since LRECs are required to state reasons if they reject a protocol approved by an MREC,[87] a cynical view is that they are a convenient way of enabling researchers and drug companies to gain approval for projects notwithstanding objections at a local level.[88] Conversely, some commentators have contended that the process for seeking MREC approval is overly complex, leading to costly delays in the process of marketing drugs.[89] It is also worth noting that with the growth of new biotechnologies, such as reproductive technologies, gene therapy and xenotransplantation, a proliferating number of committees have been established to oversee research, with consequent problems relating to the overlapping roles and functions of these various bodies.[90] In an effort to deal with this fragmentation, COREC was established in 2000 to co-ordinate the work of the various ethics committees, it was succeeded by a new National Research Ethics Service on 1 April 2007. The new research governance framework aims to eliminate variations and inconsistencies in practice. If, as expected, the recommendations of the Ad Hoc Advisory Committee on RECs are implemented, it is likely to effectively eliminate the distinction between MRECs and LRECs – leading in the view of some critics to a loss of sensitivity to local issues.[91]

A further concern about RECs relates to the inadequate resources they have to monitor research once the initial approval is granted. McNeil contends that RECs are typical of self-regulating groups in their failure to deal adequately with non-compliance,[92] especially if the researcher is not seeking overseas grants or publication in international journals.[93] Although the Declaration of Helsinki stresses the obligation on researchers to provide monitoring information to the ethical review committee and in particular to report adverse events (para. 13), there is generally no sanction for failure to do so. To address this, the Medical Research Council requires that applicants for funding include with their research protocol their plans to ensure independent supervision of the clinical trial. It recommends that a trial steering committee be set up, which should include at least one of the principal investigators conducting the research, and at least three independent members, one of whom would chair the committee. It would meet to approve the final protocol before the start of the trial, and thereafter at least annually to monitor the progress of the trial and to maximise the chances of its being completed within the agreed timescale.[94]

The Griffiths Inquiry also stressed the responsibility of research ethics committees to review past decisions and to ensure that good management processes are built into research proposals. In this regard, the Clinical Trials Directive highlights the importance of monitoring. If a Member State has objective grounds for considering that the conditions in the request for authorisation are no longer met, or has doubts about the safety or scientific validity of the clinical trial, it will have powers to suspend or prohibit the clinical trial, or inform those responsible for conducting the trial how to remedy the situation (Article 12). Member States are required to appoint investigators to inspect sites on which clinical trials are conducted (Article 15); they must report all serious adverse events (Article 16). These requirements are implemented in the Clinical Trials Regulations, which impose strict requirements for the prompt reporting of actual and suspected serious adverse events (regulations 32–5). In addition, the GAfREC guidance states that the research sponsor must ensure adequate mechanisms are in place to review significant developments as the research proceeds, and that RECS must require, as a minimum, an annual report from the researcher (para. 7.25–7). However, it remains to be seen whether these measures will constitute a meaningful form of monitoring, given Jackson's contention that '[w]hile progress reports must be submitted, the committee's role is largely confined to collecting information volunteered by the researchers, rather than investigating the extent to which there has been compliance with the original protocol'.[95] Moreover this absence of effective mechanisms for monitoring is coupled with a practice whereby RECs have approved over 90% of research proposals after asking the researchers to consider minor modifications.[96]

In the USA criticisms of the ethical review system led to the establishment of a National Bioethics Advisory Commission to provide advice and recommendations on the appropriateness of certain government policies and practices in bioethics, including principles for the ethical conduct of research.[97] Some commentators have called for a similar commission to be set up in the UK.[98] While such calls have to some extent been superseded at the supranational level by the requirement to implement the Clinical Trials Directive, it is worth noting that, notwithstanding its claims to enhance the protection of research subjects, the Directive has been criticised as industry-led and designed to promote Europe as a research location.[99] Moreover, other commentators have stressed the value of RECs having knowledge of local investigators, which is steadily being lost in the drive to centralise.[100]

12.3.3 Research fraud and deception

A further obstacle to ensuring accountability of researchers is that cases of deception and fraud have been reported with increasing frequency over the last 15 years.[101] A recent high-profile example is the scandal over stem cell scientist Woo Suk Hwang who faked data in cloning experiments in South Korea, which was exposed in 2005.[102] Since scarce funding leads to pressure to demonstrate results for money invested and to publish widely for career advancement, there is considerable temptation to falsify results in this way. Numerous prestigious journals have acknowledged the extent of research fraud.[103] Although the Royal College of Physicians has stressed the necessity of following good practice and indicated in 1991 the need for a body to investigate allegations of fraud, it is only recently that action has been taken on this proposal, with reports that Universities UK, the Department of Health and the NHS are working on a framework to establish a panel for research integrity.[104] In the meantime it is the threat of litigation that holds researchers accountable, although the establishment of the Committee on Publication Ethics (COPE) has led to increased pressure on editors of scientific journals to pursue allegations of research misconduct.[105] A more general problem with the system for publishing research is that articles are much more likely to secure publication if the conclusions are positive, so that published research provides only a very incomplete picture of research projects actually undertaken.[106]

12.4 Vulnerable groups of research subjects

Researchers must be sensitive to the fact that some groups of potential subjects may be particularly vulnerable to pressure to participate in clinical trials, either because of doubts regarding their competence to participate or because their situation means that vulnerability is exacerbated by institutional and attitudinal factors. Particular concerns have been raised regarding research on children or mentally incompetent adults, and it is widely recognised that these groups should be accorded special protection. A specific failing identified by the Griffiths Review at North Staffordshire was the lack of specific guidance to researchers on how valid consent is to be obtained in vulnerable groups. Too often it was simply assumed that researchers were aware of the useful guidance contained in the Royal College of Physicians' guidelines. Once again this highlights the need for researchers to be fully informed of their legal obligations and current professional guidance.

12.4.1 Children

Most clinical research is undertaken on competent adults. Indeed, the Nuremberg Code of 1947 and other early ethical guidance stressed that research should be carried out *only* on competent volunteers. However, in recognition of the different developmental, physiological and psychological differences in children, which make age- and development-related research important for their benefit, it is now generally accepted that children can participate in research protocols, provided strict safeguards are observed.[107] Clinical research involving child patients is important in the case of conditions that only or predominantly affect children, such as Duchenne muscular dystrophy, a rare single-gene disorder, which affects boys and typically results in death by the patient's late teens. The importance of research involving children has been highlighted recently in the wake of reports that nine out of ten drugs given to newborn babies and 50% of drugs prescribed for children of all ages have never been clinically tested on child subjects to ensure that that they are appropriate.[108] In recognition of the importance of adequate testing of drugs on children, the European commission has signalled its intention to promulgate legislation that would compel pharmaceutical companies to undertake appropriate research on children to ensure that their therapeutic needs are addressed.[109]

Guideline 14 of the CIOMS guidance provides that, prior to undertaking research involving children, the researcher must ensure that:

- the research might not equally well be carried out with adults;
- the purpose of the research is to obtain knowledge relevant to the health needs of children;
- a parent or legal representative of each child has given permission;
- the agreement (assent) of each child has been obtained to the extent of the child's capabilities;
- a child's refusal to participate in research will be respected.[110]

Thus, it seems that lawful research must relate to a condition from which the child suffers, must be designed to benefit that group, and there must be no alternative to the use of minors. Yet, beyond this, as Jackson notes, ethico-legal guidance remains inherently unclear. She suggests that it is misplaced to emphasise risk evaluation, rather than the burdens of participation, and that an assessment of the burdens should be weighed against the social benefits that may derive from involvement in research.[111]

Researchers should note that 'childhood' is a heterogeneous category and that it is important to take account of the different capabilities of children. Thus, older children who are capable of understanding the process, and better able to tolerate pain, should be selected ahead of younger children, unless there are significant age-related scientific reasons to include younger children. The Clinical Trials Directive stresses that minors should receive, from staff with experience with minors, information pertaining to the trial and its risks and benefits (Article 4(b)) – a condition implemented in the Clinical Trials Regulations.[112] As we saw in Chapter 10, English law permits a minor to consent to medical *treatment* if she is over 16 or is Gillick-competent. For some time it was unclear in English law how far this rule applied to research. The position has now been clarified by the 2004 Regulations, which define a minor as 'a person under the age of 16 years' (regulation 14). Thus, for a person younger than 16 the consent of her parents or legal representative (as defined in regulation 15) is necessary for participation in research to be lawful, regardless of whether she is Gillick-competent. The parent or legal representative should act on the basis of the minor's 'presumed will' under Article 4(a) of the Clinical Trials Directive. Thus a 'substituted judgement' test effectively replaces the Common Law test of best interests in this context. While the Directive prohibits anyone under 16 from consenting to involvement in research, it does provide that the explicit *refusal* of a minor to participate should be considered by the investigator, provided the minor is capable of assessing the information provided and refusing consent (Article 4(c)). The regulations explicitly rule out the offering of any financial inducement to the minor or those authorised to consent to her involvement.[113] Given the scope of these regulations, much will depend on how they are interpreted. Edwards and McNamee have suggested that professional guidance in the UK is generally too permissive of research.[114] For instance, they point out that the Royal College of Paediatrics and Child Health (RCPCH) guidance[115] seems to breach the requirement in the Declaration of Helsinki ruling out research that prioritises the interests of third parties over those of the research subject by stating that 'research in which children are submitted to more than minimal risk, with only slight, uncertain or no benefit to themselves deserves serious ethical consideration'. By contrast Haggar and Woods suggest that the Clinical Trials Directive and other guidance may be seen as unduly restrictive with regard to the participation of children.[116]

In practice, most research on young children and babies will involve routine interventions, such as taking blood samples. In such cases it is important that parents are informed clearly that the samples are for research purposes and can be refused without adverse consequences for the child's treatment.[117] In the case of more invasive interventions, the events at North Staffordshire indicated that particular obstacles to obtaining informed consent may be encountered in trials involving sick babies, given the emotional stress parents are likely to be under. Guidance issued as a result by the RCPCH suggests that in emergency situations (for example, where a newborn needs to be ventilated urgently), a form of provisional consent or agreement in principle should be sought by health professionals. This would allow options to be evaluated more fully after parents or legal representatives had had adequate time to reflect.[118]

12.4.2 The mentally incapacitated adult

Although incompetent adults clearly differ from children in many ways, similar issues are raised by proposals to carry out research on both groups. Once again the competence of the incapacitated person will have to be assessed carefully in relation to the particular procedure. As discussed in Chapter 7A, a patient may be competent to consent to one form of treatment but not to another. This applies equally in the research context.

The GMC guidance requires that the following criteria are met before a group of incompetent adults may participate in research:

it could be of direct benefit to their health;
it is of special benefit to the health of people in the same age group with the same state of health; or
that it will significantly improve the scientific understanding of the adult's incapacity leading to a direct benefit to them or to others with the same incapacity; and

the research is ethical and will not cause the participants emotional; physical or psychological harm; and

the person does not express objections, physically or verbally'.

Moreover, researchers must 'ensure that ... [a]ny sign of distress, pain or indication of refusal irrespective of whether or not it is given in a verbal form should be considered as implied refusal'.[119]

The CIOMS guidance stipulates that:

Before undertaking research involving individuals who by reason of mental or behavioural disorders are not capable of giving adequately informed consent, the investigator must ensure that

- such persons will not be subjects of research that might equally well be carried out on persons whose capacity to give adequately informed consent is not impaired;
- the purpose of the research is to obtain knowledge relevant to the particular health needs of persons with mental or behavioural disorders;
- the consent of each subject has been obtained to the extent of that person's capabilities, and a prospective subject's refusal to participate in research is always respected, unless, in exceptional circumstances, there is no reasonable medical alternative and local law permits overriding the objection; and,
- in cases where prospective subjects lack capacity to consent, permission is obtained from a responsible family member or a legally authorized representative in accordance with applicable law. (Guideline 15)

However, under English law, in contrast to the situation with children, there has until recently been no available proxy consent-giver for the incompetent adult, although, as we saw in Chapter 7A, according to the case of *F* v. *West Berkshire*, medical treatment could be provided on the grounds of necessity if it is in the patient's best interests.[120] F suggested that 'best interests' was to be judged by the health professional according to the *Bolam* test. However, recent cases have paid greater attention to human rights arguments in assessing best interests, and there are now compelling arguments that the *Bolam* test is a wholly inappropriate basis on which to determine whether an incompetent adult may be enrolled in a research project.[121] In the case of *Simms* v. *Simms*[122] Dame Elizabeth Butler-Sloss P was prepared to sanction the use of experimental treatment on two teenagers aged 16 and 18 who were suffering from Creutzfeldt–Jakob Disease (CJD) – a devastating brain disease, which had left them incapacitated. Clinical trials on animals suggested that the experimental drug had inhibited the progress of a similar disease in mice, but it was completely untested in humans. However, note the special conditions obtaining this case, where the disease was fatal, no cure or recognised treatment existed, and the parents wished the experimental regime to be instituted. The judge noted:

Where there is no alternative treatment available and the disease is progressive and fatal, it seems to me to be reasonable to consider experimental treatment with unknown benefits and risk, but without significant risk of increased suffering to the patient, in cases where there is some chance of benefit to the patient.[123]

Concerns over the uncertain legal position and the vulnerability of mentally incompetent adults led the Law Commission to propose that non-therapeutic research may be undertaken in certain situations but subject to additional safeguards. In particular, it suggested that any such proposal should be referred to a new mental incapacity research committee.[124] This proposal has been superseded by the enactment of the Clinical Trials Regulations 2004, which provide that for research on an incompetent adult to be lawful there must be 'grounds for expecting that administering the medicinal product to be tested in the trial will produce a benefit to the subject outweighing the risks or produce no risk at all' and that the clinical trial must be directly related 'to a life-threatening or debilitating clinical condition from which the subject suffers'.[125]

Under Article 5(a) of the Clinical Trials Directive, inclusion of an incapacitated person in research is permitted only if the informed consent of the person's legal representative is obtained, and, as in the case of enrolling children in research, this must be done on the basis of the 'presumed will' of the incapacitated person. This is the first time that proxy decision-making has been allowed in respect of health-related decisions for adults in the UK. Under Article 18 of the Clinical Trials Regulations, the legal representative may be a person who is 'suitable to act as the legal representative by virtue of their relationship with the [incapacitated] adult', who is unconnected with the trial. If no suitable person is available then the doctor primarily responsible for the person's treatment or a person nominated by the health care provider can be appointed as the professional legal representative. Doubts, however, have been raised about the adequacy of the system of legal representatives in protecting patient interests, especially as it seems in practice to rely on a form of 'fictionalised consent'.[126]

Yet, in theory at least, the involvement of the incompetent person in clinical research is tightly circumscribed. As 'clinical trial' is defined very broadly in Article 2 of the Clinical Trials Regulations,[127] these regulations will encompass most forms of clinical research. However, for any non-medical research that falls outside the 2004 regulations, such as psychological studies, sections 30–31 of the Mental Capacity Act 2005 apply.[128] These also provide that a number of conditions must be satisfied. However, as Pattinson notes, the conditions imposed by the 2005 Act are slightly more permissive than those contained in the 2004 regulations. The Act stipulates that the research must have the potential to benefit the participant or others with her condition and must pose no more than minimal risk, whereas the 2004 regulations require the research to be therapeutic or to carry *no* risk.[129] The 2005 Act seems more in line with the Convention on Human Rights and Biomedicine, which stipulates that non-therapeutic research on the incapacitated may exceptionally be carried out, provided that it entails only minimal risks and burdens for the individual concerned and has the aim of contributing:

through significant improvement in the scientific understanding of the individual's condition, disease or disorder to the ultimate attainment of results capable of conferring benefit on the person concerned or other persons in the same age category or afflicted with the same disease or disorder or having the same condition. (Article 17).

Thus, as in the case of children it can be debated whether the applicable regulations are too restrictive or too liberal.

12.4.3 Other vulnerable groups

Researchers should be conscious of the fact that other potential subject groups may feel under particular pressure to participate in research, not through doubts about their competence, but because their circumstances render them vulnerable. Nurses will typically carry out research on patients who may feel compelled to participate out of a sense of obligation to the health professionals treating them. Similar considerations apply to medical and nursing students. Great care must be taken to explain rights to refuse or withdraw consent when research is proposed for these groups.

Caution may also be necessary when enrolling pregnant women, or women of child-bearing age, in view of the possible effects on the fetus should the research subject be or become pregnant.[130] However, it is controversial to label these women as 'vulnerable', and it is equally important that women should not be excluded from research protocols, as discussed in section 12.4.5.

12.4.4 Inducements and conflicts of interest

When recruiting members of vulnerable groups for clinical research, it is important that RECs examine how far the subject may be influenced by financial inducements. The GMC guidance states that doctors must 'not offer payments at a level which could induce research participants to take risks that they would otherwise not take, or to volunteer more frequently than is advisable or against their better interests or judgement' (para. 14). Yet, in media coverage of the Northwick Park trial discussed above, it has emerged that payments in the UK routinely breach this guideline, and that certain individuals repeatedly 'volunteer' for enrolment in clinical trials.

Aside from inducements for subjects to enter trials, health care professionals also need to ensure that inducements or perks from drug companies sponsoring trials do not influence how they present benefits to potential participants. In 2000 it was reported that the outgoing editor of the prestigious *Journal of the American Medical Association* had called for restrictions on stock ownership and other financial incentives for researchers, claiming that growing conflicts of interests were tainting scientific research.[131] That this is regarded as a pressing ethical concern is reflected in the revised Declaration of Helsinki, which hitherto had been silent on the need for transparency about economic incentives in research. It now provides that all possible conflicts of interest should be disclosed (para. 22; see section 12.2.3). In its 2000 guidance, the Medical Research Council points to the potential conflicts of interest, where a researcher's scientific judgement could be unduly influenced by financial gain or personal, academic or political advancement. It recommends that researchers should automatically ask themselves,

'Would I feel comfortable if others learn about my secondary interest in this matter or perceived that I had one?' If the answer is negative, that signals that the interest must be disclosed and addressed according to the appropriate policies established by employers, peer review bodies or journals.[132]

12.4.5 The pool of available research subjects

Given the historical emphasis on protecting research subjects, the exclusion of potential subjects from consideration for clinical protocols has only recently been identified as a significant bioethical issue. Such concern signalled a paradigm shift in how enrolment in clinical trials had come to be viewed.[133] While research on human subjects was initially perceived as a necessary aspect of public health, and then as a transgression of individual rights, in some cases tantamount to torture, it has since the 1980s increasingly come to be regarded as an avenue of access to better medical care. This shift was largely prompted by the thalidomide and DES drug disasters, which led to criticisms of the policy of excluding pregnant women from trials, given the catastrophic impact of these drugs on children born to women who took them during pregnancy.[134] As noted above, pregnant women have historically been categorised as a vulnerable group, and as a result, guidance issued to researchers has in the past, explicitly excluded certain women from biomedical research if they were pregnant or of child-bearing age. Such exclusions raise important questions pertaining to autonomy and justice. While the justifications for explicit exclusions are generally couched in the rhetoric of protecting women and their unborn children, it is more likely to be attributable to fears of legal liability for any teratogenic impact on the unborn child. However, Merton has argued convincingly that such fears are more apparent than real, since no successful claim has been brought and a proper warning of known and unknown risks would in all probability extinguish the strict liability claims of both subjects and their children for either pre-natal or preconceptual harm.[135]

Explicit exclusions are now rare, and in the UK the GAfREC guidelines require ethics committees to have regard to 'the characteristics of the population from which the research participants will be drawn (including gender, age, literacy, culture, economic status and ethnicity)', how the participants were contacted and recruited, and the inclusion and exclusion criteria applied.[136] Certainly, excluding women from research may ultimately be a more dangerous legal stance; pharmaceutical researchers in particular leave themselves open to litigation by omitting women, given that their products are then aggressively marketed to women. The CIOMS guidance does advise, though, that 'a thorough discussion of risks to the pregnant woman and to her fetus is a prerequisite for the woman's ability to make a rational decision to enrol in a clinical study' (guideline 16).

The second factor responsible for changing the way in which clinical trials are viewed has been the HIV/AIDS pandemic, which has further politicised the field of clinical research. Patients with these conditions have campaigned for just allocation of access to research and have characterised clinical trials as treatment when there is no proven treatment for a medical condition (thereby further blurring the dichotomy between research and therapy, noted at the beginning of this chapter).

Stimulated by these developments, patients with other diseases, notably breast cancer and Alzheimer's disease, and their advocates, have become more vocal about access to experimental drugs and treatments and have asserted the right to participate in trials. Consequently, being a research subject is no longer viewed as an unqualified sacrifice – rather it is seen as a potentially risky opportunity. The upshot is that researchers, long sensitised to the need for protection of research subjects, must now also focus on the need to include individuals and groups. In recognition of this, guideline 12 of the CIOMS guidance states that 'groups or communities should be selected in such a way that the burdens and benefits of the research will be equally distributed. The exclusion of groups or communities that might benefit from study participation must be justified'. The commentary on this guideline stresses the injustice involved in overusing certain populations, such as the poor or the administratively convenient.

All researchers should thus bear in mind the need for increased efforts to recruit certain populations, including patients with AIDS, minorities, the elderly[137] and women. This constitutes one aspect of good experimental design of a research protocol, as well as fulfilling the general ethical obligation of fairness or justice.

12.4.6 Review of research and compensation

Until 2004 if a clinical trial was approved by a REC, then the conduct of that research was largely left up to the research team and there were limited possibilities for review. A research subject injured as a result of defective drugs or surgical appliances can theoretically bring an action under the Consumer Protection Act 1987, arguing that a defective product was supplied. However, it is likely that researchers could successfully invoke the 'state of the art' defence, i.e. that any defects in the product were not ascertainable given the state of scientific knowledge when it was marketed. Prospects of a successful negligence claim are also low, since negligence actions will probably fail if a properly conducted research programme had been approved by a REC and carried out in accordance with a responsible body of professional opinion, although in exceptional circumstances negligence claims have succeeded.[138]

Although we have seen that the 2004 Clinical Trials Regulations offer greater scope for monitoring and oversight once projects are approved, the difficulties in pursuing a legal remedy for harm suffered as a result of participation in clinical trials has focused attention on mechanisms for compensating those who suffer harm. There is no formal legal requirement that participants in research should be indemnified. Association of British Pharmaceutical Industry guidelines do provide that where commercial companies sponsor research they should give contractually binding guarantees to healthy volunteers if they should be injured, but these guidelines are not mandatory.[139] In recognition of the inadequate protection given to volunteers in clinical research, the Pearson Commission recommended years ago that 'any volunteer for medical research who suffers severe damage as a result should have a cause of action, on the basis of strict liability, against the authority to whom he has consented to make himself available'.[140] Unfortunately no government has implemented this proposal.[141] The possibility of a major claim for compensation is particularly likely in the case of new chemical compounds such as those used in the Northwick Park case described above. The interim findings of the Medicines and Healthcare products Regulatory Agency (MHRA) suggested that the severe immune reaction in this case was occasioned not by human error but the way in which genetically engineered monoclonal anti-bodies in TGN1412 acted on the immune cells of the human body – something that could not have been predicted in prior animal studies.[142] Like various bio-technologies, these 'super-antibodies' may pose serious safety concerns. The issue of how very hazardous risks, which are difficult to estimate with any degree of certainty, should be presented to research subjects is also raised in the following case study on xenotransplantation. While the EU Clinical Trials Directive now requires that ethics committees take into account the provision for indemnity or compensation in the event of injury or death when deciding whether to approve a clinical trial (Article 6(h)), concerns have been expressed about how adequate the insurance of the German pharmaceutical company – TeGenero – that created TGN1412 is.[143]

A further related source of controversy relates to health care provided in the aftermath of clinical trials. As noted above, one incentive to enrol in a clinical trial is its perception as an avenue to high quality medical care, but this raises ethical issues about the care of patients once their involvement in research is complete. Such concerns have been particularly acute where pharmaceutical companies withdraw from developing countries after the completion of a clinical trial.[144]

12.5 Case study: participating in biotechnological research projects – xenotransplantation trials

As new biotechnologies are developed, new ethical and legal dilemmas are raised for researchers. An example is offered by xenotransplantation, which potentially gives rise to incalculable risks.[145] Xenotransplantation may be defined simply as the transplant of tissue between species. Most attention to date has centred on the transplant of whole animal organs (such as hearts, kidneys and livers) into humans. Biotechnology companies are currently breeding genetically engineered pigs, which are viewed as a likely source of these organs. The ethics and safety of xenotransplantation was considered in two major reports in the mid-1990s.[146] Both concluded that xenotransplantation, using pigs as source animals, was an ethically acceptable solution to the chronic human organ shortage, although it was not deemed safe at that point to proceed to clinical trials involving humans given the huge risks the technology posed. Instead, the use of primates (effectively as 'surrogate' humans) was endorsed.

The major risk identified is that diseases will spread from the pig source to the recipient and possibly the wider population. Until December 2006, any decision to proceed to human trials had to be approved by the Xenotransplantation Interim Regulatory Authority established on the recommendation of the Depart-ment of Health review of this technology (the Kennedy Report). However, in December 2006 UKIXRA was disbanded and clinical trials of Xenotransplants will now be overseen by RECs or the Gene Therapy Advisory Committee (GTAC). In cases where the Xenogenic product is genetically modified.

Even if REC/GTAC approval were to be granted, questions remain concerning the role of health professionals involved in such trials. As with enrolment in most clinical trials, the crucial issue will be obtaining valid consent. However, xeno-transplantation raises particular problems over and above the general difficulties of obtaining informed consent. In the first place, potential recipients of pig tissue are in an especially difficult situation, where it is questionable whether their deci-sion to enter clinical trials actually represents an informed choice. If a particular class of patients realises that the only alternatives to enrolling in a potentially haz-ardous clinical trial are the slim chance of obtaining a suitable organ, or death, the likelihood is that they will be willing to take that risk regardless of the hazards it creates for them or others.

Secondly, as this is an entirely new procedure, it is arguably not possible to assess the inherent risks with any degree of accuracy. In general, little is known about pig diseases, but the history of animal–human viruses lends plausibility to the view that xenotransplantation offers a unique opportunity for prion-type diseases to jump the species barrier. This is particularly so given that, in the case of xenotransplantation, source animals are genetically engineered with human genes. Two problems arise. The first is the practical difficulty posed by the Kennedy Report's suggestion that huge amounts of information would have to be given to research subjects. It proposes that for an informed decision to be given, potential recipients should be given information regarding the psychological and social effects of xenotransplantation, the source of tissue, breeding conditions and animal suffering, as well as genetic implications.[147] It is highly questionable that many patients are equipped to fully assimilate and evaluate such quantities of information.

A still more fundamental problem is whether individual recipients should be able to consent to a procedure that has the potential to unleash unsuspected hazards on the broader population. How should this sort of risk be explained to a potential participant in a clinical trial? Additionally, given these risks, those who enrol in the first trials to be authorised must submit to surveillance and mon-itoring of their movements.[148] This gives rise to problems about how to present potentially very intrusive interferences with civil liberties (including the right to reproduce) to potential research subjects.

Xenotransplantation thus highlights the need for fuller consideration to be given to the adequacy of counselling and information provision when subjects are enrolled in clinical trials, especially where the research concerns new technolog-ies or genetically engineered compounds like TGNI421 and there is no existing or adequate way of treating the disease.[149]

This case study also raises concerns over how an effective system of scrutiny and accountability may be implemented, especially when a number of commit-tees with potentially overlapping remits exist to regulate this procedure.[150] It is somewhat unclear whether xenotransplant trials would fall within the scope of the Clinical Trials Regulations, but Beyleveld, Finnegan and Pattinson suggest that these would probably apply only to trials that involve the use of a new phar-maceutical and/or gene therapy/somatic cell therapy in addition to the transfer of organs or tissue.[151] A final issue raised by xenotransplantation is that, should the worst fears of its opponents be realised, a crucial factor is who should bear the costs of compensating victims and paying for their health care, particularly if a major new disease is unleashed on the broader population.

12.6 Conclusions

As will be apparent from the above review, the law regulating nursing research has traditionally been somewhat vague and, in the view of many commentators, loaded in favour of a pro-research agenda. In the early years of the twenty-first century, however, public concerns about many forms of research and the growing role of the European Union in regulating clinical trials,[152] combined with a political agenda that promotes research governance, has begun to impact significantly on this field. Nevertheless, it is somewhat early to judge what effect this will have on the practice of clinical research. As we have seen, some commentators see the main objective of European legislation as establishing Europe as a competitive research site rather than improving the protection of research subjects. Others point to bureaucratic inconvenience, associated costs and lengthy delays in the process of approving new treatments, which makes the conduct of trials especially difficult where they are not backed by large pharmaceutical companies.[153]

Concerns continue to be expressed about the adequacy of new monitoring arrangements and the heavy reliance on concepts such as consent and risk, which are difficult to define or judge with precision. Moreover, new arrangements aimed at protecting the interests of the incompetent and children rely on an assumption that legal representatives can second-guess what individuals would have wanted. The Griffiths Report has highlighted how, in the past, considerable disparity existed between best practice and the formal guidance available, which left considerable scope for individual latitude in how particular projects were managed. Even with more robust research governance arrangements, it will be difficult to ensure that guidance is always observed. The remit and workload of RECs is steadily increasing, leading to concerns about a loss of quality in decision-making and increased bureaucracy.

Additionally, regulation in this area remains in a state of flux. The controversial proposals contained in the Department of Health's Ad Hoc Advisory Group on RECs are likely to result in far-reaching proposals, which look set to streamline and professionalise RECs. Not only may this signal a move from the traditional dependence on volunteers and responsivity to local conditions but, arguably, it may compromise significantly the independence of RECs and subject them to greater political control, in addition to imposing accountability.

Another important and problematic aspect of the current regulatory framework is the proliferation of various forms of guidance governing a range of clinical research practices on different subjects. As demonstrated above, the tensions that exist between the numerous legal, professional and international guidelines means that, against a backdrop of growing public scepticism about clinical research, the researcher has to negotiate a complex web of regulations, which are often vague and in some cases contradictory.

As we have seen, the development of new technologies and synthetic compounds, coupled with the manner in which clinical research is increasingly dependent on private funding by pharmaceutical firms rather than government and academia, has raised new safety concerns and prompted calls for tighter regulation.[154] However, notwithstanding various doubts about the new regulatory mechanisms, and the changing nature of the research they seek to control, it is certainly the case that there is now considerable impetus (regardless of the motivations for it) to ensure that good clinical practice is observed in the conduct of research. In the meantime, the onus, as ever, is on researchers to be as truthful and clear as possible in their communications with participants about the risks and benefits of proposed research programmes, and to ensure that participants' interests are prioritised over those of society, medicine or professional advancement.

12.7 Acknowledgement

I would like to thank Jean McHale for her helpful comments on an earlier draft.

12.8 Notes and references

1. Department of Health, *Towards a Strategy for Nursing Research and Development: Proposals for Action, Department of Health* (Department of Health, London, 2000), p. 2; A. Kitson, A. McMahon, A. Rafferty & E. Scott, On developing an agenda to influence policy in health related research for effective nursing: a description of a national R&D priority setting exercise, *Nursing Times Research*, **2** (1997), p. 323.
2. Department of Health, *Making a Difference: Strengthening the Nursing, Midwifery and Health Visiting Contribution to Health and Health Care* (London, Department of Health, 1999).
3. N. Fletcher, J. Holt, M. Brazier & J. Harris, *Ethics, Law and Nursing* (Manchester, Manchester University Press, 1995), p. 185.
4. Ferguson's research has highlighted the paucity of relevant legal knowledge on the part of clinical researchers – see P. Ferguson, Legal and ethical aspects of clinical trials: the views of researchers. *Medical Law Review*, **11** (2003), pp. 48–69.
5. Royal College of Nursing, *Research Ethics: RCN Guidance for Nurses* (London, RCN, 2004).
6. M. Fox, Animal rights and wrongs: medical ethics and the killing of non-human animals. In R. Lee & D. Morgan (eds), *Death Rites: Law and Ethics at the End of Life* (London, Routledge, 1994).
7. See J. McHale and M. Fox, Health Care Law: Text and Materials, 2nd edn, 2007, London, Sweet & Maxwell, at pp. 725–37.
8. This has proven controversial in the context of suspected abuse of child patients by parents. For instance, in a review of research practices at North Staffordshire Hospital in the 1990s, considerable controversy was generated by covert video surveillance of parents suspected of abuse and the question of whether this constituted a research programme. A Review Group set up to inquire into the events recommended that the Department of Health should issue guidance to aid professionals in the identification of such abuse. See NHS Executive West Midlands Regional Office, Report of a Review of the Research Framework in North Staffordshire Hospital NHS Trust (The Griffiths

Review), para. 12.4.1. In this regard, Guideline 10 of the Council for International Organisations of Medical Sciences (CIOMS) International Guidelines for Biomedical Research Involving Human Subjects (2000) proposes that an ethical review committee must approve all research where there is an intention to deceive, and specify that the researcher must demonstrate that no other research method would suffice – see commentary on Guideline 10, http://www.cioms.ch/guidelines.html (accessed 10 April 2006). The CIOMS was formed in 1949 under the auspices of the WGO and UNESCO to promote biomedical research and offer international guidance.

9. This distinction was derived from earlier formulations of the Declaration of Helsinki – see J. Montgomery, Law and ethics in international trials, in C. Williams (ed.), *Introducing New Treatments for Cancer* (Chichester, Wiley, 1992).

10. British Medical Association, *Consent, Rights and Choices in Health Care for Children and Young People* (London, BMJ Books, 2001), pp. 207–11.

11. R. Whyte, Clinical trials, consent and the doctor–patient contract, *Health Law in Canada*, **15** (1994), p. 50; C. Grady, *Review of the Search for An AIDS Vaccine: Ethical Issues in the Development and Testing of a Preventive HIV Vaccine* (Indiana, Indiana University Press, 1995).

12. P. Alderson, Did children change or the guidelines? *Bulletin of Medical Ethics*, **150** (1999), pp. 38–44 at p. 40, cited in BMA, *Consent, Rights and Choices in Health Care for Children and Young People* (London, BMJ Books, 2001), p. 185.

13. See note 18 below.

14. H. Brody and F.G. Miller, The clinical-investigator: unavoidable but manageable tension. *Kennedy Institute of Ethics Journal*, **13** (2003), pp. 329–46.

15. S.D. Edwards & J. McNamee, Ethical concerns regarding guidelines on the conduct of clinical research on children, *Journal of Medical Ethics*, **31** (2005), pp. 351–4 at p. 354.

16. I. Oakeshott & L. Rogers, 'Earlier trials had shown that drug group was highly toxic', *Sunday Times*, 19 March 2006; M. Goodyear, Learning from the TGN1412 trial. *British Medical Journal*, **332** (2006), pp. 677–8; J. Revill, 'Drug trial firm knew of risk', *The Observer*, 9 April 2006; C. Dyer, J. Carvel & P. Curtis, 'Victims could lose out after doubts about insurance cover', *The Guardian*, 17 April 2006.

17. Declaration of Helsinki, amended 2000, with clarification 2002 and 2004, http://www.wma.net/e/policyb3.htm (accessed 17 April 2006).

18. Although the Nazi and Japanese experiments during World War II overshadow all subsequent abusive medical research on humans, other infamous examples include the Tuskegee experiments in 1932–72, which used black males to determine the natural course of syphilis, even though the treatment had existed for centuries (see J. Jones, *Bad blood: The Tuskegee Syphilis Experiment* (New York, The Free Press, 1981)); experiments to test radiation as a therapy carried out in the US until the early 1970s (see P. McNeil, *The Ethics and Politics of Human Experimentation*, Cambridge, Cambridge University Press, chapter 1); and HIV research on prostitute women in the Phillipines in the 1980s (see L. Laurence & B. Weinhouse, *Outrageous Practices: How Gender Bias Threatens Women's Health* (New Brunswick, Rutgers University Press, 1994/7), pp. 23–4). For other examples, see BMA, *The Medical Profession and Human Rights: Handbook for a Changing Agenda* (London, Zed Books, 2001), chapter 9.

19. J. Harris, Research on human subjects, exploitation, and global principles of ethics. In M. Freeman & A. Lewis (eds), *Law and Medicine: Current Issues* (Oxford, Oxford University Press, 2000), vol. 3; E. Jackson, *Medical Law: Text, Cases and Materials* (Oxford, Oxford University Press, 2006), pp. 513–21.

20. Royal College of Physicians (RCP), *Guidelines on the Practice of Ethics Committees in Medical Research Involving Human Subjects*, 3rd edn (London, RCP, 1996).

21. Royal College of Nursing, *Research Ethics: RCN Guidance for Nurses* (London, RCN, 2004).
22. Central Office for Research Ethics Committees (COREC), *Governance Arrangements for NHS Research Ethics Committees* (London, Department of Health, 2001).
23. See chapter 5 of the Convention for the articles governing scientific research. The full text of the Convention, and additional protocols is available at http://www.coe.fr/eng/legaltxt/164e.htm (last visited 17 April 2006).
24. *Consent in the Criminal Law*, Law Commission Consultation Paper No. 139, paras 8.38–8.52 (London, The Stationery Office).
25. S. Graham, 'Johns Hopkins leads changes in human studies process', *Baltimore Business Journal*, 19 July 2002. Various criticisms were made of the ethical review process by an internal investigation, although no major flaws in the trial design were found. Similar concerns were raised by a clinical trial into an experimental drug to treat Hepatitis B conducted by the National Institutes for Health in 1993 where five patient volunteers died after the drug proved toxic in humans – S. Levine, 'Five patients die of liver failure in NIH Hepatitis B drug rrial', *Washington Post*, 31 July 2001.
26. M. Brazier, *Medicine, Patients and the Law*, 3rd edn (Harmondsworth Penguin, 2003), p. 398.
27. C. Miller, Protection of human subjects of research in Canada, *Health Law Review*, 4 (1995), p. 8.
28. J.W. Berg, Legal and ethical complexities of consent with cognitively impaired research subjects: proposed guidelines, *Journal of Law, Medicine and Ethics*, 24 (1996), p. 18.
29. Nursing & Midwifery Council, *Code of Professional Conduct: Standards for Conduct, Performance and Ethics* (2004), para. 3.1.
30. P. McNeil, *The Ethics and Politics of Human Experimentation* (Cambridge, CUP, 1993), chapter 1.
31. See I. Kennedy, The law and ethics of informed consent and randomized controlled trials, in I. Kennedy, *Treat Me Right* (Oxford, OUP, 1989). Moreover, as discussed in Chapter 7A of this book, even in the context of medical treatment the Sidaway standard of disclosure seems to have been modified by subsequent cases to require much fuller answers to questions.
32. In 1965 the Saskatchewan Court of Appeal held that the subject should be informed of 'all the facts, probabilities and opinions that a reasonable man might be expected to consider before giving his consent'. See *Haluska* v. *University of Saskatchewan* (1965) 53 DLR 2d, 436, 444 per Mr Justice Hall.
33. General Medical Council, *Research: The Role and Responsibilities of Doctors* (London, GMC, 2002), available from www.gmc-uk.org/standards (accessed 17 April 2006).
34. M. Bassiouni, T. Baffes & J. Evrard, An appraisal of human experimentation in international law and practice: the need for international regulation of human experimentation. *Journal of Criminal Law and Criminology*, 72:1597 (1981), pp. 1611–12.
35. For instance, Beecher has argued that the subject's truly informed consent cannot be obtained since the results of experiments are not known beforehand, so that there is no norm for the conduct of a 'pure scientific experiment' – see H. Beecher, Research and the individual, *Human Studies*, 5 (1970).
36. J.S. Tobias, BMJ's present policy (sometimes approving research in which patients have not given fully informed consent) is wholly correct, *British Medical Journal*, 314 (1997), p. 1111.
37. E. Jackson, *Medical Law: Text, Cases and Materials* (Oxford, Oxford University Press, 2006), p. 493.

38. P. McNeil, *The Ethics and Politics of Human Experimentation* (Cambridge, Cambridge University Press, 1993), p. 135.
39. Directive 2001/20/EC of the European Parliament and of the Council of 4 April 2001.
40. For more detail on the regulatory system for licensing medicines, see E. Jackson, *Medical Law: Text, Cases and Materials* (Oxford, Oxford University Press, 2006), chapter 9; H. Teff, Products liability, in A. Grubb, *Principles of Medical Law*, 2nd edn (985–1024, 2004), pp. 985–1024; K. Mullan, *Pharmacy Law and Practice* (London, Blackstone Press, 2000), chapter 4.
41. 'GPs failing to report drug side-effects', *Independent on Sunday*, 15 April 2001; see also S. Bosley, 'Doctors urged to be more vigilant over drugs' side-effects', *The Guardian*, 12 May 2006.
42. P. McNeil, *The Ethics and Politics of Human Experimentation* (Cambridge, Cambridge University Press, 1993), p. 13.
43. R. Morehouse, Dilemmas of the clinical researcher: a view from the inside, *Health Law in Canada*, **15** (1994), pp. 52–3.
44. I. Kennedy, The law and ethics of informed consent and randomized controlled trials. In I. Kennedy, *Treat Me Right* (Oxford, Oxford University Press, 1989).
45. See M. Fox, Research bodies: feminist perspectives on clinical research. In S. Sheldon & M. Thomson (eds), *Feminist Perspectives in Health Care Law* (London, Cavendish, 1998).
46. J. Katz, Human experimentation and human rights, *Saint Louis University Law Journal*, **38**:7 (1993), p. 35.
47. R. Morehouse, Dilemmas of the clinical researcher: a view from the inside, *Health Law in Canada*, **15** (1994), p. 52. Royal College of Physicians guidelines suggest that the subject should be told the purpose, procedures, risk (including distress) and benefits (including to others), informed that she may decline to participate or withdraw at any time, and given a statement about compensation for injury. *Guidelines on the Practice of Ethics Committees in Medical Research Involving Human Subjects*, 3rd edn (London, RCP, 1996).
48. See, for example, P. Bowden, *Caring: Gender-Sensitive Ethics* (London, Routledge, 1997), chapter 4.
49. See note 8 above.
50. General Medical Council, paras 17–18; see note 33 above.
51. Medical Research Council, *Guidelines for Good Practice in Clinical Trials*, para. 5.4.6 (London, Medical Research Council, 1998).
52. See Helsinki Declaration, para. 22 – see note 9 above.
53. See J. McHale, Guidelines for medical research: some ethical and legal problems, *Medical Law Review*, **1** (1993), p. 167.
54. See, for instance, MRC, *Guidelines for Good Practice in Clinical Trials* (London, Medical Research Council, 1998), p. 3.
55. G. Rawlings, Ethics and regulation in randomised controlled trials of therapy. In A. Grubb (ed.), *Challenges in Medical Care* (Chichester, Wiley, 1992), pp. 41–2.
56. A. Oakley, Who's afraid of the randomized controlled trial. In H. Roberts (ed.), *Women's Health Counts* (London, Routledge, 1990).
57. N. Fletcher, J. Holt, M. Brazier & J. Harris, *Ethics, Law and Nursing* (Manchester, Manchester University Press, 1995), p. 187.
58. A. Oakley, Experiments in Knowing: Gender and Method in the Social Sciences (New York, The Free Press, 2000), p. 287.
59. J.S. Tobias, BMJ's present policy (sometimes approving research in which patients have not given fully informed consent) is wholly correct, *British Medical Journal*, **314** (1997), 1111.

60. I. Kennedy, The law and ethics of informed consent and randomized controlled trials. In I. Kennedy, *Treat Me Right* (Oxford, Oxford University Press, 1989).
61. See note 8 above.
62. Griffiths Review, para. 9.3.5 (see note 8 above).
63. See further the discussion of whistle-blowing in Chapter 8A of this volume.
64. See note 8 above.
65. F.G. Miller & H. Brody, What makes placebo-controlled trials unethical? *American Journal of Bioethics*, **2** (2002), pp. 3–7.
66. Council for International Organizations of Medical Sciences, *International Ethical Guidelines for Biomedical Research Involving Human Subjects*, Guideline 11 (Geneva, CIOMS, 2002), p. 287.
67. Bristol Royal Infirmary Inquiry, the Inquiry into the management of care of children receiving heart surgery at the Bristol Royal Infirmary, *Interim Report: Removal and Retention of Human Material*, May 2000; The Royal Liverpool Children's Inquiry, 30 January 2001. See M. Brazier, Human tissue retention. *Medico-legal Journal*, **72** (2004), p. 39.
68. For discussion of the specific/generic consent issue see O. O'Neill, Some limits of informed consent, *Journal of Medical Ethics*, **29** (2003), pp. 4–7.
69. For further detail see Chapter 7A of this volume, and D. Price, The Human Tissue Act 2004, *Modern Law Review*, **68** (2005), pp. 798–821.
70. Human Tissue Authority, *Code of Practice: Consent, Code 1* (London, HTA, 2006).
71. Central Office for Research Ethics Committees (COREC) (now NRES), *Governance Arrangements for Research Ethics Committees* (London, Department of Health, 2001) [hereafter GAfREC guidance].
72. J. Black, Constitutionalising self regulation, *Modern Law Review*, **59** (1996), pp. 24–56.
73. S. Kerrison & A.M. Pollock, The reform of UK research ethics committees: throwing the baby out with the bath water? *Journal of Medical Ethics*, **31**, (2005), pp. 487–9.
74. Department of Health, *Report of the Ad Hoc Advisory Group on the Operation of NHS Research Ethics Committees* (2005) [hereafter Ad Hoc Advisory Group report]. Available from COREC at http://www.corec.org.uk (accessed 12 April 2006). For a critique of these proposals, see A.J. Dawson, The Ad Hoc Advisory Group's proposals for research ethics committees: a mixture of the timid, the revolutionary and the bizarre, *Journal of Medical Ethics*, **31** (2005), pp. 435–6.
75. See Association of Research Ethics Committees (AREC), *AREC Council Response to Implementing the recommendation of the AD Hoc Advisory Group on the Operation of NHS Research Ethics Committees: a consultation* (London, AREC, 2006).
76. Ad Hoc Advisory Group Report – see note 74 above.
77. A.J. Dawson, The Ad Hoc Advisory Group's proposals for research ethics committees: a mixture of the timid, the revolutionary and the bizarre, *Journal of Medical Ethics*, **31** (2005), pp. 435–6.
78. See note 71 above.
79. S. Kerrison & A.M. Pollock, The reform of UK research ethics committees: throwing the baby out with the bath water? *Journal of Medical Ethics*, **31** (2005), pp. 487–9.
80. See note 8 above.
81. J. Neuberger, *Ethics and Health Care: The Role of Research Ethics Committees in the United Kingdom* (London, King's Fund Institute, 1992).
82. See note 71 above. For more detailed discussion of the role of, and decision-making processes, employed by RECS, see E. Gerrard & A. Dawson, What is the role of the research ethics committee? Paternalism, inducements, and harm in research ethics. *Journal of Medical Ethics*, **3** (2005), pp. 419–23.
83. J.V. McHale, Guidelines for medical research: some ethical and legal problems, *Medical Law Review*, **1** (1993), pp. 160–86.

84. M. Brazier, Liability of ethics committees and their members, *Professional Negligence*, **6** (1990), p. 186.

85. J. McHale, Clinical research. In A. Grubb, (ed.) *Principles of Medical Law*, 2nd edn (Oxford, Oxford University Press, 2004), pp. 907–8; see also the discussion in the letters page of *The Guardian* – D. Laurence, 'Ethics committees and drugs trials', 2 May 2006, and M. Levis, 'Limits of liability', 12 May 2006.

86. E. Jackson, *Medical Law: Text, Cases and Materials* (Oxford, Oxford University Press, 2006), p. 521.

87. Though see P. Glasziou & I. Chambers, Ethics review roulette: what can we learn? *British Medical Journal*, **328** (2004), p. 121.

88. K. Alberti, Multi-centre research ethics committees: has the cure been worse than the disease? *British Medical Journal*, **320** (2000), p. 1157.

89. N.R. Dunn, A. Arscott & R.D. Mann, Costs of seeking ethics committee approval before and after the introduction of multicentre research ethics committee, *Journal of the Royal Society of Medicine*, **93** (2000), pp. 511–12; K. Jamrozik, Research ethics paperwork: what is the plot we seem to have lost? *British Medical Journal*, **329** (2004), pp. 286–7.

90. M. Fox & J. McHale, Xenotransplantation: The Ethical and Legal Ramifications. *Medical Law Review*, **6** (1998), pp. 42–61.

91. *AREC Council Response to Implementing the Recommendation of the AD Hoc Advisory Group on the Operation of NHS Research Ethics Committees: A Consultation* (London, AREC, 2006).

92. P. McNeil, *The Ethics and Politics of Human Experimentation* (Cambridge University Press, 1993), p. 10.

93. P. McNeil, *The Ethics and Politics of Human Experimentation* (Cambridge University Press, 1993), p. 110.

94. Medical Research Council, *Guidelines for Good Practice in Clinical Trials* (London, MRC, 1998), chapter 6 and appendix 3.

95. E. Jackson, *Medical Law: Text, Cases and Materials* (Oxford, Oxford University Press, 2006), p. 483.

96. C. Miller, Protection of human subjects of research in Canada, *Health Law Review*, **4** (1995), p. 9.

97. *Protection of Human Research Subjects and Creation of NBAC*, Exec. Order No. 12,975, 60 Fed. Reg. 52,063 (1995). See A. Mastroianni & J. Kahn, Remedies for human subjects of Cold War research: recommendations of the Advisory Committee, *Journal of Law, Medicine and Ethics*, **24** (1996), pp. 118–26.

98. See J. McHale, Guidelines for medical research: some ethical and legal problems. *Medical Law Review*, **1** (1993), pp. 184–5.

99. E. Cave & S. Holm, New governance arrangements for research ethics committees: is facilitating research achieved at the cost of participants' interest, *Journal of Medical Ethics*, **28** (2002), pp. 318–21.

100. S. Kerrison & A.M. Pollock, The reform of UK research ethics committees: throwing the baby out with the bath water? *Journal of Medical Ethics*, **31** (2005), pp. 487–9.

101. P.J. Friedman, Mistakes and fraud in medical research, *Law, Medicine and Health Care*, **20** (1992), p. 17; D.M. Parrish, Falsification of credentials in the research setting: scientific misconduct? *Journal of Law, Medicine & Ethics*, **24** (1996), p. 260.

102. See J. Watts & I. Sample, Cloning fraud hits search for stem cell cures, *The Guardian*, 24 December 2005); I. Sample, Stem cell pioneer accused of faking all his research, *The Guardian*, 11 January 2006); E. Check & D. Cyranoski, Korean scandal will have global fallout, *Nature*, **438** (2005), pp. 1056–7; Summary of the final report on Professor

Woo Suk Hwang's research allegations by Seoul National University Investigation Committee, *New York Times*, 9 January 2006.

103. S. Lock, F. Wells & M. Farthing, *Fraud and Misconduct in Medical Research*, 3rd edn (London, BMJ Publishing Group, 2001).

104. Committee on Publication Ethics, *The COPE Report* (London, COPE, 1999).

105. F. Godlee, Dealing with editorial misconduct, *British Medical Journal*, **329** (2004), pp. 1301–2 (2002).

106. I. Chalmers, Unbiased, relevant and reliable assessments in health care, *British Medical Journal*, **318** (1999), p. 1167.

107. See preamble to Directive 2001/20/EC of the European Parliament and of the Council of 4 April 2001, para. 3. See also, BMA, *Consent, Rights and Choices in Health Care for Children and Young People* (London, BMJ Books, 2001), chapter 9; P.B. Miller & N.P. Kenny, Walking the moral tightrope: respecting and protecting children in health-related research, *Cambridge Quarterly of Healthcare Ethics*, **11** (2002), pp. 217–29.

108. M. Henderson, How drugs for adults harm children, *The Times*, 18 February 2006; N. Fleming, Scaled down drugs 'risk to the young', *Daily Telegraph*, 18 February 2006; see also E. Webb, Discrimination against children, *Archives of Disease in Childhood*, **89** (2004), pp. 804–8.

109. See L. Haggar & S. Woods, Children and research: a risk of double jeopardy? *International Journal of Children's Rights*, **13** (2005), pp. 51–72 at pp. 52–3.

110. CIOMS Guideline 14 – see note 8 above.

111. E. Jackson, *Medical Law: Text, Cases and Materials* (Oxford, Oxford University Press, 2006), p. 497.

112. Medicines for Human Use (Clinical Trials) Regulations 2004, Schedule 1, Part 4.

113. Medicines for Human Use (Clinical Trials) Regulations 2004, Schedule 1, Part 4.

114. S. Edward & M.J. McNamee, The ethical concerns regarding guidelines for the conduct of clinical research on children, *Journal of Medical Ethics*, **31** (2005), pp. 351–4. See also V. Hasner Sharav, Children in clinical research: a conflict of moral values, *American Journal of Bioethics*, W12–59 (2003).

115. Royal College of Paediatrics and Child Health (RCPCH) Guidelines of the ethical conduct of medical research involving children, *Archives of Disease in Childhood*, **82** (2000), pp. 177–82 at p. 179.

116. L. Haggar & S. Woods, Children and research: a risk of double jeopardy? *International Journal of Children's Rights*, **13** (2005), pp. 51–72.

117. See J. McHale & M. Fox, *Health Care Law: Text and Materials*, 2nd edn (London, Sweet and Maxwell, 2006), pp. 709–11.

118. Royal College of Paediatrics and Child Health, *Safeguarding Informed Parental Involvement in Clinical Research Involving Newborn Babies and Infants* (London, RCPCH, 1999).

119. General Medical Council, *Research: The Role and Responsibilities of Doctors* (London, GMC, 2002), paras 48–9.

120. *F v. West Berkshire Area Health Authority* [1989] 3 All ER 545; for the position in Scotland, see the Adults with Incapacity (Scotland) Act 2000. See further Chapter 7A.

121. See J. McHale & M. Fox, *Health Care Law: Text and Materials*, 2nd edn (London, Sweet & Maxwell, 2006), pp. 692–3.

122. *Simms v. Simms* [2003] 1 All ER 669.

123. For comment see J. Harrington, Deciding best interests: medical progress, clinical judgment and the 'good family', *Web Journal of Current Legal Issues*, **2** (2003), available at http://webjcli.ncl.ac.uk (accessed 7 April 2006).

124. Law Commission, Mental Incapacity, *Law Com.*, **231** (1995), paras 6.29–6.36.

125. Medicines for Human Use (Clinical Trials) Regulations 2004, Schedule 1, Part 4.

126. J. McHale, Clinical research. In A. Grubb (ed.), *Principles of Medical Law*, 2nd edn (Oxford, Oxford University Press, 2004), pp. 884–8; S. Pattinson, *Medical Law and Ethics* (London, Sweet & Maxwell, 2006), p. 374.

127. Article 2 a of the Clinical Trials Directive defines 'clinical trial' as 'any investigation in human subjects intended to discover or verify the clinical, pharmacological and/or other pharmacodynamic effects of one or more investigational medicinal product(s), and/or to identify any adverse reactions to one or more investigational medicinal product(s) and/or to study absorption, distribution, metabolism and excretion of one or more investigational medicinal product(s) with the object of ascertaining its (their) safety and/or efficacy'.

128. Section 30(3) of the Mental Capacity Act 2005 excludes from that Act any clinical trials regulated under the Clinical Trials Regulations, so the application of the MCA to clinical research is very limited.

129. S. Pattinson, *Medical Law and Ethics* (London, Sweet & Maxwell, 2006), p. 376.

130. Guideline 17, CIOMS guidance (see note 8 above) provides that '[i]nvestigators and ethical review committees should ensure that prospective subjects who are pregnant are adequately informed about the risks and benefits to themselves, their pregnancies, the fetus and their subsequent offspring'. However, it stresses that pregnant women should be presumed to be eligible to participate in biomedical research, although such research should be relevant to the health needs of pregnant women.

131. Reported by The Associated Press, May 17, 2000; available on www.my.aol.com/news.

132. Medical Research Council, *Good Research Practice* (London, MRC, 2000).

133. M. Fox, Research bodies: feminist perspectives on clinical research. In S. Sheldon and M. Thomson (eds), *Feminist Perspectives in Health Care Law* (London, Cavendish, 1998), pp. 122–3.

134. DES was a drug first prescribed in America in 1943, in the hope that it would avert miscarriages. Its efficacy was challenged as early as 1953, and by 1971 the FDA had banned its use during pregnancy after substantial evidence that it was associated with high rates of cervical cancer in the daughters of DES users.

135. V. Merton, The exclusion of pregnant, pregnable, and once-pregnable patients (aka women) from biomedical research, *American Journal of Law and Medicine*, **12** (1993), p. 369.

136. GAfREC guidance, para. 9.14a (see note 71 above).

137. F. Ross, Involving older people in research: methodological issues, *Health & Social Care in the Community*, **13** (2005), pp. 268–81.

138. See further Chapter 6 of this volume. Some research subjects enrolled in human growth hormone trial who became infected with CJD did mount successful negligence cases – see A. Boggio, The compensation of the victims of the Creutzfeldt-Jacob Disease in the United Kingdom, *Medical Law International*, **7**, pp. 144–67.

139. On the limitations of these discretionary payments, see J.M. Barton *et al*, The compensation of patients injured in clinical trials, *Journal of Medical Ethics*, **21** (1995), p. 166.

140. *Royal Commission on Civil Liability and Compensation for Personal Injury*, Cmnd 7054 (1978), para. 1341.

141. R. Gillon, No-fault compensation for victims of non-therapeutic research: should government continue to be exempt? *Journal of Medical Ethics*, **18** (1992), p. 59.

142. G. Vince, Drug trial horror: the official interim report, *New Scientist*, 5 April 2006; K. Archibald, It's time to test the testers, *The Guardian*, 6 May 2006.

143. C. Dyer, J. Carvel & P. Curtis, Victims could lose out after doubts over insurance cover, *The Guardian*, 17 April 2006.

144. See E. Jackson, *Medical Law: Text, Cases and Materials* (Oxford, Oxford University Press, 2006), pp. 513–21.
145. M. Fox, Reconfiguring the animal/human boundary: the impact of xenotechnologies, *Liverpool Law Review*, **26** (2005), pp. 149–67.
146. Nuffield Council on Bioethics, *Animal-to-Human Transplants: The Ethics of Xenotransplantation* (London, Nuffield Council on Bioethics, 1996); *A Report by the Advisory Group on the Ethics of Xenotransplantation* (London, Department of Health, 1997) [hereafter 'the Kennedy Report'].
147. Kennedy Report, para. 7.11.
148. United Kingdom Interim Xenotransplantation Regulatory Authority, *Draft Report of the Infection Surveillance Steering Group of the UKIXRA* (1999).
149. The Kennedy report recommended that in the case of xenotransplantation it will be particularly important to establish a system of counselling that is independent of the transplantation team: para. 7.13. See S. Fovargue, Consenting to bio-risk, *Legal Studies*, **26** (2005), pp. 404–18.
150. M. Fox & J. McHale, Xenotransplantation: the ethical and legal ramifications, *Medical Law Review*, **6** (1998), pp. 42–61; S. McLean & L. Williamson, *Xenotransplantation: Law and Ethics* (Aldershot, Ashgate, 2005).
151. D. Beyleveld, T. Finnegan & S. Pattinson (2006) The Regulation of Hybrids and Chimeras in the UK. Report produced for CHIMBRIDS (Chimera and Hybrids in Comparative European and International Research), University of Mannheim.
152. J. McHale & T. Hervey, *Health Law and the European Union* (Cambridge, Cambridge University Press, 2004), chapter 4.
153. A. Hemminki & P.K. Kellokumpu-Lehtinen, Harmful impact of EU clinical trials directive, *British Medical Journal*, **332** (2006), pp. 501–2.
154. A. Caplan, Risky Business: Human testing for a profit: new scrutiny needed after two commercial clinical trials go wrong, *MSNBC Interactive*, 24 March 2006, www.msnbc .msn.com/id/11927387/ (accessed 25 April, 2006); E. Rosenthal, When drug trials go horribly wrong, *International Herald Tribune*, 9 April 2006.

B   An Ethical Perspective – Nursing Research

Richard Ashcroft

Research is an essential element of innovation and quality improvement in health care. As such, it aims at something of great collective value. It can also be enormously personally rewarding to the researcher him- or herself. For the 'subjects' or 'participants' in research, the research process can be beneficial for their health or their well-being, both through the intervention they receive as part of the research process, and through the fact of participating in the research process itself.

Research can, however, be pursued selfishly; it can cause harm or distress to subjects; it can be irrelevant or unoriginal, and incompetently or fraudulently performed; and it can be exploitative.

There is therefore no question that research is an ethically significant activity, and that any research project must be pursued in an ethically reflective way. Merely to say this is to skate over the complexities of doing so: the diversity of research methods, settings in which research can be pursued, purposes to which the results of research are put, people who do research and relationships between them. This chapter will present the elements of the ethics of research, illustrating these with examples. It will concentrate on two kinds of nurse (and midwife and health visitor) research activity: nursing research (research into the health care work and types of care and treatment that nurses do) and the work of research nurses (the role of the research nurse in clinical trials and other kinds of bio-medical research). The nurses will also care for patients in clinical trials and other studies in which the nurse has no direct involvement, but for most purposes the ethical principles will be similar since in all circumstances the nurse's primary responsibility is for the patient. What varies between the roles of nurses with care of patients in research, research nurses and nursing researchers is the degree of responsibility for the research and control over it and the kinds of dilemma that may arise.

12.8 The sources of nursing ethics

Ethical principles for professionals have a number of sources. These include:

- the law
- professional codes of conduct
- fundamental moral principles
- the core values of
  - the individual
  - the institution
  - the profession
  - society.

This list has no special order, as it is a matter of controversy which source of ethics is most reliable, and which takes priority. However, most of us would agree that nurses have a strong obligation to abide by, and work within, the law. The law does not determine precisely what is ethical: for instance, many actions are lawful but possibly unethical, and some actions may be ethical without being lawful. Examples might include abortion and euthanasia – many people who think abortion ethical also think euthanasia ethical, while in law abortion is legal in many circumstances and active euthanasia is unlawful. Conversely, many people who think euthanasia is unethical also think that abortion is unethical.

The role of professional codes of ethics and conduct is in part to define the nature of the profession they regulate. They identify certain actions that might be permitted for lay people but are not permissible in nurses, and other actions that are permissible in nurses but not permitted for lay people. Codes set out the higher standards of competence, rights and duties that go along with being a nurse. Many of these rights and duties have an ethical character, but many are more in the nature of the requirements of professional etiquette. In identifying the roles that the law, ethics and professional codes have for nurses and others, we must turn eventually to the ethical foundations of these codes – the fundamental principles and values that are meant to underlie these codes.

An example of a fundamental moral principle is the principle of non-maleficence: individuals have a duty to refrain from harming others. This principle is particularly associated with the caring professions, but it is not specific to them alone. Rather, it has special importance for the caring professions simply because their patients or clients are particularly vulnerable, and thus at greater risk of being harmed, and because the skills and tools of the caring professions are particularly liable to being turned to harmful ends. However, saying that this principle is fundamental is not to say that it is absolute. Thus, certain actions do cause harm (e.g. venepuncture) but are justified by their being carried out with beneficent intentions (e.g. to provide pain relief). Hence, fundamental principles must be balanced against each other; in this case, non-maleficence is balanced with beneficence and with respect for autonomy (the individual must be asked for his or her consent).

The question of epistemology of values (how we know them) has exercised philosophers for generations. It appears in an interesting way in research ethics. Firstly, research ethics, like health care ethics generally, is a field that has experienced considerable historical evolution, as its principles have become more clearly articulated and ramified over time. The key scandals in the ethics of research always raise questions of whether the responsible agents knew that they were acting wrongly, and whether it was possible for them to know. Even if we can show that they did not and could not have known that they were in the wrong, we may perhaps argue that they are nonetheless culpable. Relatedly, the guilty individuals or institutions may insist that their critics and colleagues were just as guilty, and that they are unjustly escaping censure, or are being judged hypocritically. Exactly these arguments were used in their defence by the Nazi doctors at the Nuremberg Trial, for instance.

The epistemology of values and the difficulty of balancing principles lead us to consider a problem that is much discussed in the nursing ethics literature:

whether any principles exist, whether they are in any sense universal or objective, and whether the 'principles' approach is consistent with the orientation of caring, which many argue is what typifies the nursing relationship. This is a large topic, which is beyond the scope of this chapter. However, for present purposes it is important to distinguish between the genuine problems of knowledge and application of principles, and the relativist proposal that ethical principles are merely matters of stance and subjective attitude.

I suggest that moral relativism is neither a practical possibility – since in fact all nurses are regulated by a framework of law and by professional codes of conduct – nor a viable intellectual stance. Even 'situational' approaches, such as the 'ethics of care' approach, turn on judgements that certain values are non-negotiable. Where ethical approaches differ is generally in relation to how we know and apply values and principles to situations. Epistemological questions arise in another context in research ethics, as we will consider in the next section.

12.9 Ethics and the design of research

It is commonly said that 'bad science is bad ethics'. Before we consider why this is so, we must understand better what is meant by 'bad science'. I propose the following definition as a description of science: science is the activity of the disciplined, collective acquisition of reliable, generalisable knowledge; science is also the evolving set of outcomes of that activity.

The scientific activity includes a great range of methods, styles, techniques and practices, such that 'good' science is hard to define and perhaps amounts to nothing more than 'successful' science. Nevertheless, bad science is easier to define. Bad science is 'science' that contradicts the very idea of science as defined above. Hence, science that is methodologically ill-defined or likely to result in meaningless or unreliable data, unjustified knowledge claims or no significant contribution to generalisable knowledge at all is bad science. What is meant by 'generalisable' is somewhat controversial, but at least it requires the scientific experience to be communicable, that is, understandable by others and in some way usable by others. Science is about public knowledge rather than some essentially private experience. This view applies as much to qualitative or action research as to quantitative research or other 'natural science' inquiry. Likewise, scientific research that is kept secret or is unreported breaches the requirement that science be a collective enterprise.

This account of bad science is meant to cover the whole range of scientific methods, from statistical analysis of large numerical data sets to qualitative research interviews. Translated into practical terms, some obvious recommendations come out:

- The study should start with a satisfactory literature review that permits the definition of the research question in such way as to show that the question is important, that it has practical relevance and that we don't already know the answer to the question. No inquiry is so 'naive' or 'novel' that it does not build in some way on previous work or on previously developed methods, and these debts need to be brought into view and analysed, so far as this is possible.

- The design of the study must be reliable and likely to answer the research question in such a way that the validity of the answer is determinate and the findings of the study are interpretable and applicable by other practitioners and researchers.
- The results of the study must be publishable and, even if negative, must actually be published within a reasonable time from the completion of the study to permit other researchers and the public to learn from the study (its weaknesses no less than its strengths). The publication should be a fair and accurate account of the research design and results. There is an equivalent duty on the editor of the journal or book and reviewers for the journal or book to give a fair and competent assessment of the article or chapter submitted for publication.

All of these recommendations are now included in the Declaration of Helsinki, which is the most important international ethical guideline regulating biomedical research. However, they are here restated in language that shows their applicability as widely as possible to the diversity of research methods used in nursing today, including qualitative and health services research methods.

With bad science defined, it should be clear why 'bad science is bad ethics'. In the first place, research involves exposing patients or colleagues or other research subjects to the risks of the research. Hence if this research is unlikely to produce reliable results, it is arguable that the subjects are exposed to risk without this in any way being balanced by the prospect of benefit to society. To the extent that participants are taking part with altruistic motives, bad research misrepresents itself as an opportunity to benefit others, when it has no prospect of doing so. As such, it could be seen both as an insult to the altruism of the participants, and their deception. To the extent that the research offers some benefit to the participants in terms of access to new treatment, increased access to nursing or other health care services, or financial or other inducements, there is still an issue about the waste of resources bad research involves. Research always involves staff time and use of basic resources, even where there is no additional grant funding component. Hence there is always an 'opportunity cost', as the economists say, involved in doing research. The opportunity cost of bad research is at least the opportunity of using staff and other resources more effectively, in either caring for patients or carrying out bona fide research, for instance. Research ethics typically ignores the ethical issues involved in resources and facilities management in the health services, but this is morally short-sighted.

12.10 The competence of the research staff and research governance

One important exception to the requirement that the research design be 'good' science appears to be research carried out as part of the researcher's own education or training. Does 'student research' have to be judged by standards as high as those by which 'real' research is judged? There are different schools of thought here, but in essence it comes down to how the researcher (student) wishes the research to be considered. Is it an educational project, designed to instruct the student in research methods and management? Or is it primarily intended as research, that is, an attempt to add to collective knowledge? If the latter, then the research standard applies. The project must be assessed as objectively as possible in the light of existing knowledge and standards of research method. If the former, then the project must meet a different, not necessarily lower, standard.

The educational project must be evaluated as a project that aims to teach the student something about research method and management. As such, it must be evaluated in the same way that any educational intervention is – according to the aims and objectives of the teaching and the capacity this work has for permitting fulfilment of those aims and objectives. To some extent, these overlap with the aims and objectives of research; the best student research is often publishable in its own right. Moreover, at a certain standard the appropriate educational aim is to produce work that can stand the rigours of objective peer review. This is certainly the case of work produced for masters degrees by research, and for doctoral research.

The moral issues involved in educational projects are not, finally, different from those involved in research projects: the subjects must be told of the aims of the research and what it is hoped to achieve. In educational projects, they must be told that this is to help the student learn – as when a student nurse takes part in ward rounds and clinical care of patients. In research projects, they must be told that this research will aim to add to knowledge. In either case, the patient's consent should be sought (where possible) and the risks and benefits of the research explained, and so on. What differs between the educational project and the research project is simply the explicit non-clinical aim of the activity over and above its clinical aim, if any.

Just as the standard of the design may vary in the research and educational contexts, so too may the standard of competence expected of the principal investigator. However, there are limits. In research projects, there is a clear obligation for the research undertaken to lie within the competence of the investigator (or investigating team together) to carry out the work. This is clearly true in clinical negligence terms, but even where the possible incompetence has no clinical consequences for the subject, the general obligation not to do 'bad science' entails the duty to carry out only such research as can be done competently.

When the investigator is carrying out an educational project, the competence requirement obviously varies somewhat. Additionally, innovative research may well involve pushing the boundaries of the investigator's competence. What these situations illustrate is that 'competence' is as much an institutional as an individual affair. In the cases of the student or inexperienced or methodologically innovative researcher, competence must be secured by appropriate supervision and support, clear lines of accountability and, where necessary, physical oversight of the research activity. The same rules that apply to the student or inexperienced nurse in a novel situation apply also to the individual learning a new research technique. Here the emphasis must lie on 'appropriate' supervision – an otherwise experienced professional learning a new technique may not require the same kind of supervision as the greenhorn student. Nevertheless, a supervisory mechanism will be required. Supervisory mechanisms include piloting of the method, and peer review of the research design and of interim and final results, as well as more traditional means of educational supervision.

An important feature of supervision is that supervision is not identical to hierarchical reporting. So in a clinical team running a clinical trial, it may be that the principal investigator with overall responsibility for the trial, financially and administratively, is a new consultant physician. His or her research experience in this kind of clinical trial may be limited. The senior nurse on the team, acting as research nurse, may have considerable experience, however, even though from the point of trial management he or she reports to the principal investigator. (The Declaration of Helsinki requires any biomedical research project to be led by a physician, even if only nominally.) In this situation it is clear that the 'supervisory' role may in reality fall to the research nurse, rather than the designated principal investigator.

Each individual member of the clinical team is thus responsible for his or her own tasks, as well as participation in the generic task of quality oversight of the project. Hence in addition to each individual's competence (or 'supported competence' in the case of supervised work), there is 'team competence': can this group function effectively as a team to ensure that the ethical and quality obligations to carry out the research to a certain standard are met?

This is a very brief summary of the implications of 'research governance' or 'good clinical practice' for research and clinical teams.

12.11 Recruitment and consent

The voluntary informed consent of the individual research participant is essential. In certain kinds of research consent may be impossible (for instance, research with babies or young children, or incapacitated subjects who are unable to give consent). In certain circumstances consent may not be sought because the research project is of great collective importance, consent would be impractical, and the risk of harm to the participants is minimal. The details of these exceptions are complex, and cannot be covered here; the reader is referred to the excellent guidelines prepared by the UK Medical Research Council on research with the mentally incapacitated and on the use of personal medical information in research.

Consent is important because it respects the autonomy of individuals: their right to privacy, their right to determine what can be done to their bodies, and their right to choose whether or not to assist others in activities that may not benefit them directly. Justifications of departures from the consent standard may rest on legally shaky ground, but ethically two principles can be invoked. The first is that, in the case of individuals unable to consent by reason of lacking capacity to consent, medical and nursing innovations that will benefit them are required by the principle of beneficence. Research interventions that have a therapeutic component can directly benefit the individual, and enrolling an individual lacking capacity to consent would be justified by this. However, the principle of non-maleficence requires that their special vulnerability to harm and exploitation be noted, and special care be taken to minimise the possibility of harm to them.

Here, arguably, the principle of respect for autonomy is replaced by a principle of respect for the dignity of the vulnerable person.

A second justification for research without consent is that, where the harm and inconvenience caused to the individual is zero or negligible, all of us have, other things being equal, a duty to benefit others (especially if that involves no cost to us), and participation in socially useful research is one way to do that. This might be held to be supplemented in the UK by a sort of political claim that we are all members of the National Health Service, and all benefit from it, and all have an interest in its development and management. Hence, informally, we mandate it to carry out records-based research and audit, without the necessity to obtain consent provided our privacy is protected. The former version is an argument from solidarity; the latter is an argument from social contract theory. But what is clear is that both arguments rest on a claim about the importance and utility of the research, a claim that the research is minimal risk and a claim that the rational individual would not object to their consent not being sought. All of these claims need proof in each situation, and the burden of proof lies with the researcher; these claims must be adjudicated by an independent research ethics committee.

A more troubling worry about consent is the extent to which research on patients involves people who may be emotionally vulnerable, and who invest trust in health care professionals simply because they are professionals, or perhaps because they have come to like and rely on the particular individual professionals. They may not distinguish between the individual's roles as carer and as researcher, or they may think that they must somehow 'please' the member of staff in order to maintain good relationships or access to care. While this is explicitly ruled out by the Declaration of Helsinki, and patients must be told that their care will not be compromised if they refuse, this is sometimes difficult for patients to believe or accept.

A particular difficulty arises where a clinical trial is being managed by a research nurse who is requested by the principal investigator to recruit and enrol individuals in the trial. Strictly speaking, the consent must be obtained by the individual responsible for prescribing the study treatment – normally the physician principal investigator. This raises more general issues about the roles and responsibilities of the different members of the clinical team, which are beyond the scope of this chapter.

12.12 Research and care

Ethically, the issue of most profound concern about research involving patients is how research and care roles conflict. While the actions performed may be consistent with good medical and nursing care for the individual patient, there does seem to be a conflict in orientation. Research aims to benefit the community, and it must be pursued with scientific, methodical rigour. Care for the sick and vulnerable aims at benefiting the individual and is essentially personal and non-universalisable. The very idea of 'methodical care' seems to be an oxymoron, yet is implicit in the collection of clinical data and the carrying out of research procedures at regular intervals, especially in the context of busy hospital settings with the whole range of other clinical duties to be carried out by the researcher or his or her colleagues.

What is at stake here is an ethical relationship between the patient and the professional caring for them, which depends on respect for the dignity and autonomy of the patient, and maintenance of the integrity and professionalism of the carer. This can be a difficult balance to strike and is particularly acute when we reflect on the idea of the nurse as patient's advocate. To some extent this is possible where the nurse is not the principal investigator, but it is very difficult to maintain this stance where the nurse is both patient advocate and advocate of his or her own research. The risk here is that the nurse uncritically assumes that his or her goals are shared by the patient, hence that advocating the research is advocacy of the patient's interests and views. The ethical concept of most importance here is the concept of 'virtue': the researcher must maintain the virtues of the health care professional (care for the well-being of others, integrity and responsibility, for instance) at the same time as the virtues of the researcher (scrupulosity, honesty and curiosity, for instance).

This balance can be struck by many remarkable individuals, but it is more important that it is struck at the level of institutions – individuals working in teams with a shared institutional culture. The trend toward quality improvement and 'research governance' in part marks this attempt to achieve an institutional balance; there is a cultural shift in the health service to see research and treatment as complementary activities rather than activities in tension. A central question in research ethics today is whether this cultural shift is coherent, or whether it is a sort of institutional delusion.

12.13 Conclusion

Research will be an increasing part of the work of nurses in the coming years, and arguably this can only improve the care given by nurses. In this chapter I have described some of the ethical dilemmas that arise in research at a rather abstract and reflective level. As I point out at various places in this chapter, the growth in the role and importance of research outside of the narrow biomedical context that has historically shaped research ethics raises difficult philosophical and professional concerns, which guidelines alone will not solve. What is clear, however, is that attention to the core principles of good nursing – respect for the dignity and autonomy of patients, beneficence, non-maleficence, justice and integrity – will remain essential. The best research, and best practice in research, embodies and promotes these principles.

12.14 Acknowledgements

The author thanks Paul Wainwright and Heather Widdows for their helpful comments on drafts of this chapter.

12.15 Further reading

Handbooks

Baruch Brody (1998) *The Ethics of Biomedical Research*. Oxford University Press, Oxford.

Trevor Smith (1999) *Ethics of Medical Research: A Handbook of Good Practice*. Cambridge University Press, Cambridge.

Royal College of Nursing (1993) *Ethics Related to Research in Nursing*. Scutari Press, Harrow.

Principles of ethics

Donna Dickenson & Michael Parker (2001) *The Cambridge Medical Ethics Workbook*. Cambridge University Press, Cambridge.

Leslie Gelling (1999) Ethical principles in health care research. *Nursing Standard*, **13**(36), 39–42.

Raanan Gillon (1986) *Philosophical Medical Ethics*. John Wiley, Chichester.

Consent

Priscilla Alderson (1995) Consent to research: The role of the nurse. *Nursing Standard*, **9**(36), 28–31.

Len Doyal & Jeffrey S. Tobias (eds) (2000) *Informed Consent in Medical Research*. BMJ Books, London.

Sarah Edwards *et al.* (1998) Ethical issues in the design and conduct of randomised controlled trials. *Health Technology Assessment*, **2**(15), 1–128.

Recruitment

Richard Ashcroft *et al.* (1997) Implications of sociocultural contexts for ethics of clinical trials. *Health Technology Assessment*, **1**(9), 1–65.

Richard Ashcroft (2000) Human research subjects, selection of. In *Concise Encyclopedia of Ethics of New Technologies* (ed. Ruth Chadwick), pp. 255–66. Plenum Press, San Diego.

Research management

Richard Ashcroft, Ethical issues in outsourced clinical trials. In Roy Drucker & R. Graham Hughes (eds), *Outsourcing Health Care Development and Manufacturing* (Englewood, CO, Interpharm Press, 2000).

Table of Cases

Note: page numbers with suffix 'n' refer to notes

The following abbreviations are used:

A – Atlantic Reporter (USA)
AC – Law Reports, Appeal Cases
All ER (D) – All England Reports (Digest)
BMLR – Butterworths Medico-Legal Reports
CCR – Crown Cases Reserved
Ch – Law Reports, Chancery Division
CLR – Commonwealth Law Reports (Australia)
CMLR – Common Market Law Reports
Cr App Rep – Court of Appeal Reports
DLR – Dominion Law Reports (Canada)
ECJ – European Court of Justice
ECR – European Court Reports
ECtHR – European Court of Human Rights
EHRR – European Human Rights Reports
EWCA – England and Wales Court of Appeal (neutral reference)
EWHC – England and Wales High Court (neutral reference)
Fam – Family Division Law Reports
FLR – Family Law Reports
HCA – High Court of Australia (neutral reference)
KB – Law Reports, King's Bench Division
KIR – Knight's Industrial Reports
LR – Law Reports
Lloyds Rep Med – Lloyds List Medical Law Reports
LTL – Lawtel

Med LR – Medical Law Review
NSWLR – New South Wales Law Reports
OR – Ontario Reports
PIQR – Personal Injuries and Quantum Reports
QB – Law Reports, Queen's Bench Division
UKEAT – United Kingdom Employment Appeal Tribunal (neutral reference)
UKHL – United Kingdom House of Lords (neutral reference)
WLR – Weekly Law Reports
WWR – Western Weekly Reports

Table of Statutes

Note: page numbers with suffix 'n' refer to notes

Index

Note: page numbers with suffix 'n' refer to notes